ESSENTIALS of ANATOMY & PHYSIOLOGY
for Communication Disorders

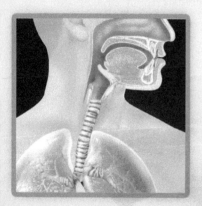
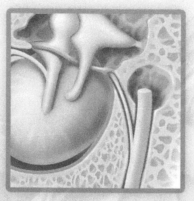
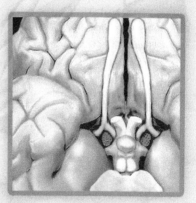

SECOND EDITION

J. Anthony Seikel, PhD
Idaho State University

David G. Drumright, BS

Paula Seikel, PhD
Idaho State University

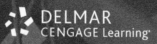

DELMAR
CENGAGE Learning·

Australia · Brazil · Japan · Korea · Mexico · Singapore · Spain · United Kingdom · United States

DELMAR
CENGAGE Learning

Essentials of Anatomy and Physiology for Communication Disorders, Second Edition
J. Anthony Seikel, David Drumright, and Paula Seikel

Vice President, Careers & Computing:
Dave Garza

Director of Learning Solutions:
Matthew Kane

Associate Acquisitions Editor: Tom Stover

Managing Editor: Marah Bellegarde

Senior Product Manager: Juliet Steiner

Editorial Assistant: Anthony Souza

Director, Market Development Manager:
Debbie Yarnell

Market Development Manager:
Jonathan Sheehan

Production Director: Wendy Troeger

Production Manager: Andrew Crouth

Senior Content Project Manager:
Andrea Majot

Senior Art Director: David Arsenault

For product information and technology assistance, contact us at
Cengage Learning Customer & Sales Support, 1-800-354-9706

For permission to use material from this text or product,
submit all requests online at **www.cengage.com/permissions.**
Further permissions questions can be e-mailed to
permissionrequest@cengage.com

Library of Congress Control Number: 2012949114

ISBN-13: 978-1-133-01821-6

ISBN-10: 1-133-01821-1

Delmar
5 Maxwell Drive
Clifton Park, NY 12065-2919
USA

Cengage Learning is a leading provider of customized learning solutions with office locations around the globe, including Singapore, the United Kingdom, Australia, Mexico, Brazil, and Japan. Locate your local office at:
International.cengage.com/region

Cengage Learning products are represented in Canada by
Nelson Education, Ltd.

To learn more about Delmar, visit **www.cengage.com/delmar**

Purchase any of our products at your local college store or at our preferred online store **www.cengagebrain.com**

Printed in the United States of America
3 4 5 6 7   20 19 18 17 16

Contents

Chapter 3 Anatomy and Physiology of Phonation 119

Preface to the Second Edition

We are pleased to present the new second edition of *Essentials of Anatomy and Physiology for Communication Disorders*. With this text we provide you with the tools you need to move forward in your career working with communication disorders. Understanding the anatomy and physiology of the speech, language, and hearing mechanisms is at the heart of all disorders you will study that have a physical origin, and it is our goal to make the information as accessible to you as possible.

As you will soon see, the physical systems of communication are extraordinarily complex. We hope that, through reading this text, you will gain the same awe we have for the communicative act.

CHANGES IN ESSENTIALS OF ANATOMY AND PHYSIOLOGY FOR COMMUNICATION DISORDERS

As we developed this text we were attempting to work with the "essential" elements of anatomy and physiology related to our chosen professions, while not burdening you with excessive detail. The balance is a delicate one, because anatomy and physiology are very detail-centered. In this revised edition we have added more detail about respiratory and articulatory physiology, and have added some information about new models of motor speech learning and production. Perhaps the most striking changes for this edition are the new, technically detailed figures and full-color presentation. We hope that this makes learning easier, and perhaps more fun.

ORGANIZATION OF ESSENTIALS OF ANATOMY AND PHYSIOLOGY FOR COMMUNICATION DISORDERS

This text takes a systemic approach to the study of anatomy and physiology. The first chapter sets the stage, providing you with terminology and background necessary to comprehend the world of anatomy. The succeeding chapters progress through the systems of communication, beginning with the energy source for speech (Chapter 2, Anatomy and Physiology of Respiration), and followed by the sound source for speech (Chapter 3, Anatomy and Physiology of Phonation). We have combined articulation and resonance (Chapter 4, Anatomy and Physiology of Articulation, Resonation, and Deglutition) with the philosophy that the resonatory system appropriately fits in the domain of moveable resonance systems (articulation). Chapter 5 (Anatomy and Physiology of Hearing) presents the essentials of hearing, and Chapter 6 (Neuroanatomy and Neurophysiology) focuses on essential components of the nervous system, again with particular attention to the elements most likely to be of use to the clinician. At the back of the text, you'll find a complete glossary of the terms defined in the margins and an index to make this text an even more valuable resource.

SPECIAL FEATURES OF ESSENTIALS OF ANATOMY AND PHYSIOLOGY FOR COMMUNICATION DISORDERS

We have tried to link the anatomical structures with clinical reality whenever possible. You will notice that we provide frequent "side trips" in the form of clinical notes that illuminate the relevance of the structures under study to your career, and we have added some new ones for the second edition. We have also included many figures and photographs to help you gain a multidimensional view of anatomy. The figures were chosen to illustrate vital points and areas of discussion, while the photographs provide dimension to the information presented in the drawings.

Anatomy has its own vocabulary, and you will make it yours before the course is through. As new terms are presented in text, they are highlighted in boldface type and defined in the margins as well as in the complete glossary at the back of the book. By inserting key terms in the margins, we hope that you can quickly and easily become familiar with new terms without having to take time to flip to a glossary. However, should you need it, there is a complete glossary for your use.

In addition, we are proud to provide ANATESSE, Software for *Essentials of Anatomy and Physiology for Communication Disorders*. We have found that study software is critical to retention of the dense information in anatomy, and we think that this will be very helpful in your studies.

The ANATESSE Software

We have provided a very powerful study tool to use with your computer. The ANATESSE software that accompanies this text gives you one more way to learn the material. It will walk you through the anatomy and physiology, quiz you, and be a virtual laboratory where you can learn at your own pace. Updated for the new second edition with improved navigation and a reader-friendly user guide, this free self-study software reinforces the concepts in the book and makes learning fun and interactive.

NEW TO THIS EDITION

As previously noted, the second edition of *Essentials of Anatomy and Physiology for Communication Disorders* has some exciting new features added to improve the learner's experience.

- Full-Color Design: Beautiful new interior design in full color supports learning and student engagement.
- Detailed Full-Color Artwork: New full-color illustrations bring the topics to life, reinforcing visual content and making abstract details more tangible.
- New Clinical Notes: These new boxed features add depth to discussions about important therapies and modern clinical approaches.
- Hearing Updates: All-new discussions of auditory physiology and motor control guide readers through this complex and fascinating subject.
- Swallowing Physiology: An enhanced discussion of the neural control of swallowing demonstrates its impact on speaking, and fuels discussions about related disorders and therapies.

HOW TO USE THIS INSTRUCTIONAL PACKAGE

We believe that experience is the key to understanding. Needless to say, we can't provide you with a fully equipped cadaver laboratory, but we can guide you to an understanding of how the various components of anatomy fit together. We offer "guided tours" of your own body's structures and we hope that these tours will bring your knowledge of anatomy into a cohesive unit.

If you supplement your reading with the relevant computer activities, you will give yourself the best opportunity to gain the knowledge of the anatomy and physiology of communication! We hope that this text and the accompanying software serve you well.

Instructor Companion Site to Accompany *Essentials of Anatomy and Physiology for Communication Disorders,* Second Edition
ISBN 13: 978-1-1330-1822-3

For instructors interested in resources to support this text, please visit www.CengageBrain.com and add the Instructor Resources to your bookshelf. Resources include:

- **Instructor Slides in PowerPoint** A robust presentation of slides created in PowerPoint provides a chapter-by-chapter outline of the concepts from the text to assist the instructor with lectures.

- **Instructor's Manual** Valuable instructor resources are provided including a class syllabus, lesson plans, lecture discussion questions, classroom activities, terminology worksheets, and labeling quizzes. These ready-to-use resources are provided in Microsoft Word® format so you can also modify them to meet your individual instructional goals.

- **Animations** Thirteen multimedia animations in fantastic detail demonstrate various unique processes of the speech, language, and hearing systems. Available to show in class, animations include the processes of phonation, respiration, swallowing, hearing, and more.

ACKNOWLEDGMENTS

We wish to acknowledge the assistance of Juliet Steiner, Laura Woods, Andi Majot, David Arsenault, Chris Catalina, Sherry Dickinson, and Tom Stover in their dedicated work on this project at Cengage Learning. We are grateful for the massive, accumulated wisdom and knowledge of all the authors referenced in this text. We are awed by the efforts of reviewers of our first draft who gave us such excellent feedback, and wish to thank each of them for their contribution to this effort. And finally, we thank our students and clients for inspiring us to educate the next generation of speech and hearing professionals.

About the Authors

J. Anthony (Tony) Seikel, PhD

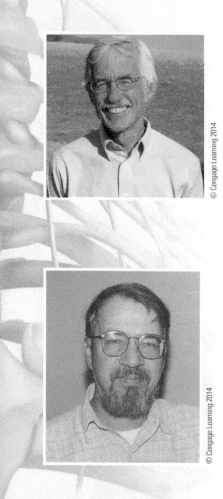

Tony Seikel, PhD, is a Professor in the Department of Communication Sciences and Disorders at Idaho State University. His background in speech and hearing sciences, oromyofunctional therapy, and neurogenics has drawn him to study the use of speech acoustics for prediction of disease in neurogenic conditions. He has been active in the development of computerized instructional materials for both speech pathology and audiology. His 30-year collaboration with David Drumright has resulted in numerous contributions to instruction in the field, and he has written many papers and given presentations on the topic of instructional pedagogy.

David G. Drumright, BS

David Drumright, BS, has created many nationally distributed software programs for instruction and measurement of speech and hearing as a result of collaborations at the University of Kansas, Pennsylvania State University, Washington State University, and Idaho State University. He is the coauthor of numerous papers and articles on software and measurement technology in the field. Prior to his work with Washington State University and collaboration with Idaho State University, he worked as a research technician at the Noise Control Laboratory at Pennsylvania State University. He has also taught electronics at DeVry University in Kansas City. His most recent software creation has been distributed for use by audiologists and audiology students who are learning instrumentation.

Paula Seikel, PhD

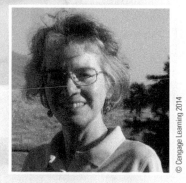

Paula Seikel, PhD, earned her Doctorate in Clinical Psychology from the University of Kansas and completed her predoctoral internship at the Veterans Administration Hospital in Leavenworth, Kansas. She has worked in community mental health and in university counseling for 26 years. With her husband, Tony, she has coauthored a paper on speech science instruction. Her contribution to this text was writing and editing for clarity and maintaining an awareness of the person, not just the bones.

Reviewers

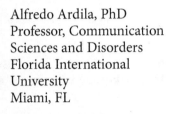

Alfredo Ardila, PhD
Professor, Communication
Sciences and Disorders
Florida International
University
Miami, FL

Angela D. Brown, MEd,
CCC-SLP
Adjunct Instructor
Shaw University
Wendell, NC

Sandra R. Ciocci, PhD,
CCC-SLP
Professor
Bridgewater State University
Bridgewater, MA

Janis H. Deane, MEd,
CCC-SLP
Adjunct Faculty,
Department of Speech and
Hearing Sciences, UNT
Clinical Center for Voice
Care, Department of
Otolaryngology Head and
Neck Surgery, UT South-
western Medical Center
Denton, TX

Virginia A. Hinton, PhD,
CCC-SLP
Associate Professor,
Department of
Communication Sciences
and Disorders
The University of North
Carolina at Greensboro
Greensboro, NC

Jerry K. Hoepner, PhD,
CCC-SLP
Assistant Professor,
Communication Sciences
and Disorders
University of
Wisconsin—Eau Claire
Eau Claire, WI

Gail B. Kempster, PhD,
CCC-SLP
Associate Professor,
Communicative Disorders
and Sciences
Rush University
Oak Park, IL

Lisa R. LaSalle, PhD,
CCC-SLP
Professor
University of
Wisconsin—Eau Claire
Eau Claire, WI

Bridget Russell, PhD,
CCC-SLP
Associate Professor
SUNY-Fredonia
Fredonia, NY

Mark Stimley, PhD,
CCC-SLP
Professor, Communication
Disorders Program,
CDCSEP
Indiana State University
Terre Haute, IN

ESSENTIALS of ANATOMY & PHYSIOLOGY
for Communication Disorders

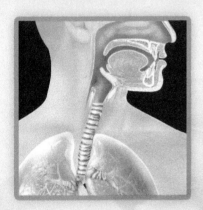
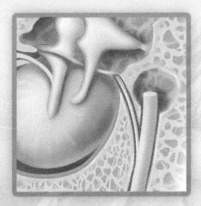
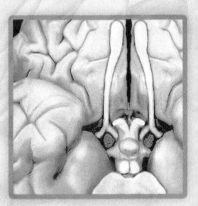

SECOND EDITION

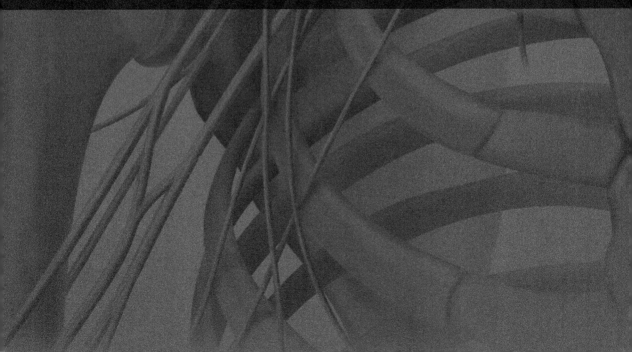

1

Basic Elements of Anatomy

OUTLINE

2. Connective tissue: Supportive tissue
   a. Areolar tissue (loose connective tissue)
   b. Adipose tissue
   c. White fibrous tissue
   d. Yellow elastic tissue (in cartilage)
   e. Lymphoid tissue
   f. Blood
   g. Bone: spongy, compact
B. Muscle Tissue
   1. Striated muscle
   2. Smooth muscle
   3. Cardiac muscle
C. Neural tissue
   1. Neurons
   2. Glial cells

III. Tissue Combinations

A. Fascia
B. Perimysium
C. Ligaments
   1. Visceral ligaments
   2. Skeletal ligaments
D. Tendons
   1. Aponeurosis
   2. Periosteum
E. Cartilage
   1. Hyaline cartilage
   2. Fibrocartilage
F. Joints
G. Operation of muscles
   1. Functional unity
   2. Origin
   3. Insertion
   4. Agonists (prime movers)
   5. Antagonists
   6. Synergists

IV. Innervation and Sensation of Muscles

A. Innervation
B. Sensation and muscle activation
C. Motor unit

ANATOMY AND PHYSIOLOGY

The term anatomy refers to the study of the structure of an organism. Applied anatomy, also known as clinical anatomy, is the study of anatomy for diagnosis and treatment of disease as it relates to surgical procedures. Descriptive anatomy, also known as systemic anatomy, is involved in the description of individual parts of the body without reference to disease conditions. Descriptive anatomy views the body as a composite of systems that function together. Gross anatomy studies structures visible without the aid of microscopy.

Electrophysiology measures the electrical activity of single cells or groups of cells, including muscle and nervous system tissue. Auditory physiology includes procedures involved in measurement of auditory function. Respiratory physiology is concerned with all processes involved in breathing.

We rely heavily on descriptive anatomy to guide our understanding of the physical mechanisms of speech and to aid our discussion of its physiology. We call on pathological anatomy as we deal with the results of conditions, such as emphysema, that change how systems work.

TERMINOLOGY OF ANATOMY AND PHYSIOLOGY

The human body and its parts have been studied for centuries, and a rich vocabulary has developed as a result. Many terms will seem foreign at first, but you will want to make this vocabulary your own. A good medical dictionary will help you develop your knowledge. In this chapter, we present the basic elements to prepare you for your study of the anatomy and physiology of speech, including a broad picture of the field of anatomy and the basic tissues of the human body. We also set the stage for your understanding of the new and foreign terminology of anatomy.

SYSTEMS OF VERBAL COMMUNICATION

Verbal communication is a very complex process that capitalizes on the anatomical systems of the body. The systems of verbal communication are defined according to function, and the systems combine organs and structures in a unique fashion. A classical categorization of the systems of verbal communication includes the nervous, respiratory,

anatomy: *The study of structure of an organism.*

applied, or clinical, anatomy: *The subdiscipline of anatomy concerned with diagnosis, treatment, and surgical intervention.*

descriptive, or systemic, anatomy: *The description of individual parts of the body without reference to disease.*

gross anatomy: *The study of structures visible without the aid of microscopy.*

electrophysiology: *Measurement and study of the electrical activity of cells.*

auditory physiology: *The procedures involved in measurement of auditory function.*

respiratory physiology: *The study of all processes involved in breathing.*

pathological anatomy: *The study concerned with diseased tissue.*

phonatory, articulatory, resonatory, and auditory systems. In this text, we combine the articulatory and resonatory systems.

The definition of systems of verbal communication is really just a convenience, because no system operates in isolation. Speech and hearing require the integrated action of all of the systems. The nervous system for communication includes the motor and sensory control of all the various structures involved in speech. This is the most essential communication system because without it we would have neither hearing nor speech. The respiratory system for communication is a precise match with the anatomical respiratory system, including the respiratory passageway and lungs. The phonatory system is the system involved in production of voiced sound through vibration of vocal folds (or vocal cords). This system uses components of the respiratory system (the larynx and other structures). The articulatory system is the combination of structures that are used to shape the sounds of speech. It includes parts of the digestive and respiratory systems (the tongue, lips, teeth, soft palate, etc.). The resonatory system includes the nasal cavity and soft palate and portions of the anatomically defined respiratory and digestive systems. It is responsible for one component of articulation, the use of the nasal cavity to produce sounds of speech. Although some speech scientists view the resonatory system as separate from the articulatory system, we take an alternative view in this text and combine the two systems as the articulatory-resonatory system of verbal communication. The auditory system includes the outer, middle, and inner ears, as well as the auditory pathways to the brain. This system provides a mechanism for processing auditory verbal information that we receive.

- In the discipline of speech pathology, there are five functionally defined systems of speech production: respiratory, phonatory, articulatory-resonatory, auditory, and nervous systems.
- The nervous system includes sensory and motor control of the various structures involved in speech.
- The respiratory system is concerned with respiration.
- The phonatory system is made up of the components of the respiratory and digestive systems associated with production of voiced sounds (the larynx).
- The articulatory-resonatory system includes the structures of the face, mouth, and nose.
- The auditory system is responsible for receiving and processing auditory stimuli.

UNDERSTANDING LATIN AND GREEK TERMS

The names of muscles, bones, and other organs were mostly set down at a time in history when medical people spoke Latin and Greek as universal languages. The intention was to name parts unambiguously rather than to make things mysterious. Many of the Latin and Greek morphemes are worth learning separately. When you come across a new term, you will often be able to determine its meaning from these components. For instance, when a text mentions an "ipsilateral" course for a nerve tract, you can see *ipsi* ("same") and *lateral* ("side") and conclude that the nerve tract is on the same side as something else.

While you are studying the nomenclature of the field, do not let the formation of plurals confuse you. A few general rules will assist you in sorting through terminology. If a singular word ends in "-a," the plural is most likely "-ae" (*pleura, pleurae*). If the word ends in "-us" the plural word ends with "-i" (*locus, loci*). (The pronunciation sometimes changes as well. For instance, *locus* is pronounced with a hard "c," but *loci* changes to a soft "c"). When the singular form ends in "-um" (as in *datum* or *stratum*), the plural ends with "-a" (*data* or *strata*). Often you will hear the anglicized version of plurals (*hiatuses*), but they are technically incorrect. Another common mistake is the use of *data* as a singular noun, as in "the data *is* inconclusive," rather than the correct plural form ("the data are inconclusive").

Many terms use a possessive form, denoting ownership (the genitive case, in linguistic jargon): *corpus*, "body," *corporum*, "of the body." The English pronunciation of these forms is unfortunately less predictable; the pronunciation presented in the dictionary often does not agree with the pronunciations common among medical personnel. Even among health professionals, though, pronunciation varies widely. Be prepared to adapt to the environment in which you work!

DESCRIPTIVE ANATOMICAL TERMS

The study of anatomy is extremely hierarchical—what you learn today will be the basis for what you learn tomorrow. The terms are the bedrock for understanding anatomical structures, and by mastering terms as they are presented, you will gain the maximum benefit from new material.

Terms of Orientation

Specific terminology lets us communicate relevant information concerning location and orientation of body parts and organs. In the **anatomical position**, the body is erect and the palms and arms face forward, as shown in Figure 1–1. Whenever we discuss terms of direction, we are referring to this position.

Some terms are relevant to the physical orientation of the body (such as *vertical* and *horizontal*). Other terms (such as *frontal, coronal,* and *longitudinal*) refer to **planes** or **axes** of the body and are therefore not relevant to the position of the body (Figure 1–1A).

With the anatomical position in mind, let us turn to planes of reference. You may think of the following planes as referring to sections of a standing body, but they are actually defined relative to imaginary axes of the body.

If you were to divide the body into front and back sections you would have a **frontal section**, or frontal view. A frontal section is also called a coronal section because the

anatomical position: *The body is erect and the palms and arms face forward.*

plane: *A flat or relatively smooth surface.*

axis: *The real or imaginary line running through the center of a body or structure.*

frontal section: *Section that divides the body into front and back portions.*

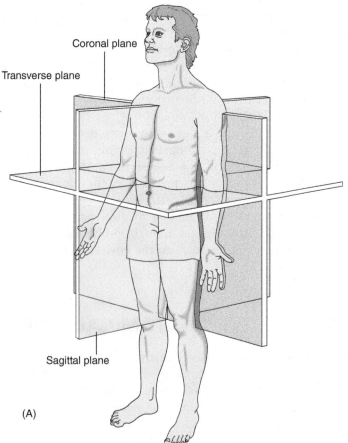

Coronal plane

Transverse plane

Sagittal plane

Figure 1–1. Terms of orientation. (A) Planes of orientation.
(continues)

(A)

© Cengage Learning 2014

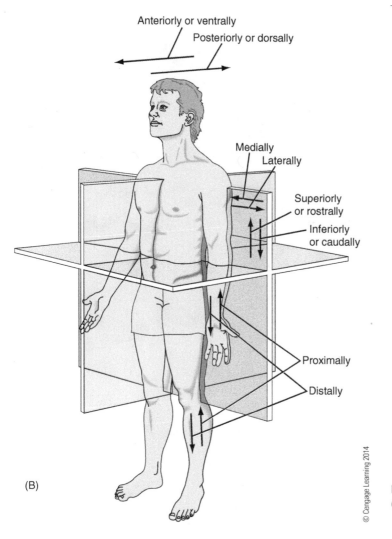

(B)

© Cengage Learning 2014

Figure 1–1. continued
(B) Terms of movement.
                    (continues)

coronal suture of the skull divides the head roughly into front and back halves. If you cut the body into left and right halves you would have **midsagittal sections**. A **sagittal section** is any cut that divides the body into left and right portions, and the cut is in the **sagittal plane**. A **transverse section** produces upper and lower halves of a body. Figure 1–1 illustrates these sections.

Note that these are midline sections, which provide equal halves. Sections can also be made off midline. Armed with these basic planes of reference, you could rotate a structure in space and still discuss the relative orientation of its parts.

The next group of items (Figure 1–1B and 1–1C) describes the position of parts of the body in relation to other parts. **Anterior** means "in front of" and is used to describe the front surface of the human body. We also use

midsagittal section: *Section that cuts the body into left and right halves.*

sagittal section: *Section that divides the body into left and right parts.*

sagittal plane: *Plane created by a sagittal section.*

transverse section: *Section that divides the body into upper and lower halves.*

anterior: *In front of.*

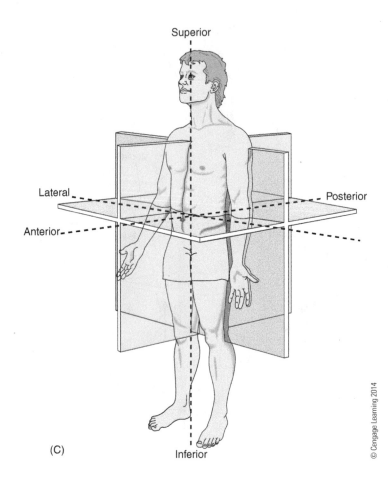

Figure 1–1. continued
(C) Terms of spatial orientation.

(C)

© Cengage Learning 2014

it to describe the relative position of one organ or structure to another, such as "the central incisors are anterior to the tongue." (Those of you who play cards may say "ante up," meaning "put your money up front!" You may also know the term *antebellum*, meaning "before the war"). **Ventral** also refers to the front surface of the human body. Ventral and anterior are synonymous for the standing human, but have different meanings for animals that walk on four legs (quadrupeds). The ventral aspect of a standing dog includes its abdominal wall, which happens to be directed toward the ground. **Posterior** is the opposite of anterior, meaning "toward the back" for dogs and humans. **Dorsal** refers to "back," as in "dorsal fin" on a fish. For humans dorsal is synonymous with posterior.

Figure 1–1B may help with these terms: **Rostral** is often used to mean "toward the head." If it is used to refer to structures in the cranium, *rostral* refers to a structure superior to another. **Caudal** means "toward the tail."

ventral: *Referring to the front surface of a body.*

posterior: *Toward the back; behind.*

dorsal: *Referring to the back surface of a body.*

rostral: *Toward the head.*

caudal: *Toward the tail.*

These terms are "body-specific:" Regardless of the body's position, anterior is "toward the front" of that body. When discussing the course of a muscle, we often need to clarify its orientation with reference to the surface of the body. A **peripheral** structure is one that is that placed *away* from the center of the body. For instance, the "peripheral nervous system" refers to the portion of the nervous system outside the skull bone or vertebral column. **Superficial** means "confined to the surface." **Deep** means "closer to the central axis of the body." When we say one organ is "deep to another," we mean that it is closer to the body's or limb's center. A wound that is superficial is confined to the surface and does not involve deep structures. A structure can also be referred to as **external** or **internal**, but these terms are generally reserved for cavities within the body.

Distal means "away from the midline." **Medial,** or **mesial**, means "toward the midline." These terms are used for appendiceal structures, such as arms and legs.

A few terms refer to the *present position of an actual body* rather than a description based on the anatomical position. As you can see in Figure 1–1C, **superior** (above, farther from the ground) and **inferior** (below, closer to the ground) are used when gravity is important. The terms **prone** (lying on the belly) and **supine** (lying on the back) describe the present actual position.

Often we describe the orientation of a structure relative to another structure, and so we disregard the anatomical position. **Lateral** means "to the side," as in football's "lateral pass." **Proximal** means "near," as in "approximate." *Lateral* and *proximal* are usually reserved for discussion of the relationship between limbs and trunk.

The concept of axis is important to add here. The body and brain (and many other structures) are said to have axes or midlines. The **axial skeleton** is the head and trunk, with the spinal column being the axis. The **appendicular skeleton** includes only the lower and upper limbs. The **neuraxis**, or axis of the brain, is slightly less straightforward, because of morphological changes of the brain during development. The embryonic nervous system is essentially tubular, but as the cerebral cortex develops, a flexure occurs and the telencephalon (the region that will become the cerebrum) folds forward. As a result, the neuraxis takes a T-formation. The spinal cord and brainstem have dorsal and ventral surfaces corresponding to those of the surface of the body. Because the cerebrum folds forward, the dorsal surface is also the superior surface, and the ventral surface is the inferior surface. Most anatomists avoid this confusion by referring to the superior and inferior surfaces.

peripheral: *Away from the center of the body.*

superficial: *Confined to the surface.*

deep: *Closer to the central axis of the body.*

external: *Outside a cavity or body.*

internal: *Within a cavity or body.*

distal: *Away from midline.*

medial, mesial: *Toward midline.*

superior: *Above, farther from the ground.*

inferior: *Below, closer to the ground.*

prone: *Lying on the belly.*

supine: *Lying on the back.*

lateral: *To the side.*

proximal: *Near a body or structure.*

axial skeleton: *The portion of the skeleton that is the head and trunk, with the spinal column being the axis.*

appendicular skeleton: *The portion of the skeleton that includes only the lower and upper limbs.*

neuraxis: *The axis of the nervous system, including spinal cord, brainstem, and cerebrum.*

flexion: *Bending at a joint, usually toward the ventral surface.*

extension: *The act of pulling two ends farther apart; the opposite of flexion.*

hyperextension: *Extension that continues to the point where the dorsal surfaces approach each other.*

dorsiflexion: *Hyperextension.*

plantar: *Referring to the sole of the foot, the flexor surface.*

plantar flexion: *Extension of the toes.*

plantar grasp reflex: *Reaction to stimulation of the sole of the foot that causes the toes of the feet to "grasp."*

inversion: *Turning the sole of the foot inward.*

eversion: *Turning the foot outward.*

palmar: *Referring to the palm of the hand.*

palmar grasp reflex: *Reaction to stimulation of the palm that causes the fingers to grasp.*

pronation: *Rotation of the hand so the palmar surface is directed inferiorly.*

supination: *Rotation of the hand so the palmar surface is directed superiorly.*

thorax: *The chest region.*

abdomen: *The region represented externally as the front (anterior) abdominal wall.*

dorsal trunk: *The region commonly referred to as "the back."*

pelvis: *The area of the hip bones.*

cranium: *The part of the skull that houses the brain.*

upper extremity: *The region consisting of the arm, forearm, wrist, and hand.*

There are specialized terms associated with movement. Flexion refers to bending at a joint, usually toward the ventral surface. That is, flexion usually results in two ventral ("belly") surfaces coming closer together. Sit-ups are an act of flexion, because you are bending at the waist. Extension is the opposite of flexion, being the act of pulling two ends farther apart. Again, having completed a sit-up, you return to the extended condition. Hyperextension, as in arching your back at the end of your sit-up, is sometimes called dorsiflexion. It occurs when extension continues to the point where the dorsal surfaces approach each other.

Use of flexion and extension with reference to feet and hands is a little more complex. Plantar refers to the sole of the foot, the flexor surface. If you rise on your toes, you are extending your foot, but the gesture is referred to as plantar flexion. A plantar grasp reflex is one in which stimulation of the sole of the foot causes the toes of the feet to "grasp." The term *dorsiflexion* may be used to denote elevation of the dorsum (upper surface) of the foot. You may turn the sole of your foot inward, in inversion. A foot turned out is in eversion. Palmar refers to the palm of the hand, that is, the ventral (flexor) surface. A palmar grasp reflex is elicited by lightly stimulating the palm of the hand. The response is to flex the fingers to grasp. The side opposite the palm is the dorsal side.

If the hand is rotated so that the palmar surface is directed inferiorly, it is pronated. Remember that in the prone position one is lying on the stomach or ventral surface. Supination refers to rotating the hand so that the palmar surface is directed superiorly.

Terms for Regions of the Body

The human body can be defined in terms of regions. The thorax is the chest region. The abdomen is the region represented externally as the front (anterior) abdominal wall. Together these two components make up the trunk, or torso. The dorsal trunk is the region we commonly refer to as "the back" (*dorsal* refers to back). The area of the hip bones is known as the pelvis. The head, or caput, rests atop the trunk. The cranium is the part of the skull that houses the brain. The upper and lower extremities are appended to the trunk. The upper extremity consists of the arm (from the shoulder to the elbow), forearm, wrist, and hand. The lower extremity is made up of the thigh, knee, leg (from the knee to the ankle), calf, ankle, and foot. These and other useful terms and their definitions are in the glossary at the end of the book.

Summary

- The axial skeleton consists of the trunk and head, whereas the appendicular skeleton comprises the upper and lower extremities.
- The trunk consists of the abdominal and thoracic regions.
- Anatomical terminology is the specialized set of terms used to define position and orientation of structures.
- A frontal section divides the body into front and back halves, whereas a midsagittal section divides the body into right and left halves.
- A transverse section divides the body into upper and lower portions.
- *Anterior* and *posterior* refer to the front and back surfaces of a body, as do *ventral* and *dorsal* for the erect human.
- *Superficial* refers to the surface of a body, and *deep* refers to directions away from the surface.
- *Superior* means "above," whereas *inferior* is closer to the ground.
- *Prone* means on the belly, and *supine* means on the back.
- *Lateral* refers to the side, *proximal* means close to the central axis, *distal* means farther from the center, and *medial* refers toward the midline of a free extremity.
- *Flexion* and *extension* refer to bending at a joint, whereas *flexion* refers to bringing ventral surfaces closer together and *extension* is moving them farther apart.
- *Plantar* refers to the sole of the foot, and *palmar* refers to the palm of the hand, both ventral surfaces.
- The neuraxis, or axis of the brain, is slightly less straightforward, because of morphological changes of the brain during development.
- Anatomy is the study of an organism's structure, whereas physiology is the study of function.
- Several subspecializations of anatomy interact to provide the detailed knowledge required to understand the anatomy and physiology of speech.
- Descriptive anatomy relates the individual parts of the body to functional systems.
- Pathological anatomy relates to changes in structure as a result of disease.
- Gross and microscopic anatomy refer to levels of visibility of structures under study.
- Developmental anatomy studies the growth and relevant changes of the organism.

arm: *The region from the shoulder to the elbow.*

lower extremity: *The region including the hip, thigh, ankle, and foot.*

leg: *The portion of the lower extremity from the knee to the ankle.*

microscopic anatomy: *The study of structures not visible to the unaided eye.*

developmental anatomy: *The study of development of the organism's anatomy from conception to adulthood.*

BUILDING BLOCKS OF ANATOMY: TISSUES

In the sections that follow, we present the building blocks of the human physical system. These blocks include the basic tissues and organs, the structures made up of the tissues, and the systems made up of the organs.

Introduction

Depending on the type of cell, every human cell is specialized to perform different functions. Cells combine to form tissues.

Four basic tissues comprise the human body: epithelial, connective, muscular, and neural. **Epithelial tissue** provides a protective lining for the surface of the body and internal surfaces of cavities. **Connective tissue** is supportive, and **muscular tissue** is capable of contraction. **Neural tissue** is specialized to transmit information. The subcategories of these tissues are shown in Table 1–1.

epithelial tissue: *Tissue that provides a protective lining for the surface of the body and internal surfaces of cavities.*

connective tissue: *Tissue that supports and connects other tissue.*

muscular tissue: *Tissue that is capable of contraction.*

neural tissue: *Tissue that is specialized to transmit information.*

Table 1–1. Tissues, Descriptions, and Locations

I. Epithelial
  A. Simple Epithelium: Single layer of cells
    1. Squamous (pavement) epithelium: Flat; linings of blood vessels, heart, alveoli, lymph vessels
    2. Cuboidal (cubical) epithelium: Cube-shaped; secretory function in some glands, such as thyroid
    3. Columnar epithelium: Cylindrical; inner lining of stomach, intestines, gallbladder, bile ducts
    4. Ciliated epithelium: Cylindrical with cilia; lining of nasal cavity, larynx, trachea, bronchi
  B. Compound Epithelium: Different layers of cells
    1. Stratified epithelium: Flattened; on bed of columnar cells; epidermis of skin, lining of mouth, pharynx, esophagus, conjunctiva
    2. Transitional epithelium: Pear-shaped; lining of bladder
  C. Basement Membrane (baseplate)
    Made predominantly of collagen; underlies epithelial tissue; serves stabilizing and other functions, including joining epithelial and connective tissues

II. Connective
  A. Areolar: Elastic; supports organs, between muscles
  B. Adipose: Cells with fat globules; between muscles and organs   *(continues)*

C. **White Fibrous:** Strong, closely packed; ligaments binding bones; periosteum covering bone; covering of organs; fascia over muscle

D. **Yellow Elastic:** Elastic; in areas requiring recoil, such as trachea, cartilage, bronchi, lungs

E. **Lymphoid:** Lymphocytes; make up lymphoid tissue of tonsils, adenoids, lymph nodes

F. **Cartilage:** Firm and solid
   1. Hyaline: Bluish white; smooth; on articulating surfaces of bones, costal cartilage of ribs, larynx, trachea, bronchial passageway
   2. Fibrocartilage: Dense, white, flexible; intervertebral disks, between surfaces of knee joints
   3. Yellow (elastic): Firm; pinna, epiglottis

G. **Blood:** Corpuscles (blood cells: red, white), platelets, blood plasma

H. **Bone:** Hardest connective tissue
   1. Compact: Has haversian canal, lamellar structure
   2. Cancellous (spongy): Spongy appearance, larger haversian canal, red bone marrow producing red and white blood cells and plasma

III. **Muscular**
   A. **Striated:** Skeletal, voluntary muscle
   B. **Smooth:** Muscle of internal organs, involuntary
   C. **Cardiac:** Combination of striated and smooth, involuntary

IV. **Nervous**
   A. **Neurons:** Transfer information; communicating tissue
   B. **Glial cells:** Nutrient transfer; blood-brain barrier

Source: Adapted from Ross, J. S. & Wilson, K. J. W. (1966). *Taxonomy from foundations of anatomy and physiology* (pp. 1–32). Baltimore: Williams & Wilkins.

Tissues

Epithelial Tissue

Epithelial tissue is composed of the superficial layer of mucous membranes and the cells that make up the skin. Epithelial tissue has little material between the epithelial cells so that it forms a tight, compact sheet. It is a protective barrier, keeping whatever is covered from seeping out and keeping some foreign material from getting in. There may be many layers of epithelium for added protection. Some forms of epithelium secrete fluids, and these tissues are called glandular epithelium.

A baseplate, or basement membrane, made predominantly of collagen underlies epithelial tissue, providing a number of functions, depending on the location of the epithelium. Basement membrane may serve as a filter (for instance, in the kidneys) or may stabilize the epithelial tissue (as in the juncture of connective tissue with epithelium). The

glandular epithelium: *Epithelium that secretes fluids.*

baseplate (basement membrane): *Thin, membranous subsurface of epithelial tissue that serves structural, functional, and developmental purposes, depending on its location.*

beating ciliated epithelium: *Epithelial cells with hairlike protrusions that actively beat to remove contaminants from the epithelial surface.*

matrix: *Intercellular material of connective tissue.*

areolar tissue (loose connective tissue): *Supportive connective tissue.*

adipose tissue: *Areolar tissue that is richly impregnated with fat cells.*

lymphoid tissue: *Specialized connective tissue in tonsils and adenoids.*

fibrous tissue: *Tissue that binds structures together.*

white fibrous tissue: *Connective tissue that is strong, dense, and highly organized.*

yellow elastic tissue: *Connective tissue in cartilage.*

basement membrane is important in the process of directing growth patterns for epithelial cells.

Other types of epithelium have cilia, which are hairlike protrusions that actively beat to remove contaminants from the epithelial surface (beating ciliated epithelium). Epithelial tissue lines nearly all of the cavities of the body as well as the tubes that connect them.

Connective Tissue

Connective tissue is perhaps the most complex type of tissue. The body has a great deal of connective tissue, which provides support for other structures. Connective tissue is made up mostly of intercellular material, known as the matrix, within which the cells of connective tissue are bound. Connective tissue may be solid, liquid, or gel-like. The major types of connective tissue are as follows: Areolar tissue (also known as loose connective tissue) is supportive. Areolar fibers join to form an area like an elastic woven mat. They form a thin sheet between muscles and organs and fill the space between organs. Adipose tissue is areolar tissue that is richly impregnated with fat cells. Lymphoid tissue is specialized connective tissue found in tonsils and adenoids. Fibrous tissue binds structures together, and it may contain combinations of fiber types. White fibrous tissue is strong, dense, and highly organized. It is found in ligaments that bind bones together, as well as in the fascia that encases muscle. Yellow elastic tissue is found in cartilage.

Osteoporosis

Osteoporosis is a condition wherein bone becomes increasingly porous owing to loss of calcium. The reduction in calcium may be the result of aging, vitamin D deficiency, disuse (as found in individuals confined to bed during illness), or other causes. Osteoporosis makes a person susceptible to bone fractures. Breaks of osteoporotic bones may go undetected. For example, an elderly person may "fall and break a hip," when actually the hip might have been broken before the fall, as a result of the fragility and porousness of the bone. An individual with osteoporosis can break ribs while coughing. Osteoporosis can be localized, as seen in the skull bones of a person with Paget's disease (osteitis deformans). Osteoporosis can have a large effect on the bones related to mastication, or chewing. Degeneration of the mandible and maxilla can result in tooth loss, and because of this bone loss the surgeon will be unable to perform surgical procedures to correct misalignment of these structures. Osteoporosis can also result in fracture of the ossicles of the middle ear, resulting in significant conductive hearing loss.

Blood is a connective tissue. Blood cells (including red and white corpuscles) are suspended in blood plasma, which is the liquid matrix of this connective tissue. Plasma has numerous functions, among them the precipitation of clotting when cells are damaged. The blood cells develop in the marrow of another type of connective tissue, bone.

Bone is the hardest connective tissue. The hardness comes from the inorganic salts that make up a large portion of it. Bone is generally described as compact or spongy. Compact bone has a sheetlike (lamellar) structure, and spongy bone appears porous. Spongy bone contains the marrow that produces both blood cells and blood plasma.

blood: *Connective tissue that contains plasma and blood cells.*

plasma: *Fluid component of blood.*

bone: *Dense, inelastic connective tissue.*

compact bone: *Sheetlike bone.*

spongy bone: *Porous bone.*

Muscle Tissue

Muscle fibers can be stimulated to contract. Muscle is generally classified as striated, smooth, or cardiac (Figure 1–2).

(A) Striated muscle tissue

(B) Smooth muscle tissue

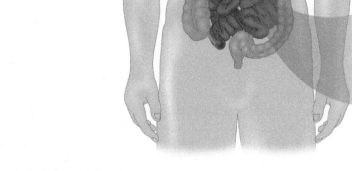
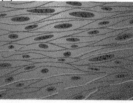

© Cengage Learning 2014

Figure 1–2. Striated (A) and smooth muscle (B).

striated muscle: *Skeletal muscle, voluntary muscle.*

smooth muscle: *Includes the muscular tissue of the digestive tract and blood vessels not under voluntary control.*

cardiac muscle: *Muscle of the heart, composed of cells that interconnect like a net.*

neurons: *Cells specialized for communication.*

Striated muscle is named for the striped appearance of the tissue when viewed through a microscope. Striated muscle is also known as skeletal because it is the muscle used to move skeletal structures. It is also described as voluntary or somatic muscle because it can be moved in response to conscious, voluntary stimulation. **Smooth muscle** includes the muscular tissue of the digestive tract and blood vessels, and it is sheetlike, with spindle-shaped cells. **Cardiac muscle** is composed of cells that interconnect like a net. Smooth and cardiac muscle are generally outside voluntary control and are controlled through the autonomic (involuntary) nervous system.

Neural Tissue

Neurons, which take on a variety of forms, are specialized for communication. They transmit information from one neuron to another, from neuron to muscle, and from sensory receptors to other neural structures.

Summary

- Four types of tissue compose the human body: epithelial, connective, muscular, and neural (nervous).
- Epithelial tissue includes the surface covering of the body and linings of body cavities and passageways.
- Connective tissue varies as a function of the intercellular material (matrix) surrounding it.
- Areolar connective tissue is loose and thin, and adipose tissue is areolar tissue with significant fat deposits.
- White fibrous connective tissue and yellow elastic connective tissue are found in ligaments, tendons, and cartilage.
- Blood is a fluid connective tissue, whereas bone is a dense, inelastic connective tissue.
- Muscle tissue consists of voluntary (striated), involuntary (smooth), and cardiac muscle.
- Neural tissue is specialized for communication.

Tissue Combinations

The four basic types of body tissue (epithelial, connective, muscular, and nervous) combine to provide structure to the body. The following structures are formed from basic connective tissues.

fascia: *Sheetlike membrane of connective tissue that surrounds organs.*

A **fascia** (pl. fasciae) is a sheetlike membrane of connective tissue that surrounds organs. Fasciae may take many forms, but the fibers are typically woven together for compressive strength. Compressive strength is the ability of a material to resist being crushed. **Perimysium** is a special type of fascia that surrounds muscle.

Ligaments are bands of connective tissue that are responsible for binding structures together. **Visceral ligaments** bind organs together and hold structures in place. **Skeletal ligaments** bind bone to bone and must withstand great pressure. Ligaments generally do not stretch.

Tendons are bands of connective tissue that are part of the muscle; they are the means by which muscle is attached to bone or cartilage (Figure 1–3). The fibers of tendons run longitudinally (as opposed to interwoven or matted, as in fascia). This gives them great **tensile strength** but reduced compressive strength. Tensile strength gives a material resistance to being pulled apart. Tendons tend to have the **morphology** (or form) of the muscles they serve. Compact, tubular muscles tend to have long, thin tendons. Flat muscles, such as the diaphragm, have flat tendons. An **aponeurosis** is a sheetlike tendon.

Bones are dense connective tissue providing the structure for most of the body. Bones are broadly characterized by length (long or short) and shape (flat) or are irregular. The **periosteum** is the fibrous membrane covering of a bone that extends along its entire surface except where there is cartilage. The outer periosteum layer is tough and fibrous but the inner layer of periosteum contains cells that facilitate bone repair.

Cartilage is a particularly important connective tissue combination. Cartilage has three qualities that make it ideally suited for several structural purposes: great tensile strength, great compressive strength, and **elasticity**, which means that when it is moved or displaced it will tend to return to its original position. Bones often have a cartilaginous portion in areas where they need to have flexibility, such as in the nose, or in areas where two bones **articulate** (join together). Cartilage is smoother than

compressive strength: *The ability of a material to resist crushing.*

perimysium: *Special fascia surrounding muscle.*

ligaments: *Bands of connective tissue responsible for binding structures together.*

visceral ligaments: *Connective tissue that binds organs together or holds structures in place.*

skeletal ligaments: *Connective tissue that binds bone to bone.*

tendons: *Connective tissue bands that are part of the muscle and attach muscle to bone or cartilage.*

tensile strength: *The ability of a material to resist being pulled apart.*

morphology: *Form.*

aponeurosis: *Sheetlike tendon.*

periosteum: *Fibrous membrane covering of a bone.*

cartilage: *Connective tissue that is elastic.*

elasticity: *Having the ability and tendency to return to original position.*

articulate: *Join together.*

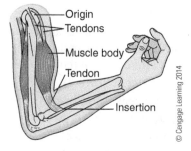

Origin
Tendons
Muscle body
Tendon
Insertion

© Cengage Learning 2014

Figure 1–3. Tendon attaching muscle to bone.

bone, so many joints between bones have cartilage on the two surfaces so that they can glide across each other with reduced friction.

hyaline cartilage: *Smooth, glassy, blue cartilage for surfaces of bones that come together in joints.*

There are three basic subtypes of cartilage. Hyaline cartilage is smooth and has a glassy, blue cast. It gives a smooth surface for mating of bones that come together in joints. It is also a primary form of cartilage for the larynx, trachea, and bronchial passageway. It makes up the cartilaginous portion of the rib cage. Fibrocartilage contains collagen fibers that provide the cushion between bones. For instance, it makes up the disks between the vertebrae, as well as the mating surface for the temporomandibular joint between the lower jaw and the skull. Fibrocartilage is a shock absorber and provides a relatively smooth surface for gliding. Yellow (elastic) cartilage has less collagen but more elastic fibers. It is found in the pinna (the visible portion of the ear), the nose, and the epiglottis.

fibrocartilage: *Smooth cartilage made up of a mixture of white fibrous and collagen tissue.*

yellow (elastic) cartilage: *Cartilage that has greater elasticity than other forms of cartilage.*

Joints

diarthrodial, or synovial, joints: *Highly mobile joints lubricated with synovial fluid.*

A joint is the means by which two bones articulate. Although there is a wide variety of joints, we discuss only one type in this overview. Diarthrodial, or synovial, joints are highly mobile and have a cavity in which synovial fluid, a lubricating substance, is found. Hyaline cartilage covers the surface of each bone of the joint, providing a smooth, strong mating surface.

Summary

- Tissues combine to form larger structures.
- Fascia is a sheetlike membrane surrounding organs.
- Ligaments bind organs together and hold bone to bone or cartilage.
- Tendons attach muscle to bone or to cartilage, and a flat tendon is referred to as an aponeurosis.
- Bones and cartilage provide the structure for the body, articulating by means of joints.
- Cartilage has both tensile and compressive strength and is elastic (fibers of cartilage resist being torn apart or crushed, and cartilage tends to return to its original shape after being deformed).
- Hyaline cartilage is smooth, and fibrocartilage provides a cushion between structures.
- Yellow cartilage is very elastic.
- Diarthrodial (synovial) joints are highly mobile and lubricated by synovial fluid.

Muscles

You can look at muscles in terms of either their anatomy or their physiology. The role of muscle is to move the structures to which it is attached closer together. Anatomically, muscles are groups of muscle fibers with a single functional purpose (**functional unity**). The form of the muscle (morphology) varies widely, depending on its function. Fibers of wide, flat muscles tend to radiate from a broad point of origination to a more focused insertion. More cylindrical muscles have single points of attachment on either end.

Muscle fiber can only actively shorten. A muscle can contract to approximately one half its original length, so long muscles can contract greater distances than short muscles. The diameter of a muscle is directly related to its strength. The more fibers a muscle has, the greater the force the muscle can exert to do work. Muscles can contract only in a straight line, with the exception of sphincter muscles, which act like a drawstring on a purse.

Muscles are attached to some structures at both ends. The point of attachment that is immobile when a muscle contracts is the **origin**. The point of attachment that moves as a result of muscle contraction is the **insertion**. When referring to limbs, the insertion point is more distant from the body. Muscles that move a structure are referred to as **agonists** or **prime movers**. Muscles that oppose a given movement are **antagonists**. Muscles used to stabilize structures are **synergists**.

A muscle attached closer to a joint will move the bone farther and faster than one attached farther from the joint, and it will provide greater range of movement. A muscle attached farther from the joint will be able to exert more force through its range because of the greater leverage and will have an advantage for lifting (Figure 1–4).

Neural Innervation

Innervation is communication between neurons or between neurons and muscle. Muscle innervation provides the means for a muscle to contract. Sensory information is also transmitted by neurons, so regions or structures of the body receive afferent (sensory) innervation. Muscles are innervated by a single nerve that is responsible for activating the muscle. Another nerve is responsible for monitoring the muscle's length and state of tension.

Innervation is either **sensory** (generally termed **afferent**) or **motor** (**efferent**, or **excitatory**). A sensory nerve from a muscle sends information about the state of the muscle (for instance, how much it has been stretched) to the central nervous system. A **motor nerve** sends impulses

functional unity: *Groups of tissues working for a single functional purpose.*

origin: *The point of attachment of a muscle that is immobile when a muscle contracts.*

insertion: *The point of attachment of a muscle that is mobile when a muscle contracts.*

agonists (prime movers): *Muscles that move a structure.*

antagonists: *Muscles that oppose a prime mover or agonist.*

synergists: *Muscles used to stabilize structures.*

innervation: *Distribution of nervous tissue to serve communication between brain and muscles.*

sensory (afferent) innervation: *Innervation that provides the central nervous system with information about the state of the body or tissues.*

motor (efferent/excitatory) innervation: *Innervation that causes muscles to contract or glands to secrete.*

motor nerve: *Nerve that activates muscle or gland.*

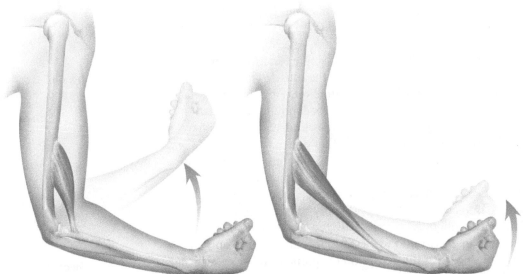

© Cengage Learning 2014

Figure 1–4. Mechanical advantage derived from point of insertion. On the left, the muscle inserts closer to the point of rotation, and the movable point will undergo a greater excursion on contraction of the muscle. On the right, the muscle is attached a greater distance from the point of rotation so that the bone will move a smaller distance, but the muscle is capable of exerting greater force in the direction of movement.

Neuromuscular Diseases

A host of neuromuscular conditions prey on the muscular system and the nerve components that supply it with energy. Amyotrophic lateral sclerosis (ALS, or Lou Gehrig's disease) is a condition in which the motor neuron of the nerve is destroyed, resulting in loss of muscle function. Myelin destruction occurs in multiple sclerosis (MS), with manifestation of the disease varying by site of lesion. Myasthenia gravis is a condition in which the nerve-to-muscle junction is destroyed as a result of an immune system response. The result is weakness and loss of muscle range because nerve and muscle cannot communicate.

motor unit: Tissue consisting of one motor nerve fiber and the muscle fibers to which it attaches.

from the nervous system to muscles to make them contract. A **motor unit** consists of one motor neuron (nerve) and the muscle fibers to which it attaches.

Summary

- Muscle is contractile tissue, with muscle bundles capable of shortening to about half their length.

- The point of attachment with the least movement is the muscle's origin, and the insertion is the point of attachment of relative mobility.
- Muscles that move a structure are agonists and those that oppose movement are antagonists.
- Muscles that stabilize structures are synergists.
- A muscle is innervated by a single nerve.
- Motor nerves communicate excitatory impulses to muscle fibers.
- Sensory nerves communicate sensation from regions of the body to the central nervous system.
- A motor unit is the motor nerve fiber and the muscle fibers it innervates.

CHAPTER SUMMARY

Anatomy and physiology are the study of the structure and function of an organism. The discipline of speech pathology includes five functionally defined systems of speech production: respiratory, phonatory, articulatory-resonatory, auditory, and nervous. The respiratory system is concerned with respiration. The phonatory system is made up of the components of the respiratory and digestive systems associated with production of voiced sounds (the larynx). The articulatory system includes the structures of the face, mouth, and nose. The auditory system is responsible for receiving and processing auditory stimuli. The nervous system includes the sensory and motor control of the various structures involved in speech.

The axial skeleton supports the trunk and head, and the appendicular skeleton refers to the extremities. Anatomical terminology relates position and orientation of the body and its parts. A frontal plane cuts the body into front and back halves, a sagittal plane divides the body into left and right halves, and a transverse plane divides the body into upper and lower halves. *Anterior* and *posterior* refer to front and back of a body, as do ventral and dorsal for the human. *Peripheral* refers to a direction toward the surface or superficial region, while *deep* refers to direction away from the surface. *Distal* means away from a central structure, and *proximal* means to the side of a structure. *Superior* and *inferior* refer to upper and lower regions. *Lateral* means to the side, and *medial* refers to the midline. *Flexion* refers to bending ventral surfaces toward each other at a joint, and *extension* is moving those surfaces farther apart. *Plantar* and *palmar* refer to ventral surfaces of the feet and hands, respectively.

The four basic types of tissue of the human body are epithelial, connective, muscular, and nervous. Epithelial tissue comprises the surface covering of the body and the linings of cavities and passageways. Connective tissue includes the variety of tissues linking structures together, including ligaments, tendons, cartilage, bone, and blood. Muscular tissue is contractile, comprising striated, smooth, and cardiac muscle. Nervous tissue is specialized for communication. Tissues combine to form structures and organs. Fascia surrounds organs, ligaments bind bones and cartilage, tendons attach muscle to bone or to cartilage, and bones and cartilage provide the structure for the body. Diarthrodial, or synovial, joints are those in which lubricating synovial fluid is contained in a capsule.

Muscle bundles can shorten to about half their length. The origin of a muscle is the point of attachment with the least movement, and the muscle's insertion is the relatively mobile point of attachment. Agonists are muscles that move a structure, antagonists oppose movement, and synergists stabilize a structure. Muscles are innervated by a single nerve, and innervation can be sensory or motor. A motor unit is the motor nerve fiber and the muscle fibers it innervates.

STUDY QUESTIONS

1. _____ is the study of the structure of an organism.
2. _____ is the study of the function of a living organism and its parts.
3. _____ anatomy is anatomical study for diagnosis and treatment of disease.
4. _____ anatomy is involved in the description of individual parts of the body without reference to disease, viewing the body as a composite of systems that function together.
5. Skin and mucous membrane are made up of _____ tissue.
6. _____ is a particularly important connective tissue because it is both strong and elastic.
7. _____ is contractile tissue.
8. _____ bind organs together or hold bones to bone or cartilage.
9. _____ is a sheetlike membrane surrounding organs.
10. _____ attach muscle to bone or to cartilage.
11. _____ is the relatively immobile point of attachment of a muscle.

12. _____ is the relatively mobile point of attachment of a muscle.

13. Identify the anatomical systems from their definitions:

  A. _____ This system includes smooth, striated, and cardiac muscle of the body.

  B. _____ This system includes the bones and cartilage that form the structure of the body.

  C. _____ This system includes the passageways and tissues involved in gas exchange with the environment, including the oral, nasal, and pharyngeal cavities, the trachea and bronchial passageway, and the lungs.

  D. _____ This system includes the esophagus, liver, intestines, and associated glands.

  E. _____ This system includes the nerve tissue and structures of the central and peripheral nervous systems.

14. Identify the systems of speech from their definitions:

  A. _____ This system includes the passageways and tissues involved in gas exchange with the environment, including the oral, nasal, and pharyngeal cavities, the trachea and bronchial passageway, and the lungs.

  B. _____ This system is involved in production of voiced sound and uses components of the respiratory system (the laryngeal structures).

  C. _____ This system is the combination of structures used to alter the sounds of speech, including parts of the anatomically defined digestive and respiratory systems (the tongue, lips, teeth, soft palate, etc.).

  D. _____ This system includes the nasal cavity and soft palate and portions of the anatomically defined respiratory and digestive systems.

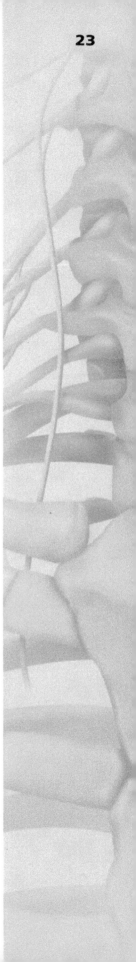

15. On the accompanying figure, identify the descriptive terms indicated.

A. _____ plane

B. _____ plane

C. _____ plane

D. _____ aspect

E. _____ aspect

F. _____ (movement away from midline)

G. _____ (movement toward midline)

H. _____ (located away from midline)

I. _____ (located near midline)

J. _____ (related to the side)

K. _____ (above)

L. _____ (below)

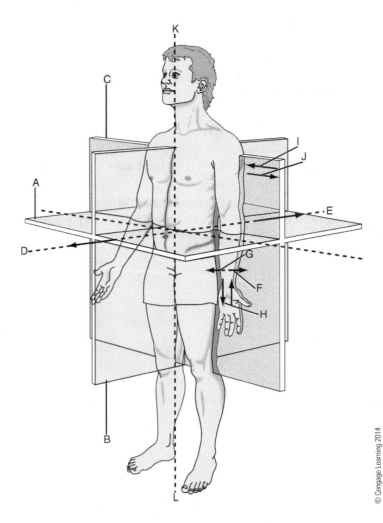

16. As our field has developed, the professionals working with speech and language became known as "speech-language pathologists." Reflecting on the terminology you have just reviewed, to what does the term *pathologist* refer?

REFERENCES

Barnett, H. L. (1972). *Pediatrics*. New York: Appleton-Century-Crofts.

Basmajian, J. V. (1975). *Grant's method of anatomy*. Baltimore: Williams & Wilkins.

Bateman, H. E. (1977). *A clinical approach to speech anatomy and physiology*. Springfield, IL: Charles C. Thomas.

Bateman, H. E., & Mason, R. M. (1984). *Applied anatomy and physiology of the speech and hearing mechanism*. Springfield, IL: Charles C. Thomas.

Duffy, J. R. (1995). *Motor speech disorders*. St. Louis, MO: Mosby.

Fink, B. R., & Demarest, R. J. (1978). *Laryngeal biomechanics*. Cambridge, MA: Harvard University Press.

Gosling, J. A., Harris, P. F., Humpherson, J. R., Whitmore, I., Willan, P. L. T. (1985). *Atlas of human anatomy*. Philadelphia: J. B. Lippincott.

Gray, H., Bannister, L. H., Berry, M. M., & Williams, P. L. (Eds.) (1995). *Gray's anatomy*. London: Churchill Livingstone.

Grobler, N. J. (1977). *Textbook of clinical anatomy* (Vol. 1). Amsterdam: Elsevier Scientific.

Kaplan, H. (1960). *Anatomy and physiology of speech*. New York: McGraw-Hill.

Kuehn, D. P., Lemme, M. L., & Baumgartner, J. M. (1991). *Neural bases of speech, hearing, and language*. Boston: Little, Brown.

Moore, K. L., Persaud, T. V. N., & Chabner, D.-E.B (2003). *The developing human*. Philadelphia: W. B. Saunders.

Rahn, H., Otis, A., Chadwick, L. E., & Fenn, W. (1946). The pressure-volume diagram of the thorax. *American Journal of Physiology, 146*, 161–178.

Rohen, J. W., & Yokochi, C. (1993). *Color atlas of anatomy*. New York: Igaku-Shoin.

Ross, J. S., & Wilson, K. J. W. (1966). *Foundations of anatomy and physiology*. Baltimore: Williams & Wilkins.

Williams, P., & Warrick, R. (1980). *Gray's anatomy* (36th Brit. Ed.). Philadelphia: W. B. Saunders.

Zemlin, W. R. (1998). *Speech and hearing science: Anatomy and physiology* (4th ed.). Needham Heights, MA: Allyn & Bacon.

2

Anatomy and Physiology of Respiration

OUTLINE

I. Introduction
   A. Respiration is exchange of gas between an organism and its environment
   B. Pressure is force distributed over area
   C. Boyle's law
   D. Pressure increase and decrease

II. Support Structure for Respiration
   A. Vertebral column
      1. Five vertebral segments form a strong but flexible column
      2. Vertebrae labels are based on their levels: C1 to C7 (cervical), T1 to T12 (thoracic), L1 to L5 (lumbar), S1 to S5 (sacral)
      3. Coccyx
      4. Spinous and transverse processes
      5. Vertebral column houses the spinal cord
      6. Spinal nerves
      7. Ribs articulate with the vertebral column

III. Pelvic and Pectoral Girdle
   A. Pelvic girdle
      1. Ilium
      2. Sacrum

    3. Pubic bone
    4. Ischium
  B. Pectoral girdle
    1. Scapula
    2. Clavicle
    3. Sternum

IV. Ribs and Rib Cage
  A. Total of 12 ribs: 7 true ribs, 3 false ribs, and 2 floating ribs
  B. Cartilaginous attachment of ribs to the sternum
  C. Elevation of rib cage
  D. Sternum

V. Soft Tissue of the Thorax and Respiratory Passageway
  A. Right and left lungs
  B. Trachea and bronchial tree
  C. Oxygen and carbon dioxide exchange
  D. Cleansing action of beating epithelia

VI. Movement of Air through the System
  A. Pleural linings of lungs
  B. Association between the pleurae and the diaphragm
  C. Action of diaphragm in respiration

VII. Muscles of Inspiration
  A. Primary muscle of inspiration
  B. Interaction of diaphragm and central tendon

VIII. Accessory Muscles of Inspiration
  A. Anterior thoracic muscles of inspiration
    1. External intercostal
    2. Interchondral portion, internal intercostal
  B. Posterior thoracic muscles of inspiration
    1. Levatores costarum (brevis and longus)
    2. Serratus posterior superior
  C. Accessory muscles of the neck
    1. Sternocleidomastoid
    2. Scalenes (anterior, middle, posterior)
  D. Muscles of Upper Arm and Shoulder
    1. Pectoralis major
    2. Pectoralis minor
    3. Serratus anterior
    4. Levator scapulae

       5. Rhomboideus major
       6. Rhomboideus minor
       7. Trapezius

IX. Muscles of Forced Expiration

  A. Muscles of thorax: anterior/lateral thoracic muscles
     1. Internal intercostal (interosseous portion)
     2. Transversus thoracis
  B. Posterior thoracic muscles
     1. Subcostals
     2. Serratus posterior inferior
  C. Abdominal muscles of expiration
     1. Anterolateral abdominal muscles
       a. Transversus abdominis
       b. Internal oblique abdominis
       c. External oblique abdominis
       d. Rectus abdominis
     2. Posterior abdominal muscles: quadratus lumborum
  D. Muscles of upper limb: latissimus dorsi

X. Physiology of Respiration

  A. Measurement of respiration
     1. Flow, volumes, and capacities
     2. Pressure
     3. Volume measured in liters, milliliters, and cubic centimeters
  B. Respiration for life
     1. Respiratory cycle
       a. Adults, 12–18 cycles per minute
       b. Adults quiet respiration, about 500 cc per cycle
     2. Developmental processes of respiration
       a. Conducting airway complete at birth
       b. As they grow, the lungs are stretched to fill the thorax
  C. Volumes
     1. Tidal volume (TV)
     2. Inspiratory reserve volume (IRV)
     3. Expiratory reserve volume (ERV)
     4. Residual volume (RV)
     5. Dead space air
  D. Capacities
     1. Vital capacity (VC)
     2. Functional residual capacity (FRC)
     3. Total lung capacity (TLC)
     4. Inspiratory capacity (IC)

INTRODUCTION

The human body depends on regular oxygen exchange to stay alive. As communicating organisms, humans have "hijacked" the respiratory system to provide the energy source for oral communication. As you will see in our discussion of respiratory physiology, we exercise a great deal of external control over the respiratory mechanism while working within the bounds of the biological requirements for life. First, we will discuss respiration, which is essential to sustain life.

Respiration is defined as the exchange of gas between an organism and its environment. We bring oxygen to the cells of the body to sustain life by breathing in (inspiration) and eliminate waste products by breathing out (expiration). A close look at the mechanics of gas exchange will provide an understanding of how a deficit in this area can impair speech.

Gas exchange happens in the alveoli, the minute air sacs located deep in the lungs, only after gas has been drawn into the system. The basic mechanism of inspiration can be

respiration: *Exchange of gas between an organism and its environment.*

inspiration: *The process of bringing air into the lungs for respiration.*

expiration: *The process of eliminating air from the lungs for respiration.*

(A)

(B)

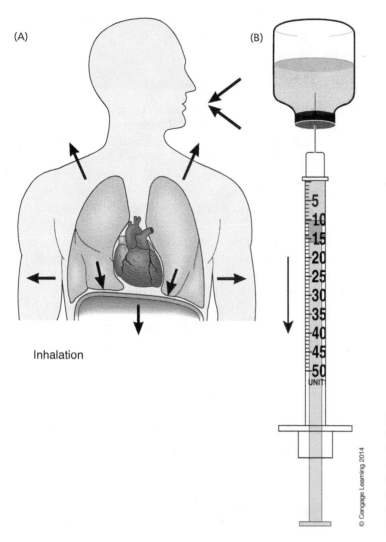

Inhalation

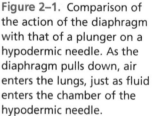

Figure 2–1. Comparison of the action of the diaphragm with that of a plunger on a hypodermic needle. As the diaphragm pulls down, air enters the lungs, just as fluid enters the chamber of the hypodermic needle.

likened to that of a hypodermic needle. If the plunger on the hypodermic needle in Figure 2–1 is pulled out, whatever is near the opening will enter the tube and be drawn into the awaiting chamber. If you envision the respiratory system as a hypodermic needle, with your mouth or nose as the tip of the needle, you will realize that pulling on the plunger (your diaphragm) causes air to enter the chamber (your lungs). Although the rest of this chapter is devoted to the structures and functions of the respiratory process, let us first examine in more detail the physical principles involved.

Before we can talk about the forces that drive respiration, you need an intuitive feel for what air pressure really is. Air pressure is the force exerted on walls of a chamber by molecules of air. Because of their molecular charge, air molecules tend to keep their distance from other air molecules. If the chamber is open to the atmosphere, the pressure exerted

Muscle Weakness and Respiratory Function

Many disease processes cause reduced respiratory function, which can have a remarkable effect on other systems as well. Diseases that produce spasticity can result in paradoxical contraction of the muscles of expiration during inspiration, greatly reducing the vital capacity. Likewise, some individuals have flaccid or hypotonic (low muscle tone) conditions that reduce the degree and strength of muscular contraction. When you think about it, it makes perfect sense that diseases that cause muscular weakness can reduce respiratory capacity.

We must be cautious about quickly blaming the muscles of respiration for apparent deficits in vital capacity, inspiratory reserve, and so forth. When observing an individual with a compromised motor system, remember that you are observing the whole system. An individual with weak labial (lip) muscles might have difficulty getting an adequate seal around the mouthpiece of the spirometer or manometer, so that readings from these instruments will imply respiratory deficits when, in reality, the problem is with the articulatory system! Likewise, insufficiency of the soft palate, whether due to muscular weakness or inadequate tissue, can result in nasal leakage during respiratory tasks. Again, this can result in an apparent respiratory deficit.

on the inner walls of the chamber is the same as that exerted on the outer walls.

The action starts when you close the chamber and change the air volume. Making the chamber smaller does not change the forces that are keeping molecules apart. Rather, it lets those forces be manifest on the walls of the chamber. Although the forces have not changed, the area on which they can exert themselves has, and that results in increased pressure on the walls. That is, Pressure is Force exerted on Area, or $P = F/A$. You have just increased pressure by decreasing area.

Boyle's law states that given a gas of constant temperature, if you increase the volume of the chamber in which the gas is contained, pressure will decrease. When volume increases, pressure decreases, and natural air will flow to equalize that pressure. Thus, air flows into the chamber, in our case, the lungs.

Figure 2–2 shows the same effect graphically. Each chamber has 11 molecules in it. On the left, the volume of the chamber has been reduced, the 11 molecules are much closer together, and the pressure has increased (known as positive pressure). Likewise, when you pull the plunger back so the

Boyle's law: *Given a gas of constant temperature, increasing (or decreasing) the volume of the chamber in which the gas is contained will cause a corresponding decrease (or increase) in pressure.*

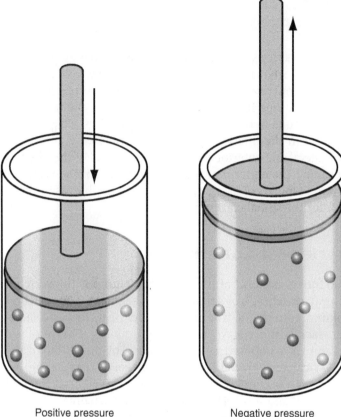

Positive pressure   Negative pressure

Figure 2–2. The piston on the left has been depressed, compressing the air in the chamber and increasing the air pressure. On the right, the piston has been retracted, increasing the space between the molecules and creating a relatively negative pressure.

© Cengage Learning 2014

molecules are farther apart than the forces dictate, the pressure decreases, and the pressure is now referred to as negative pressure. The forces that draw air into the lungs also are responsible for drawing carbon dioxide out. We should also mention that we are not discussing other relevant physical laws that govern gases, such as laws related to volume changes when gases are heated (Charles's law). These laws aren't like the speed limit . . . you can't disobey them, even if you want to!

Summary

■ Pressure is defined as force distributed over area.
■ Boyle's law tells us that as the volume of a container increases, the air pressure in the container decreases.
■ This relatively negative pressure will cause air to enter the container until the pressure is equalized.
■ If volume is decreased, pressure increases and air flows out until the pressure inside and outside are equal.
■ This principle forms the basis for movement of air into and out of the lungs.

SUPPORT STRUCTURE FOR RESPIRATION

The respiratory system consists of a gas-exchanging mechanism supported and protected by a bony cage. Gas exchange is carried out by the lungs while the rib cage protects them.

The lungs are housed in the rib cage in the thorax, an area bounded in the superior aspect by the first rib and clavicle and in the inferior by the twelfth rib (see Figure 2–3). The lateral and anterior aspects are composed of the ribs and sternum. The entire thorax is suspended from the vertebral column (spinal column), a structure that doubles as the conduit for the spinal cord.

Vertebral Column

The functional unit of the vertebral column is the vertebra (plural, vertebrae), or spinal column segment. The vertebral column consists of five divisions: cervical, thoracic, lumbar, sacral, and coccygeal (see Figure 2–4). The vertebral column is composed of 33 segments of bone. There are 7 cervical vertebrae, 12 thoracic vertebrae (paralleling the 12 ribs of the thorax), 5 massive lumbar vertebrae, 5 sacral vertebrae, and 3 (or 4) fused coccygeal vertebrae. The vertebrae are numbered sequentially from superior to inferior

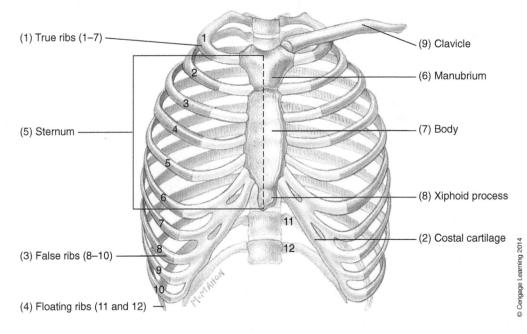

(1) True ribs (1–7)

(9) Clavicle

(6) Manubrium

(5) Sternum

(7) Body

(8) Xiphoid process

(2) Costal cartilage

(3) False ribs (8–10)

(4) Floating ribs (11 and 12)

© Cengage Learning 2014

Figure 2–3. Anterior view of the thorax.

by section, so that the uppermost cervical vertebra is C1, the second is C2, and so forth to C7. Likewise, the first thoracic vertebra is T1 and the last is T12. Lumbar vertebrae include L1 through L5, sacral vertebrae include S1 through S5, and the coccygeal vertebrae are considered a fused unit, known as the coccyx.

The general structure of the vertebrae includes a prominent *spinous process* and *transverse processes* on both sides (Figures 2–5 and 2–6). The *corpus* of the vertebra makes up the anterior portion, with a prominent hole or *vertebral foramen* just posterior to that. The tracts of the nervous system (spinal cord) that supply the body's periphery pass through the vertebral foramen. The spinal nerves exit and enter the spinal cord through the *intervertebral foramina* on either side of the vertebra. Vertebral segments ride one atop another to form the vertebral column, and this articulation is completed by means of the *superior* and *inferior articular*

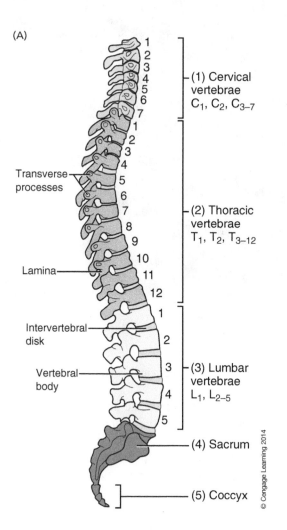

(A)

Transverse processes

Lamina

Intervertebral disk

Vertebral body

1
2
3
4
5
6
7

(1) Cervical vertebrae
C_1, C_2, C_{3-7}

1
2
3
4
5
6
7
8
9
10
11
12

(2) Thoracic vertebrae
T_1, T_2, T_{3-12}

1
2
3
4
5

(3) Lumbar vertebrae
L_1, L_{2-5}

(4) Sacrum

(5) Coccyx

© Cengage Learning 2014

Figure 2–4. (A) Components of the vertebral column consist of 7 cervical (C), 12 thoracic (T), 5 lumbar (L), and 5 sacral (S) vertebrae, as well as the 3 or 4 fused coccygeal vertebrae (the coccyx).   *(continues)*

(B)

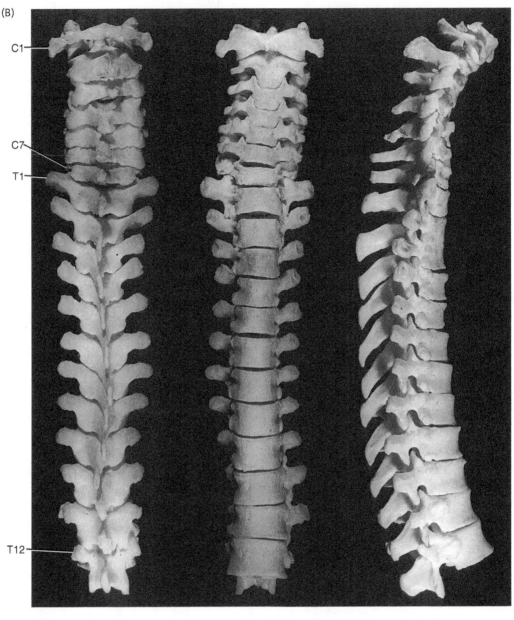

C1

C7

T1

T12

Posterior   Anterior   Lateral

Figure 2–4. continued
(B) Articulated cervical and thoracic vertebrae.

facets. The uppermost cervical vertebra, C1, is the *atlas* and C2 is the *axis.*

The 12 thoracic vertebrae are the base of the respiratory framework because they form the posterior point of attachment for the ribs of the bony thorax. The superior and inferior costal facets are the points of attachment for the ribs, as seen in Figures 2–7 and 2–8.

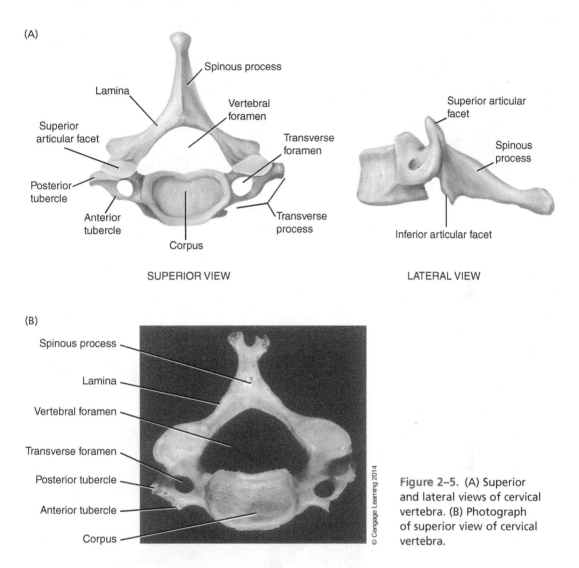

(A)

Spinous process

Lamina

Vertebral foramen

Superior articular facet

Transverse foramen

Posterior tubercle

Anterior tubercle

Transverse process

Corpus

SUPERIOR VIEW

Superior articular facet

Spinous process

Inferior articular facet

LATERAL VIEW

(B)

Spinous process

Lamina

Vertebral foramen

Transverse foramen

Posterior tubercle

Anterior tubercle

Corpus

© Cengage Learning 2014

Figure 2–5. (A) Superior and lateral views of cervical vertebra. (B) Photograph of superior view of cervical vertebra.

The five lumbar vertebrae are quite large compared with those of the thoracic and cervical regions. They provide direct or indirect attachment for a host of back and abdominal muscles, as well as for the posterior fibers of the diaphragm.

The five sacral vertebrae are actually a fused mass known as the *sacrum*. The sacrum and its ossified intervertebral disks retain vestiges of the vertebrae from which they are formed, with remnants of spinous and transverse processes. The *coccyx* is composed of the fused *coccygeal vertebrae*, and it articulates with the inferior sacrum by means of a small disk (see Figure 2–9).

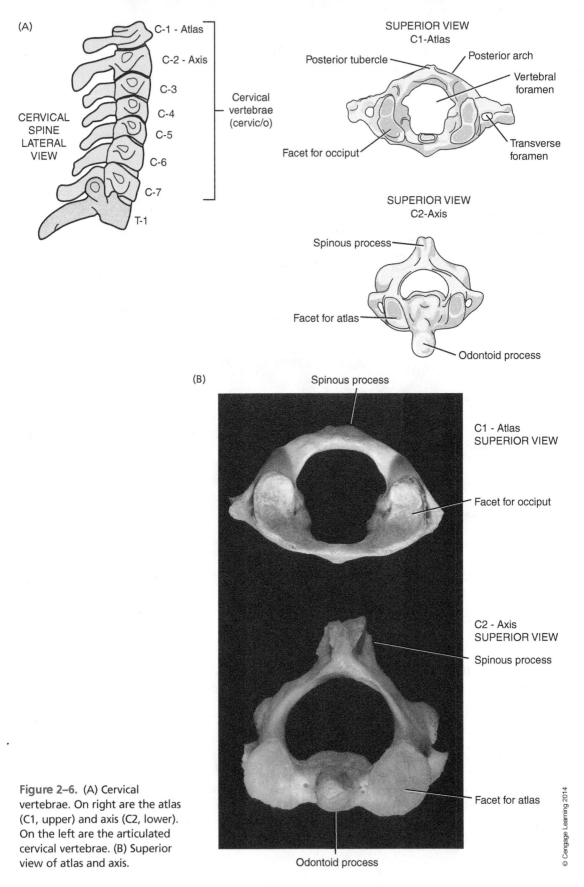

Figure 2–6. (A) Cervical vertebrae. On right are the atlas (C1, upper) and axis (C2, lower). On the left are the articulated cervical vertebrae. (B) Superior view of atlas and axis.

© Cengage Learning 2014

38

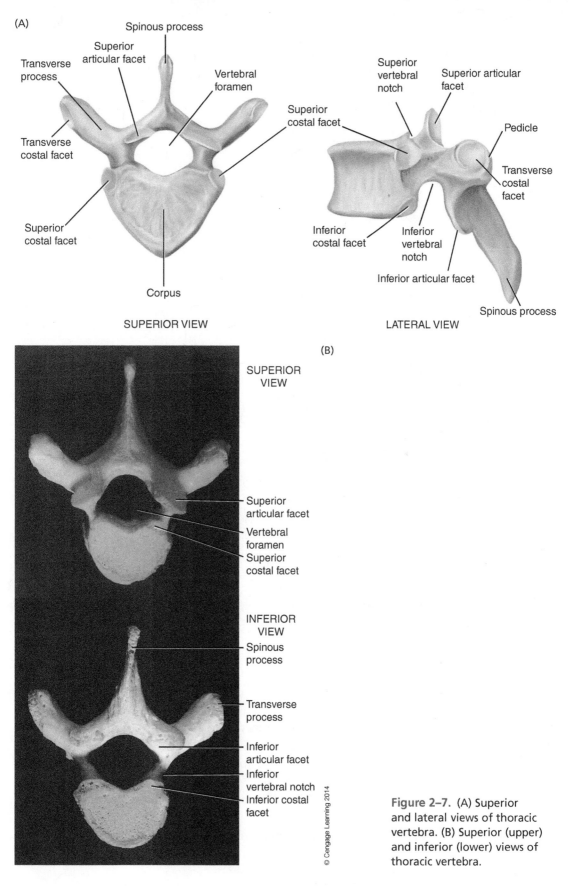

(A)

Spinous process

Superior
articular facet

Transverse
process

Vertebral
foramen

Superior
costal facet

Transverse
costal facet

Superior
costal facet

Corpus

SUPERIOR VIEW

Superior
vertebral
notch

Superior articular
facet

Pedicle

Transverse
costal
facet

Inferior
costal facet

Inferior
vertebral
notch

Inferior articular facet

Spinous process

LATERAL VIEW

(B)

SUPERIOR
VIEW

Superior
articular facet

Vertebral
foramen

Superior
costal facet

INFERIOR
VIEW

Spinous
process

Transverse
process

Inferior
articular facet

Inferior
vertebral notch

Inferior costal
facet

© Cengage Learning 2014

Figure 2–7. (A) Superior
and lateral views of thoracic
vertebra. (B) Superior (upper)
and inferior (lower) views of
thoracic vertebra.

39

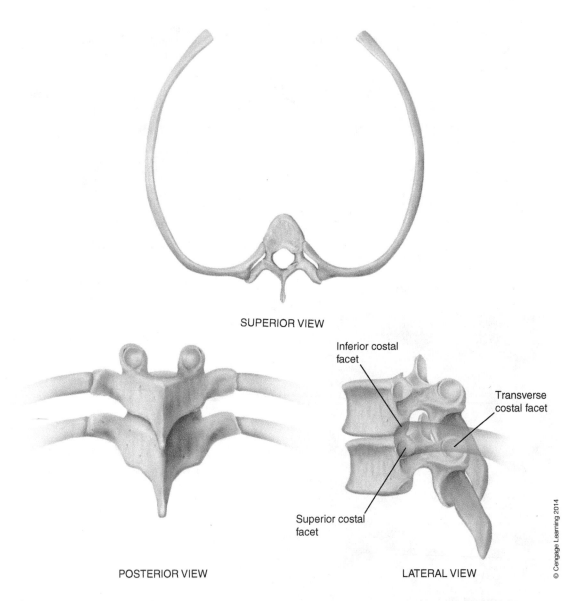

SUPERIOR VIEW

Inferior costal
facet

Transverse
costal facet

Superior costal
facet

POSTERIOR VIEW

LATERAL VIEW

© Cengage Learning 2014

Figure 2–8. Articulation of ribs
and vertebrae.

Summary

- The vertebral column is composed of vertebral segments combined to form a strong but flexible column.
- Vertebrae are labeled, based on their level: C1 to C7 (cervical), T1 to T12 (thoracic), L1 to L5 (lumbar), S1 to S5 (sacral).
- The fused coccygeal vertebrae are referred to as the coccyx.
- The vertebral column provides the points of attachment for numerous muscles by means of the spinous and transverse processes.

(A)

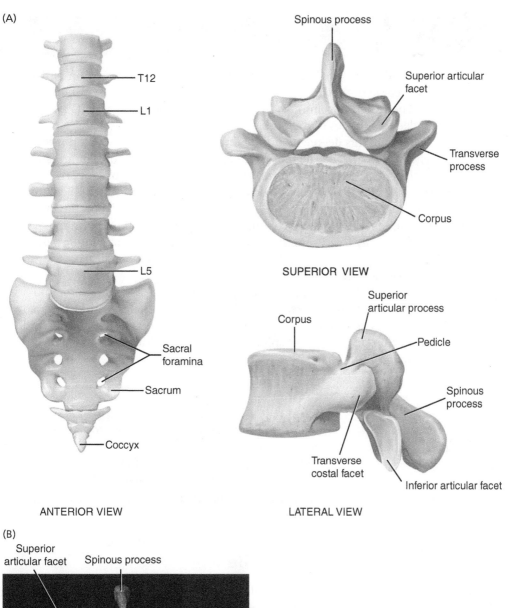

T12

L1

L5

Sacral
foramina

Sacrum

Coccyx

ANTERIOR VIEW

Spinous process

Superior articular
facet

Transverse
process

Corpus

SUPERIOR VIEW

Corpus

Superior
articular process

Pedicle

Spinous
process

Transverse
costal facet

Inferior articular facet

LATERAL VIEW

(B)

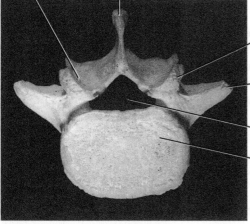

Superior
articular facet

Spinous process

Superior
articular process

Transverse
process

Vertebral foramen

Corpus

Lumbar vertebra
SUPERIOR VIEW

© Cengage Learning 2014

Figure 2–9. (A) Lumbar
vertebrae articulated with
sacrum and coccyx (left).
Upper right shows superior
view of lumbar vertebra, and
lower right shows lateral view.
(B) Superior view of lumbar
vertebra.

Spinal Cord Injury

The spinal cord is well protected by the osseous vertebral column in that the vertebrae fit together in a partial lock-and-key fashion to inhibit motion. The vertebral column is richly bound together by ligaments and surrounded by muscles of the back.

Despite this degree of redundant protection, the spinal cord is frequently traumatized. The most frequent cause of spinal cord injury is vehicle accidents, especially those in which the occupant is not properly restrained. When a person is ejected from a vehicle, the vertebral column can undergo rotatory stresses that can tear the spinal cord, and the impact can compress the vertebral column, resulting in distention of the spinal cord. (Typically the compression occurs in the corpus, implying hyperflexion of the neck.) Significant transverse forces can cause a shearing of the spinal cord as well.

The result of spinal cord injury is frequently the loss of motor and sensory function to the area below the spinal cord injury, with subsequent paraplegia (legs paralyzed) or quadriplegia (both arms and legs paralyzed). For an exhaustive review of spinal cord injury, see Mackay, Chapman, and Morgan (1997).

- The vertebral column houses the spinal cord, with spinal nerves emerging from and entering the spinal cord through spaces between the vertebrae.
- The ribs of the rib cage articulate with the spinal column in a fashion that permits the rib cage limited movement for respiration.

Pelvic Girdle

The pelvic girdle provides a strong structure for attaching the legs to the vertebral column (see Figure 2–10). The pelvic girdle is made up of the ileum, sacrum, pubic bone, and ischium. The ilium is a large, winglike bone (similar in this way to the scapula, or shoulder blade, of the upper body) that provides the bulk of support for the abdominal musculature and the prominent hip bone. The iliac bones articulate with the sacrum laterally, forming the sacroiliac joints.

Pectoral Girdle

The pectoral, or shoulder, girdle includes the scapula and clavicle. The clavicle, also known as the collarbone, is attached to the superior sternum, running laterally to join the scapula. The clavicle provides the anterior support for the shoulder by its articulation with the scapula (see Figure 2–11). The scapula has its only skeletal attachment via the clavicle, which in turn has its only skeletal attachment at the sternum. From the scapula are slung several muscles that hold it in a dynamic tension that facilitates flexible upper body movement while not compromising strength.

Summary

- The bony support structure of the respiratory system is composed of the rib cage and vertebral column.
- At the base of the vertebral column is the pelvic girdle, composed of the ilium, sacrum, pubic bone, and ischium.
- The pectoral girdle comprises the scapula and clavicle, which attach to the sternum, and is the superior counterpart to the pelvic girdle.

Ribs and Rib Cage

Ribs are capable of a degree of movement, so that the rib cage can rock up in front and flare out via lateral rotation,

(A)

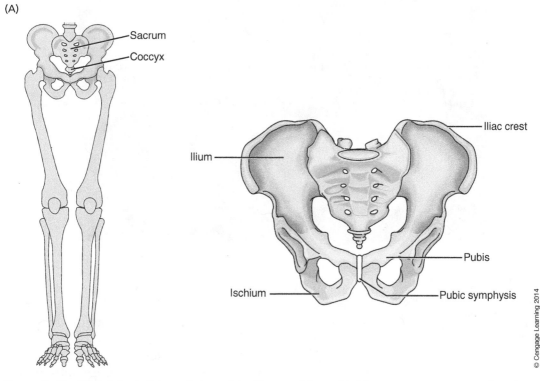

Figure 2–10. (A) Pelvic girdle, consisting of the ilium, pubis, and ischium.   *(continues)*

(B)

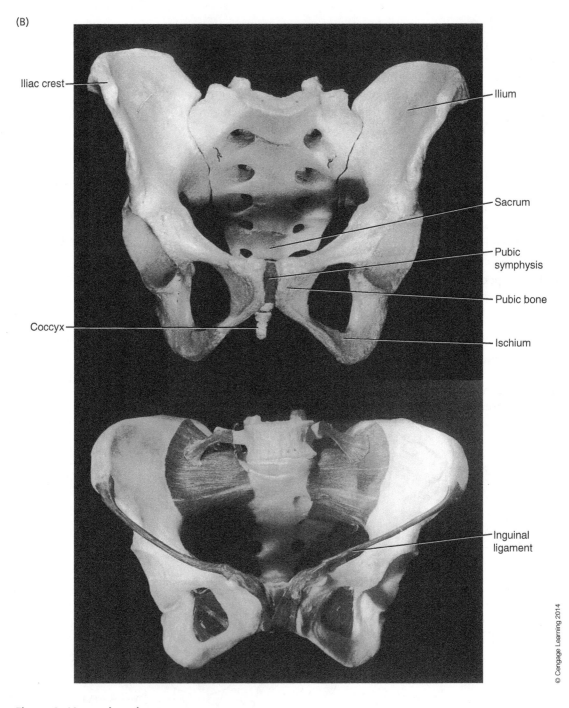

Iliac crest

Ilium

Sacrum

Pubic symphysis

Pubic bone

Coccyx

Ischium

Inguinal ligament

Figure 2–10. continued
(B) Anterior view of pelvis. Lower view shows location of the inguinal ligament.

hinged on the vertebral articulation with the rib cage. The rib cage is made up of 12 ribs, with all but the lowest two attached by means of cartilage to the sternum in the front aspect of the rib cage.

The rib cage tends to slant down in front, as shown in Figure 2–12. With the mobility of the rib cage granted by the articulation of the vertebrae and ribs, the rib cage is quite capable of elevating during inspiration to increase the size of the thorax.

Ribs are of three general classes: true ribs, false ribs, and floating ribs. The *true ribs* consist of ribs 1 through 7, all of which form more or less direct attachment with the sternum. Their actual attachment is by means of a cartilaginous

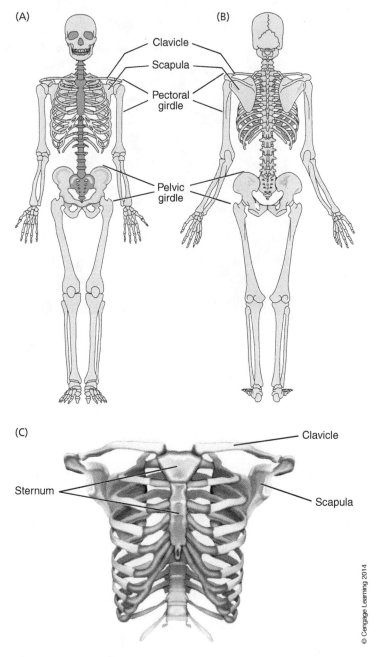

Figure 2–11. (A) Anterior view of skeleton, showing components of pelvic and pectoral girdle. (B) Posterior view. (C) Isolated pectoral girdle. *(continues)*

(D)

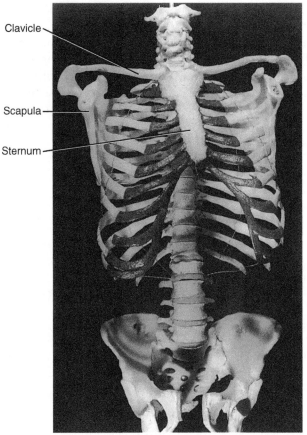

Clavicle

Scapula

Sternum

© Cengage Learning 2014

PELVIC AND PECTORAL GIRDLES

Figure 2–11. continued
(D) Articulated thorax with pelvic and pectoral girdles.

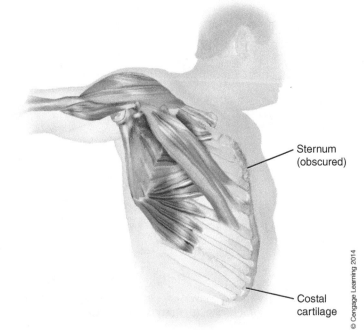

Sternum (obscured)

Costal cartilage

© Cengage Learning 2014

Figure 2–12. Lateral view of rib cage showing relationships among ribs and sternum. Note that the rib cage slants down in the front.

union through the cartilaginous (*chondral*) portion of the rib. The *false ribs* (ribs 8, 9, and 10) also are attached to the sternum through cartilage, although this chondral portion must run superiorly to attach to the sternum. The *floating*, or *vertebral, ribs* (ribs 11 and 12) articulate only with the vertebral column.

The chondral attachment is particularly useful because the elastic properties of cartilage permit the rib cage to be expanded without breaking. Thus, the rib cage is quite strong (being made predominantly of bone) but capable of movement (being well-endowed with resilient cartilage).

The rib cage provides the basis for respiration, and the general structure of the "barrel" deserves some attention here. The ribs make their posterior attachment along the vertebral column. The ribs course posterolaterally and then arch around to the anterior aspect of the body. This provides the bony structure for most of the posterior, lateral, and anterior aspects of the thorax. The ribs slope downward when the rib cage is inactive and at equilibrium. We should note that for a long time the field held the trilogy of torque, elasticity, and gravity to be the components that governed passive expiration, but we have gained new insight into this

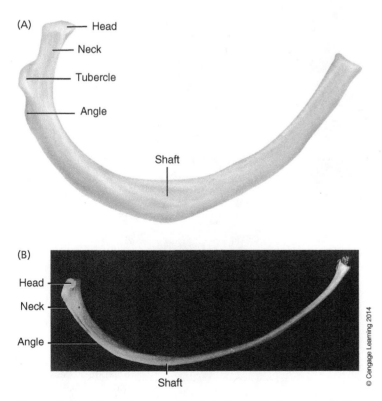

Figure 2–13. (A) Landmarks of typical rib. (B) Photograph of rib showing landmarks.

function and realize that torque most likely is not a player in expiration (Hixon, 2006).

The posterior attachment of the rib is made through a *gliding* (arthrodial) *articulation* with the thoracic vertebrae (see Figure 2–13). This permits the rib to rock up in both lateral and anterior directions during inspiration.

Sternum

The sternum has three components: the *manubrium sterni*, the *corpus* (body), and the *xiphoid*, or *ensiform, process* (see Figure 2–14). The clavicle and first rib are attached to the

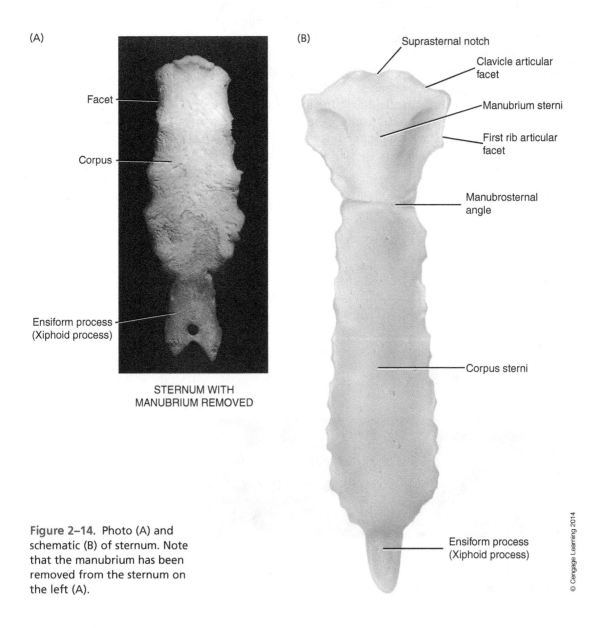

(A)

Facet

Corpus

Ensiform process
(Xiphoid process)

STERNUM WITH
MANUBRIUM REMOVED

(B) Suprasternal notch

Clavicle articular facet

Manubrium sterni

First rib articular facet

Manubrosternal angle

Corpus sterni

Ensiform process
(Xiphoid process)

© Cengage Learning 2014

Figure 2–14. Photo (A) and schematic (B) of sternum. Note that the manubrium has been removed from the sternum on the left (A).

manubrium sterni, and the second rib articulates at the juncture of the manubrium and corpus, known as the *manubrosternal angle*. The next five ribs (3 through 7) articulate directly with the corpus, and the remaining (false) ribs (8, 9, and 10) are attached by means of more indirect costal cartilage. The floating ribs (11 and 12) are free in the anterior.

Summary

- The rib cage is composed of 12 ribs (7 true ribs, 3 false ribs, and 2 floating ribs).
- The cartilaginous attachment of the ribs to the sternum permits the ribs to rotate slightly during respiration, allowing the rib cage to elevate.
- The construction of the ribs provides the characteristic curved barrel shape of the rib cage.
- At rest the ribs slope downward, but they elevate during inspiration.

SOFT TISSUE OF THE THORAX AND RESPIRATORY PASSAGEWAY

Deep inside the rib cage lies the core of respiration. Gas exchange for life occurs within the lungs, which are spongy, elastic tissue that is richly perfused with vascular supply and air sacs. Healthy, young lungs are pink; older lungs that have undergone the stresses of modern, polluted life are gray. The lungs communicate with the external environment by means of the respiratory passageway, which includes the oral and nasal cavities, larynx, trachea, and bronchial tubes.

Turbulence and Respiration

The respiratory passageway offers relatively low resistance to airflow, a fact that works in favor of efficient respiration with little effort. As resistance to airflow increases, the effort required to draw air into the lungs increases as well, causing rapid fatigue. You may remember the exhaustion you felt the last time you had a respiratory infection that caused excessive secretions in your respiratory passageway. Part of the fatigue you felt was caused by the turbulence produced by the mucus in the passageway. The extra drag caused by these elements has to be overcome to keep the body oxygenated, and the muscles of respiration have to work overtime to do the task.

bifurcates: *Divides into two parts.*

The trachea is a flexible tube composed of a series of 16 to 20 hyaline cartilage rings that are open in the posterior aspect. This tube runs from the inferior border of the larynx for about 11 cm, where it bifurcates (divides) to become the left and right mainstem bronchi (or bronchial tubes), which serve the left and right lungs, respectively (see Figure 2–15).

The cartilaginous rings of the trachea are particularly well suited for the task of air transport. Because the process involves drawing air into the lungs and expelling it, pressures (negative and positive) must be generated to get that gas moving, but the same pressures will tend to collapse

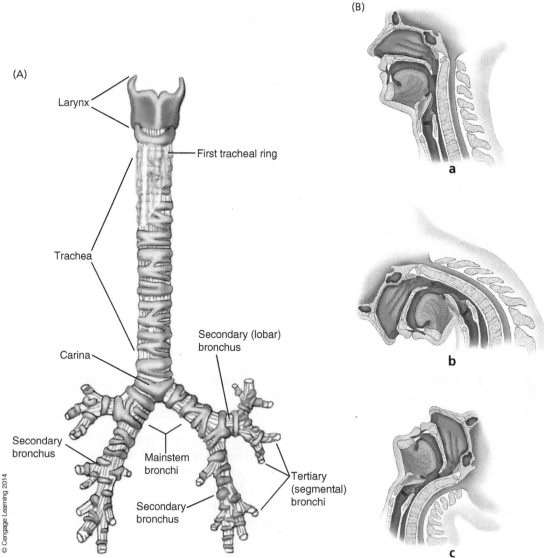

Figure 2–15. (A) Bronchial passageway, including trachea, mainstem bronchi, secondary (lobar) bronchi, and tertiary (segmental) bronchi. (B) Effect of head posture on airway patency.   *(continues)*

Modified from Moser, K. M., & Spragg, R. G. (1982). *Respiratory emergencies.* St. Louis: Mosby.

© Cengage Learning 2014

(C)

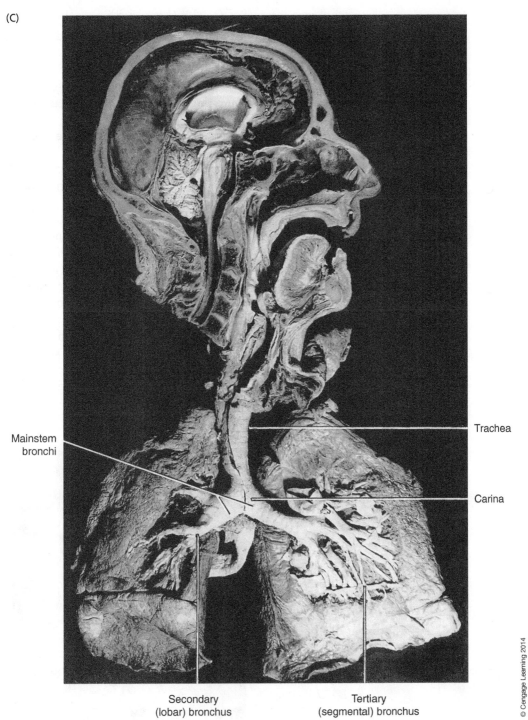

Mainstem
bronchi

Trachea

Carina

Secondary
(lobar) bronchus

Tertiary
(segmental) bronchus

© Cengage Learning 2014

Figure 2–15. continued (C) Respiratory passageway from oral cavity to segmental bronchi. Note that lungs have been dissected to reveal the bronchi within.

or expand tissue that is not reinforced for strength. On the other hand, a strictly rigid tube would restrict body movements. Thus, the trachea must be both rigid and flexible. In response to this need, the trachea is built of hyaline cartilage rings connected by fibroelastic membrane. The cartilage provides support while the membrane permits freedom of movement.

Posterior to the trachea is the esophagus. The *esophagus* is a long, collapsed tube that runs behind and adjacent to the trachea and is the conduit to the digestive system.

The lungs are a composite of tissues, including blood, arterial and venous network, connective tissue, respiratory pathway, and tissue specialized for gas exchange. The bronchial tree is characterized by increasingly smaller tubes as it progresses into the depths of the lungs. The *mainstem bronchi* serve the left and right lungs, and the *lobar* (intermediate) *bronchi* supply the lobes of the lungs. Further branchings occur, down to the final *terminal respiratory bronchioles.*

The right lung is composed of three lobes, separated by fissures. The left lung has only two lobes (see Figure 2–16). The right mainstem bronchus divides to supply the superior, middle, and inferior lobes of the right lung. The left mainstem bronchus bifurcates to serve the superior and inferior

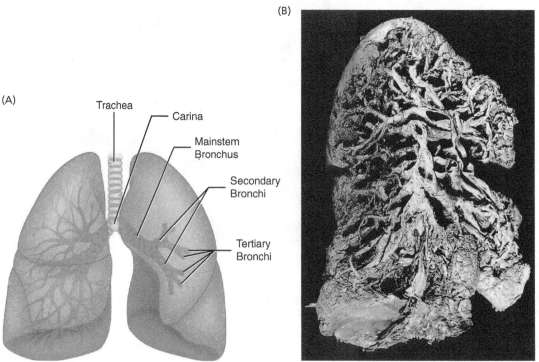

(B)

(A)

Trachea

Carina

Mainstem Bronchus

Secondary Bronchi

Tertiary Bronchi

© Cengage Learning 2014

Figure 2–16. (A) Bronchial tree within lungs. (B) Lung dissected to reveal bronchial passageway.

lobes of the left lung, and there is a vestigial middle lobe (called the lingula). The space vacated by the missing lobe is taken up by the heart and mediastinum, or "middle space," structures (see Figure 2–17).

The next level of branching serves the segments of each lobe. At this level of division, the bronchi divide repeatedly into smaller and smaller cartilaginous tubes, with the final tube being the terminal (end) bronchiole (see Figure 2–18).

(A)

Right lung		Left lung	
Superior lobe		Superior lobe	
Apical	1	Upper division	
Posterior	2	Apical/Posterior	1 & 2
Anterior	3	Anterior	3
Middle lobe		Lower division (lingular)	
Lateral	4	Superior lingula	4
Medial	5	Inferior lingula	5
Inferior lobe		Inferior lobe	
Superior	6	Superior	6
Medial basal	7	Anterior medial basal	7 & 8
Anterior basal	8	Lateral basal	9
Lateral basal	9	Posterior basal	10
Posterior basal	10		

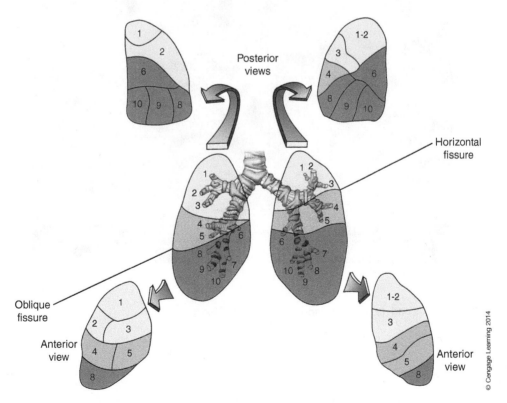

Figure 2–17. (A) Schematic representation of lungs, showing lobes and segments.   *(continues)*

© Cengage Learning 2014

(B)

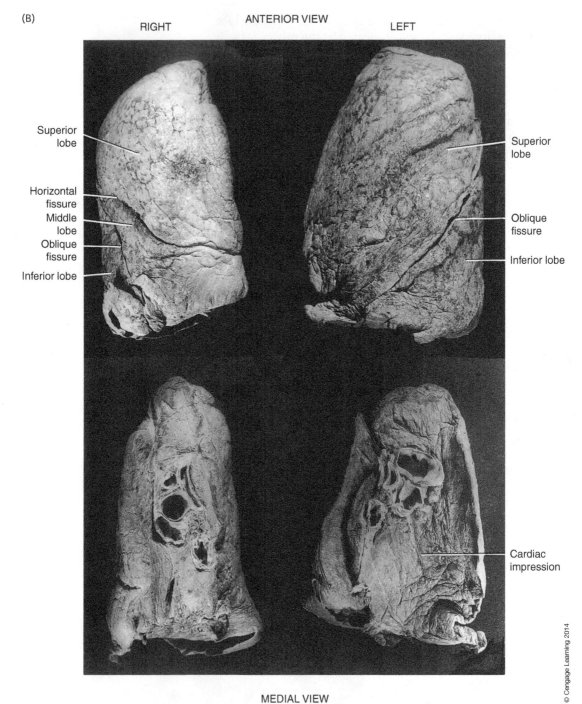

ANTERIOR VIEW

RIGHT   LEFT

Superior
lobe

Superior
lobe

Horizontal
fissure

Oblique
fissure

Middle
lobe

Oblique
fissure

Inferior lobe

Inferior lobe

Cardiac
impression

MEDIAL VIEW

© Cengage Learning 2014

Figure 2–17. continued (B) Anterior and medial view of lungs.

(C)

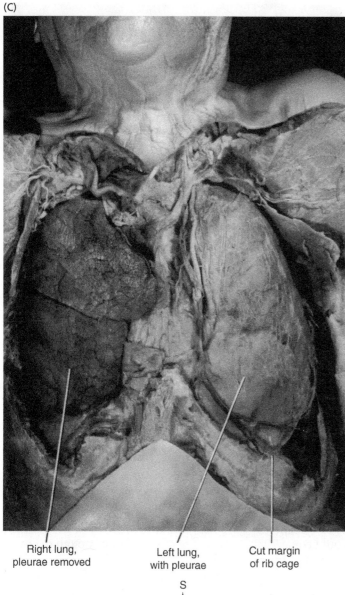

Right lung,
pleurae removed

Left lung,
with pleurae

Cut margin
of rib cage

S

R ←——→ L

I

© Cengage Learning 2014

Figure 2–17. continued
(C) Anterior view of lungs
in situ.

 This repeated branching has an important effect on re-spiratory function. There are 28 generations of subdivisions in the respiratory tree, providing a truly amazing amount of surface area for respiration. Although the cross-sectional area of the trachea is about 5 cm^2 (about the diameter of a quarter), the cross-sectional area of the 300 million alveoli

Muscular Weakness and Respiration

Individuals with diseases that weaken the muscles of inspiration are at significant respiratory risk for a number of reasons. Although gravity is the friend of respiration in a person with normal function, inspiration requires muscular effort, and that effort is aimed very specifically at overcoming gravity.

Individuals in the later stages of motor neuron diseases such as amyotrophic lateral sclerosis (ALS) suffer from extreme muscular weakness as a result of the disease but are still faced with the oxygenation demands typically met with respiratory work. If a person with such a disease is placed in the supine position (on the back), gravity will conspire against his or her respiratory effort, and this "resting" position will actually put the person at risk for respiratory distress. Here's why: when supine, gravity is pushing on the abdominal viscera, forcing the viscera toward the person's back. When the individual attempts to inhale, the abdomen should protrude, but with compromised muscular strength, that will require more effort than the person can accomplish. When supine, the abdominal viscera are one more thing to overcome, and that is one thing too many.

To overcome this, people in the later stages of ALS often remain in a semireclined position to permit rest but capitalize on gravity to assist with respiration. By the way, this might also give you a clue as to why individuals with weakened musculature are more prone to pneumonia than healthy individuals. It takes a great deal of work to clear the lungs and to keep them clear.

would equal 70 m^2, or the area of a rug large enough to cover a 10 ft × 24 ft room!

The terminal bronchiole is small (about 1 mm in diameter), and at its end becomes the alveolar duct, which in turn communicates with the alveolus. The alveoli are extremely small (approximately 0.25 mm in diameter) but extremely plentiful. There are approximately 300 million alveoli in mature lungs.

alveoli: *Air sacs in the lungs.*

The **alveoli** at this terminal point do the real work of respiration by virtue of their architecture and relationship with the vascular supply (see Figure 2–18). The alveolus is an extremely thin membrane (about one third the thickness of a red blood cell) that is permeable to both oxygen and carbon dioxide in the proper circumstances.

The rich investment with alveoli make the lungs spongy because the surfactant (a substance that lowers surface tension) at that level promotes inflation of the alveoli.

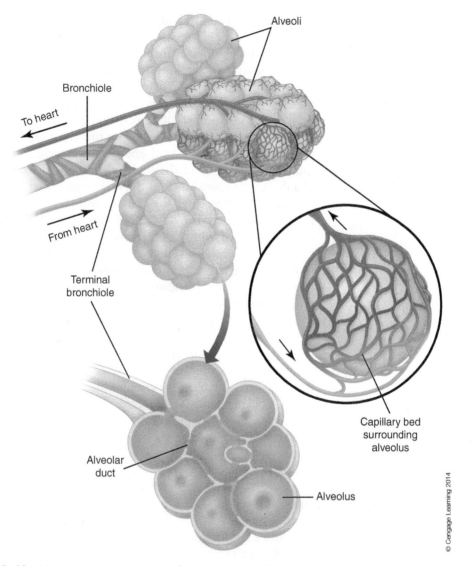

Figure 2–18. Schematic representation of cluster of alveoli with capillary bed. Lower portion shows a cross section through alveoli and terminal bronchiole.

Each alveolus is richly supplied with blood for gas exchange from more than 2000 capillaries. A little multiplication will reveal that there are more than 600 billion capillaries involved in gas exchange, reminding us of the amount of vascular tissue in the lungs. The lungs also have an intricate lacework of cartilage; the bronchial tree is invested with this supportive tissue and most branches of this tree contain cartilage. At the terminal point in the bronchial tree the marvel of gas exchange takes place. Attached to the final cartilaginous bronchiole is the alveolus, or air sac, the point at which oxygen and carbon dioxide are transferred to and from the bloodstream.

The respiratory pathway has multiple filtering functions to safeguard the lungs against pollutants. The nostril hairs are the first line of defense, catching most particulate matter greater than 10 microns (a micron is one millionth of a meter, also known as a micrometer, μm) before they enter the trachea. The moist mucous membrane of the upper respiratory system provides another receptacle for foreign matter. Goblet cells in the mucosal lining and submucosal glands secrete lubricant into the respiratory tract that traps pollutants as they enter the trachea and larynx. The respiratory passageway from the nose to the beginning of the bronchi is lined with tall columnar epithelium covered by cilia (hairlike processes) that beat more than 1000 times per minute. In the lower pathway, the beating action drives pollutants upward, and beating drives nasal-passage contaminants posteriorly.

The beating epithelial cilia progressively move the material up the bronchi to the level of the vocal folds in the larynx, at which time the breathing person feels the stimulation of secretion at the vocal folds and "clears her throat." That "ahem" is just enough force to blow the mucus off the folds (mucus is the dense fluid product of mucous membrane tissue), where it can be swallowed without further ado. Unfortunately, these beating epithelial cells can be damaged by pollutants such as cigarette smoke, resulting in the failure of this system. Particles in the 2 to 10 micron range will settle on the walls of the bronchi, where they are eliminated by these beating epithelial cilia. If a particle is smaller than 2 microns, it will generally reach the alveolus but will be eliminated by microphages, the cells that destroy foreign matter.

The lymphatic system provides a final cleaning stage for the respiratory tissue. The upper respiratory passageway effectively removes normal levels of particulate pollution down to diameters of approximately 5 microns, but smaller particles are not filtered. These particles down to the level of the terminal bronchiole are eliminated by the lymphatic system. Pollutants are suspended in mucus and through coughing migrate to the bronchioles, where they can be eliminated by the lymphatics and macrophages.

The respiratory passageway also protects the lungs by warming and humidifying the air as it enters. The mucous membrane is highly vascularized, permitting rapid transfer of heat from blood to air.

Summary

- The respiratory system is composed of right and left lungs, which have three and two lobes, respectively.
- Communication between the external and internal environments is by means of the trachea and bronchial tree.
- Repeated subdivisions of this bronchial tree ends with the alveoli, the site of gas exchange.
- These highly vascularized alveoli provide the mechanism by which oxygen enters the bloodstream and carbon dioxide is removed.
- Pollutants entering the respiratory tract are removed through the cleansing action of beating epithelia that line the bronchial passageway.

MOVEMENT OF AIR THROUGH THE SYSTEM

Recall that the cavity holding the lungs is supported by muscle and bone, which cover every centimeter of the thoracic wall. Likewise, the bottom of the thoracic cavity is completely sealed by the diaphragm, making the thorax almost impervious to the outside world, were it not for the respiratory passageway. The only way air can normally enter or leave the lungs is through the tubes connected to them (the bronchial tree, continuous with the upper respiratory passageway).

Pneumothorax

Pneumothorax (*pneumo* = air) is aggregation of air in the pleural space between the lungs and the chest wall with subsequent loss of the negative intrapleural pressure. It can arise through one of several means, but the product is always a "collapsed" lung. In "open" pneumothorax, air is introduced into the space through a breach of the thoracic wall, typically by means of a puncture wound (e.g., knife wound, automobile accident). Air introduced into the intrapleural space causes a loss of the constant negative intrapleural pressure. If you recall that this pressure maintains the close bond between the visceral pleural lining of the lungs and that of the inner thorax, it may not surprise you to learn that when that bond is broken by the open wound, the lungs collapse. This collapse occurs because the lungs are in a state of constant distention, owing to the difference between the size of the thorax and the smaller lungs.

Now comes the tricky part. The lungs are simply placed inside this cavity, not held to the walls by ligaments or cartilage. It is as if you placed a too-small sponge in a too-large bottle, because the thoracic volume is greater than that of the lungs at rest.

The lungs and inner thoracic wall are completely covered with a *pleural lining* (see Figure 2–19), and this lining is a smooth contact for rough tissue, as well as a mechanism for translating the force of thorax enlargement into inspiration. The lungs are encased in linings referred to as the *visceral pleurae*, and the thoracic linings are the *parietal pleurae*. The visceral and parietal pleurae are actually continuous with each other. These wrappings completely encase both the lungs and inner thorax. This continuous sheet provides the airtight seal required to permit the lungs to follow the movement of the thorax.

To understand how these pleurae help us breathe will take a little thought. You have probably experienced the difficulty involved in separating two pieces of plastic food wrap, especially if there is fluid between the two sheets. There is a degree of surface tension arising from the presence of fluid and highly conforming surfaces that helps keep the sheets together. Likewise, cuboidal cells in the pleural lining produce a mucous solution that is released into the space between the parietal and visceral pleurae. This surfactant

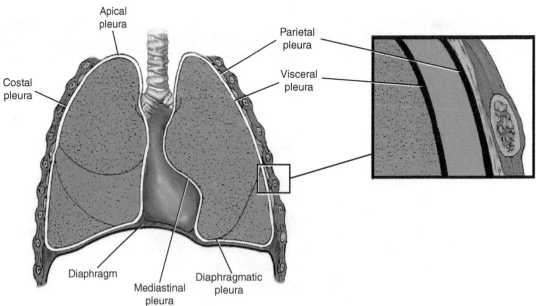

Figure 2–19. Pleural linings of the lungs and thorax. Parietal pleurae include costal, diaphragmatic, mediastinal, and apical pleurae. Visceral pleurae line the lungs.

reduces the surface tension in the lungs and provides a slippery interface between the lungs and the thoracic wall, permitting easy, low-friction gliding of the lungs within the thorax. The lung and rib cage surfaces conform to each other as a result of the fluid bond between them, and a negative pressure is maintained by lack of contact with the outside atmosphere. When you contract the diaphragm, the pleural lining of the diaphragm (diaphragmatic pleura) maintains its contact with the visceral pleurae of the two lungs above it, and the lungs expand.

The heart is encased in the mediastinal pleurae, along with nerves, blood vessels, thymus gland, the esophagus, and lymph vessels (see Figure 2–20). The mediastinum is the most important and best protected region of the body.

The left and right *phrenic nerves* serving the diaphragm pass along the lateral surfaces of the pericardium (the membranous sac enclosing the heart) to innervate the diaphragm.

mediastinal: *Referring to the mediastinum or middle space of the thorax, which contains the heart.*

pericardium: *The membranous sac enclosing the heart.*

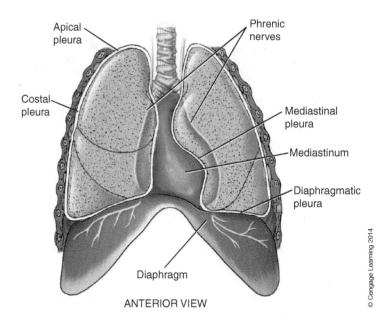

Apical pleura

Phrenic nerves

Costal pleura

Mediastinal pleura

Mediastinum

Diaphragmatic pleura

Diaphragm

ANTERIOR VIEW

© Cengage Learning 2014

Figure 2–20. Relationships among mediastinum, diaphragm, and lungs. Note the phrenic nerve innervation of the diaphragm.

Summary

■ The lungs are covered with pleural linings that, in conjunction with the lungs, provide the mechanism for air movement through muscular action.

- When the diaphragm contracts, the lungs are pulled down as a result of the association between the pleurae and the diaphragm.
- Diaphragmatic contraction expands the lungs, drawing air into them through the bronchial passageway.

MUSCLES OF INSPIRATION

As with many voluntary bodily functions, inspiration is a graded activity. Depending on your body's needs, you are capable of quiet inspiration, which requires only one muscle, and forced inspiration, which calls on many more muscles. We enlist the help of increasingly larger numbers of muscles as our respiratory needs increase. Refer to Table 2–1 for a summary of the muscles of respiration.

palpation: *Feeling a structure using one's hands.*

Palpation of Sternal Landmarks

Palpation of structures (feeling them with your hands) on your own body will improve your awareness of these structures and their organization into systems. First, palpate the sternal notch. To identify its location, find your "Adam's apple," the prominence of the larynx about which you will learn a great deal in future chapters. Now draw your finger down until you reach a prominent horizontal ledge. That ledge is the sternal notch. Now draw your finger to either side and you will feel a significant bump. This is the clavicle.

Now move your fingers laterally to feel the clavicle itself as it projects to its union with the scapula. Identify the lower margin of the clavicle at the sternoclavicular joint; if you press deeply into the muscle at that point, you may be able to palpate the first rib. Move your fingers back to the sternal notch, and then draw them down the sternum about an inch. You should easily feel a prominent ridge, the manubrosternal angle or joint. Placing one finger on your sternal notch and another on the manubrosternal angle will show you the upper and lower limits of the manubrium sterni.

If you draw your finger down another couple of inches below the manubrosternal angle, you will feel the lower margin of the corpus sterni, and beneath this the xiphoid or ensiform process.

The union of the sternum and clavicle is the sternoclavicular joint, and it occurs at the manubrium sterni, lateral to the sternal notch.

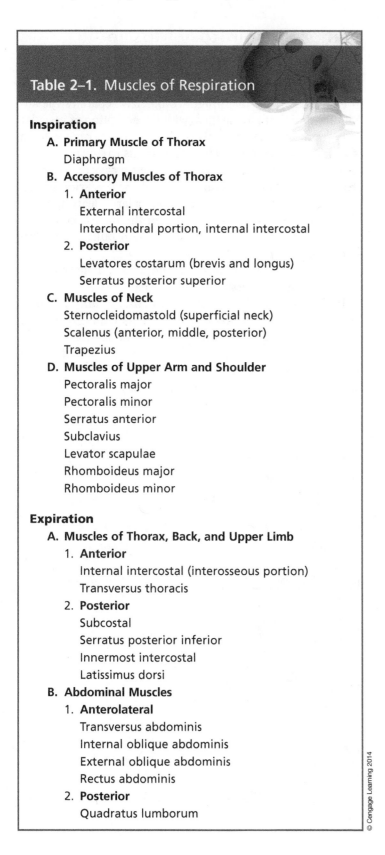

Table 2–1. Muscles of Respiration

Inspiration
  A. **Primary Muscle of Thorax**
     Diaphragm
  B. **Accessory Muscles of Thorax**
     1. **Anterior**
        External intercostal
        Interchondral portion, internal intercostal
     2. **Posterior**
        Levatores costarum (brevis and longus)
        Serratus posterior superior
  C. **Muscles of Neck**
     Sternocleidomastold (superficial neck)
     Scalenus (anterior, middle, posterior)
     Trapezius
  D. **Muscles of Upper Arm and Shoulder**
     Pectoralis major
     Pectoralis minor
     Serratus anterior
     Subclavius
     Levator scapulae
     Rhomboideus major
     Rhomboideus minor

Expiration
  A. **Muscles of Thorax, Back, and Upper Limb**
     1. **Anterior**
        Internal intercostal (interosseous portion)
        Transversus thoracis
     2. **Posterior**
        Subcostal
        Serratus posterior inferior
        Innermost intercostal
        Latissimus dorsi
  B. **Abdominal Muscles**
     1. **Anterolateral**
        Transversus abdominis
        Internal oblique abdominis
        External oblique abdominis
        Rectus abdominis
     2. **Posterior**
        Quadratus lumborum

© Cengage Learning 2014

Primary Inspiratory Muscle of Thorax: The Diaphragm

The primary muscle of inspiration is the *diaphragm*. As seen in Figure 2–21, the diaphragm completely separates the abdominal and thoracic cavities (with the exception of vascular and esophageal hiatus). This striated muscle takes the form of a large inverted bowl. The edges of this irregular bowl attach along the inferior boundary of the rib cage and xiphoid process and to the vertebral column in the posterior aspect. The intermediate region is made up of a large, leafy aponeurosis called the *central tendon*. When the muscle contracts, muscle fibers shorten and the diaphragm pulls the central tendon down and back (see Figure 2–22).

The muscle fibers of the diaphragm radiate out from the central tendon, forming the sternal, costal, and vertebral attachments. The anterior-most *sternal attachment* is made at the xiphoid process, with fibers coursing up and back to insert into the anterior central tendon. Lateral to the xiphoid, the fibers of the diaphragm attach to the inner borders of ribs 7 through 12 and to the costal cartilages to form the *costal attachment*. In the posterior aspect,

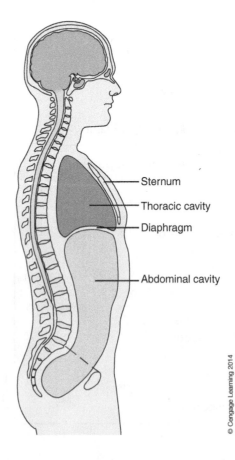

Sternum

Thoracic cavity

Diaphragm

Abdominal cavity

© Cengage Learning 2014

Figure 2–21. Lateral view schematic of diaphragm and thorax. Notice that the diaphragm courses markedly down from the sternum to the vertebral attachment, completely separating the thorax from the abdomen.

the *vertebral diaphragmatic* attachment is made with the lumbar vertebrae.

The actual muscle fibers of the diaphragm radiate out from the imperfect center formed by the central tendon. Careful examination of the forces of muscular contraction will be most helpful in later discussion of muscular contraction and action. Remember that muscle can perform only one task, and that is to shorten. If a muscle is attached to two points, shortening tends to bring those two points closer together or simply tense the muscle if neither point is capable of moving. Although the principles of muscle action and result still hold, movement of the diaphragm will not make a great deal of sense until you realize where the points of attachment really are.

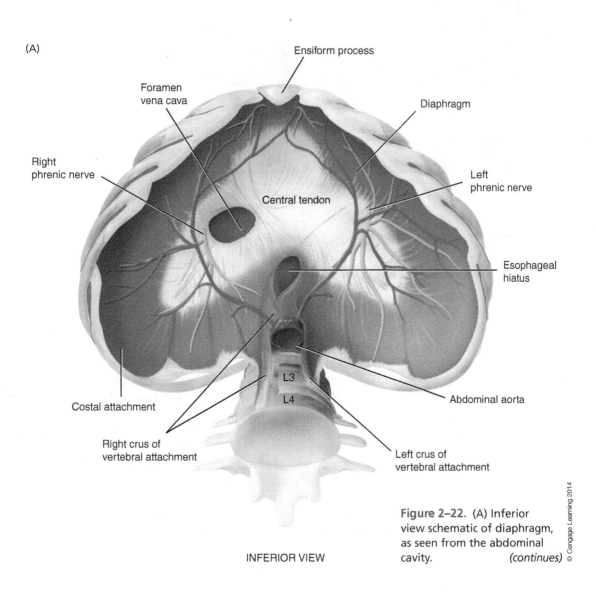

(A)

Ensiform process

Foramen vena cava

Diaphragm

Right phrenic nerve

Left phrenic nerve

Central tendon

Esophageal hiatus

L3

L4

Costal attachment

Abdominal aorta

Right crus of vertebral attachment

Left crus of vertebral attachment

INFERIOR VIEW

Figure 2–22. (A) Inferior view schematic of diaphragm, as seen from the abdominal cavity.   *(continues)*

© Cengage Learning 2014

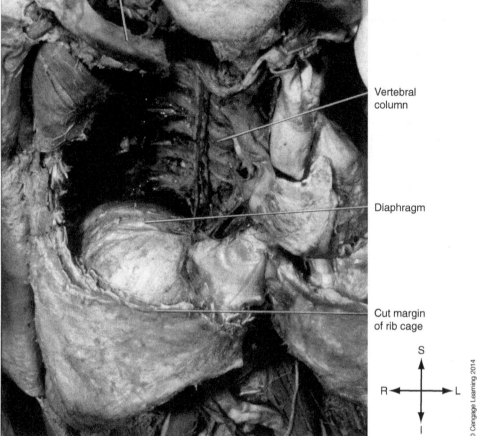

Clavicle (cut)

Vertebral column

Diaphragm

Cut margin of rib cage

S

R ← → L

I

© Cengage Learning 2014

Figure 2–22. continued (B) Photograph of superior view of diaphragm.

Palpation of Rib Cage

Although you cannot palpate your diaphragm, you can identify its margins easily enough. First, find your xiphoid process. This point marks part of the origin of the rectus abdominis, but the diaphragm attaches on the inner surface. Place your fingers on the xiphoid process and the muscle below, and breathe deeply in and out once. You can feel the rectus abdominis being stretched during inspiration. Now place the fingers of both hands at the bottom of the rib cage on both sides of the sternum, so that your fingers are pressing into your abdominal muscles. Breathe out as deeply as you can and hold that posture while you bend slightly forward. Your fingers are marking the margin of the diaphragm, although you are palpating abdominal muscles.

Bring your fingers up to feel your ribs. Place your fingers between the ribs, with your little finger of each hand on the abdominal muscles below the rib cage. Breathe in a couple of times and feel the abdominal muscles first draw in and then tighten up as you reach maximum inspiration. Feel your rib cage elevate as you do this.

Contraction of the diaphragm has the result of pulling the central tendon down. It is directly analogous to placing someone in the middle of a blanket while a host of friends pull on the corners of the blanket. When the friends pull together, the person in the middle flies up. Because the diaphragm has the shape of an inverted bowl, pulling on the edges (muscular contraction) draws the center down (see Figure 2–23). Innervation of the diaphragm is by means of the phrenic nerve. The diaphragm can be placed under voluntary control, but it is under primary control of the autonomic system.

Summary

- The primary muscle of inspiration is the diaphragm, the dividing point between the thorax and the abdomen.
- The fibers of the diaphragm pull on the central tendon, resulting in downward motion of the diaphragm during inspiration, and this movement expands the lungs in the vertical dimension.

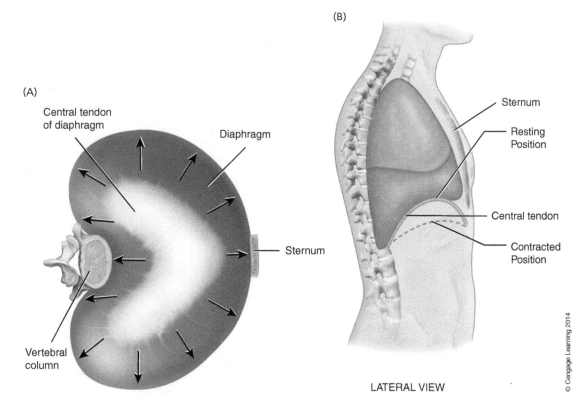

Figure 2–23. (A) Schematic of transverse view of the diaphragm with central tendon. The arrows depict the direction of force on contraction of the diaphragm. (B) This lateral view of the diaphragm shows that contraction of the diaphragm pulls the central tendon down.

ACCESSORY MUSCLES OF INSPIRATION

Although the diaphragm is the major contributor to inspiration, it needs help to meet your body's needs for forced inspiration. If you look at Figure 2–24, you will see the rib cage from the side. Direct your attention first to the way the ribs run. They are directed distinctly downward as they make their path to the front of the skeleton. Next, imagine raising the ribs in front. When you do that, the front of the rib cage expands as a result. Swinging those ribs up means that they will swing out a bit, thereby increasing the volume of the rib cage.

To put this function in everyday terms, look at Figure 2–24 showing venetian blinds from the side. When they are closed, they are similar to the rib cage at rest, and when they are opened, they are similar to ribs being elevated. That elevation brings the ribs more nearly horizontal, just like the blinds, and that change increases the overall front-to-back dimension. We will differentiate these muscles that are responsible for elevation based on their locations.

Anterior Thoracic Muscles of Inspiration

Internal and External Intercostal Muscles. The *external intercostal* muscles are among the most significant respiratory muscles for speech. They not only provide a significant

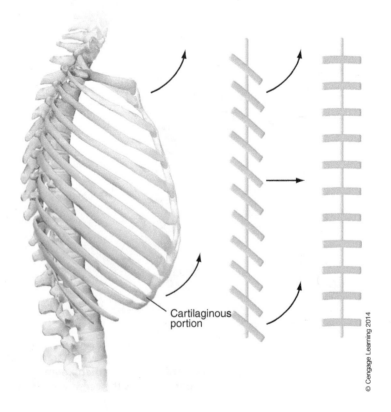

Figure 2–24. Schematic of rib cage from the side. Notice that the ribs slant down as they run forward. During inspiration the rib cage elevates, as shown by the arrows. On the right side, the venetian blinds shown from the side demonstrate the change in volume achieved by elevation of the rib cage.

Cartilaginous portion

© Cengage Learning 2014

proportion of the total respiratory capacity, but they also perform functions that are uniquely speech-related.

As you can see in Figure 2–25, the 11 external intercostal muscles reside between the 12 ribs of the thorax, providing the ribs with both unity and mobility. The external intercostal muscles originate on the lower surface of each rib (except rib 12) and course downward and inward to insert into the upper surface of the rib immediately below. These muscles provide a unified surface of diagonally slanting striated muscle on all costal surfaces of the rib cage with the exception of the region near the sternum. Contraction of external intercostal fibers in that region would provide little benefit (and perhaps some negative effect) to the job of increasing cavity size.

The internal intercostal muscles are predominantly muscles of expiration, with the exception of the chondral portion. The **parasternal** ("near the sternum") portion of the internal intercostal muscles encompassing the chondral aspect of the ribs is active during forced inspiration.

parasternal: *Near the sternum.*

The external intercostal muscles elevate the rib cage. As the rib cage is elevated, the flexible coupling of the costosternal attachment permits the chondral portion of the ribs to rotate. The net result is that the sternum remains relatively parallel to the vertebral column even as the rib cage expands, increasing the anterior dimension and thus the volume of the lungs. Innervation of the external intercostal

(A)

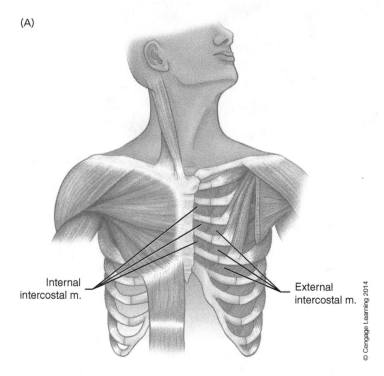

Internal intercostal m.

External intercostal m.

© Cengage Learning 2014

Figure 2–25. (A) Rib cage with external and internal intercostal muscles. External intercostals are absent near the sternum, and thus one can see the deeper internal intercostals in that region. Note that on the left rib cage the fascia covering the internal intercostals has been removed. *(continues)*

(B)

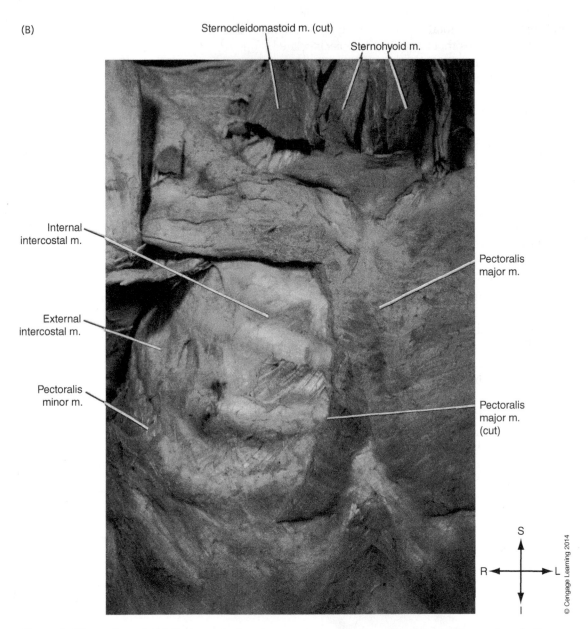

Sternocleidomastoid m. (cut)

Sternohyoid m.

Internal intercostal m.

External intercostal m.

Pectoralis minor m.

Pectoralis major m.

Pectoralis major m. (cut)

S

R ←——→ L

I

© Cengage Learning 2014

Figure 2–25. continued (B) Photograph showing some accessory muscles of inspiration and expiration.

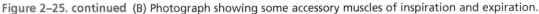

muscles is achieved by the intercostal nerves arising from spinal nerves T1 through T11.

Although the external intercostals account for most of the second dimensional change (the anterior-posterior dimension), there are other muscles that help. Any muscle that attaches to the rib cage or sternum could feasibly elevate either the rib cage or sternum. Some other possible assistants in respiration are the *levatores costarum* (*brevis* and *longus*) and *serratus posterior superior*, as shown in Figure 2–26. You can imagine that they would elevate the rib cage on contraction, as would the serratus posterior superior.

Keeping the Airway Open in Respiratory Emergency

Sometimes in a respiratory emergency it is necessary to ensure that the respiratory pathway remains patent ("open"). In a conscious patient, the normal head and neck orientation places the mouth at a 90° angle to the airway above the larynx (pharynx). If an unconscious individual's head drops forward (see Figure 2–15B(b)), the airway can become occluded and limit respiration.

In some cases, there is concern that the vocal folds or airway above that level will not remain open, so an emergency tracheostomy is performed (*tracheo* = trachea; *stoma* = mouth). This medical procedure involves opening an artificial passageway into the trachea.

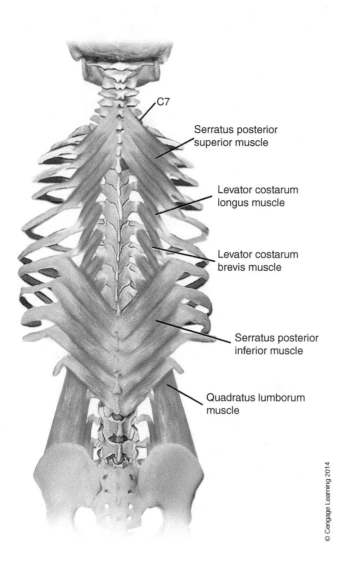

C7

Serratus posterior superior muscle

Levator costarum longus muscle

Levator costarum brevis muscle

Serratus posterior inferior muscle

Quadratus lumborum muscle

© Cengage Learning 2014

Figure 2–26. Posterior thoracic muscles. Note that the levatores costarum muscles are present on all ribs, but in the superior aspect they are deep to the serratus posterior muscles, and these are muscles of inspiration. Quadratus lumborum and serratus posterior inferior are considered to be muscles of expiration. *(continues)*

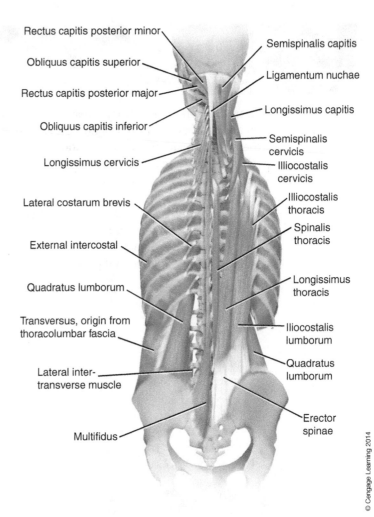

Rectus capitis posterior minor

Obliquus capitis superior

Rectus capitis posterior major

Obliquus capitis inferior

Longissimus cervicis

Lateral costarum brevis

External intercostal

Quadratus lumborum

Transversus, origin from
thoracolumbar fascia

Lateral inter-
transverse muscle

Multifidus

Semispinalis capitis

Ligamentum nuchae

Longissimus capitis

Semispinalis
cervicis

Illiocostalis
cervicis

Illiocostalis
thoracis

Spinalis
thoracis

Longissimus
thoracis

Iliocostalis
lumborum

Quadratus
lumborum

Erector
spinae

© Cengage Learning 2014

Figure 2–26. continued

Posterior Thoracic Muscles of Inspiration

Levatores Costarum. Shortening the levatores costarum (brevis and longus) tends to elevate the rib cage. Although these muscles would appear to be muscles of the back, they are considered thoracic muscles. The brevis ("brief") portions of the levator costarum originate on the transverse processes of vertebrae C7 through T11, for a total of 12 levator costarum brevis muscles. Fibers course obliquely down and out to insert into the tubercle of the rib below.

The longus portions originate on the transverse processes of T7 through T11, with fibers coursing down and obliquely out. The fibers bypass the rib below the point of origin, inserting instead into the next rib. You can see that the longus portion will have a greater effect on elevation of the rib cage. The levatores costarum muscles are innervated by the intercostal nerves.

Serratus Posterior Superior. In Figure 2–26, you can see that, given their course, contraction of the serratus posterior superior muscles could easily contribute to elevation of the rib cage. The serratus posterior superior muscles have their origins on the spinous processes of C7 and T1 through T3. Fibers from these muscles course down and laterally to insert just beyond the angles of ribs 2 through 5. Innervation of the serratus posterior superior is completed by means of the ventral intercostal portion of the spinal nerves T1 through T4 or T5.

Accessory Muscles of the Neck

Sternocleidomastoid. The *sternocleidomastoid muscle* courses from its origin on the mastoid process of the temporal bone to its insertion at the sternum (sterno) and clavicle (cleido) (see Figure 2–27). When a sternocleidomastoid muscle is contracted separately, it will rotate the head toward the side of contraction. When both left and right sternocleidomastoid muscles are contracted simultaneously, the thoracic cavity will be the beneficiary because these muscles have the capacity to elevate the sternum and subsequently the anterior rib cage. The sternocleidomastoid and trapezius muscles derive their innervation from the eleventh cranial nerve, spinal branch (XI) accessory.

Scalenus Anterior, Middle, and Posterior. The *scaleni*, or scalenes, are muscles of the neck that provide stability to the head and facilitate rotation and, by virtue of their attachment on the first and second ribs, can increase the superior-inferior dimension of the thorax (see Figure 2–27). Neck

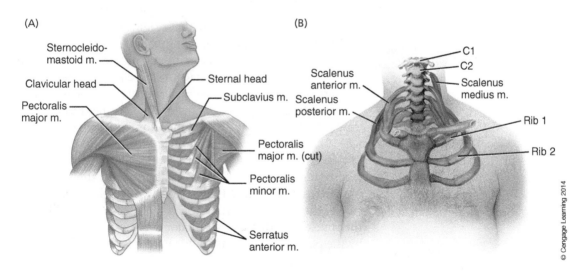

Figure 2–27. (A) Schematic of pectoralis major, pectoralis minor, sternocleidomastoid, subclavius, and serratus anterior muscles. (B) Schematic of scalenus anterior, medius, and posterior muscles.

stability and control are essential ingredients for normal development of speech.

The *anterior scaleni* originate on the transverse processes of vertebrae C3 through C6, with fibers coursing down to insert into the superior surface of the first rib. The *middle scaleni* take their origins on transverse processes of vertebrae C2 through C7, also inserting into the first rib. The *posterior scaleni* insert into the second rib, having coursed from the transverse processes of C5 through C7. The scaleni anterior are innervated by spinal nerves C4 through C6.

Muscles of Upper Arm and Shoulder

The accessory muscles of the arm may assist the external intercostal in elevation of the thorax by virtue of their attachment to the sternum and ribs. Although not confirmed through physiological study, the action of each of the following muscles has the potential to increase the anterior-posterior dimension of the thorax. As we talk about these muscles, it's important to note that reference to "origin" and "insertion" will differ from classical anatomical description, *because we are talking about different functions.* When *our field* discusses the pectoralis major, for instance (in the following discussion), we are less interested in the fact that it draws the arm forward and down (its classic function) than that it helps us expand the rib cage. If we focus on arm movement, the origin is the margin of the sternum, whereas if we focus on rib cage movement, the origin is the humerus. This is because origin and insertion are defined by their function: If the sternum moves more than the arm (as in respiration), it will be considered the insertion point.

Pectoralis Major and Minor. The *pectoralis major* muscle is a large, fan-shaped muscle that originates from two heads (see Figure 2–27). The *sternal head* attaches along the length of the sternum at the costal cartilages, and the *clavicular head* arises from the anterior surface of the clavicle. The muscle converges at the crest of the greater tubercle of the humerus. In respiration, the pectoralis major elevates the sternum and thus increases the transverse dimension of the rib cage.

The *pectoralis minor* originates on the anterior surface of ribs 2 through 5, with fibers coursing up to converge on the coracoid process of the scapula. As with the pectoralis major, respiratory function would involve elevation of the rib cage, although this function has not been verified for either muscle. Both pectoralis major and minor are innervated by the pectoral nerves, arising from the brachial plexus.

Serratus Anterior. Fibers of the *serratus anterior* muscle arise from ribs 1 through 9 along the side of the thorax, coursing up to converge on the inner vertebral border of the scapula. Contraction may elevate the ribs to which it is attached and subsequently the rib cage (see Figure 2–27). The serratus anterior receives innervation by spinal nerves C5 through C7.

Back Muscles of Inspiration

Levator Scapulae. The *levator scapulae* muscle provides neck support secondarily as a result of its function as an elevator of the scapula. This muscle originates from the transverse processes of C1 through C4 and courses down to insert into the medial border of the scapula (see Figure 2–28). The levator scapulae derives its innervation from the brachial plexus.

Rhomboideus Major and Minor. The *rhomboids* (*major* and *minor*) lie deep to the trapezius, originating on the spinous processes of T2 through T5 (rhomboideus major) and from C7 and T1 (rhomboideus minor). The rhomboid muscles course down and laterally to insert into the medial border of the scapula. Primary speech function of the rhomboids is the support they provide for the upper body,

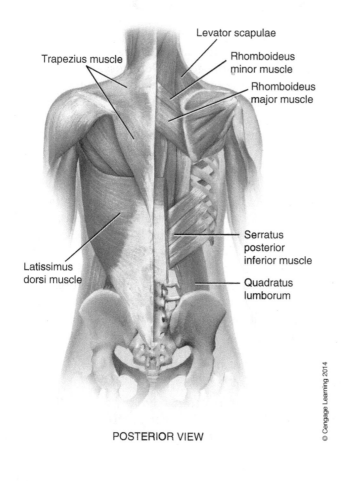

POSTERIOR VIEW

© Cengage Learning 2014

Figure 2–28. Accessory muscles of respiration: trapezius, levator scapulae, rhomboideus minor, rhomboideus major, serratus posterior inferior, latissimus dorsi, and quadratus lumborum.

especially the shoulder girdle. The rhomboids receive their innervation from the dorsal scapular nerves arising from spinal nerve C5.

Trapezius. The *trapezius* (Figure 2–28) is a massive muscle making up the superficial upper back and neck, originating along the spinous processes of C2 to T12. Fibers of this muscle fan laterally to insert into the acromion of scapula and superior surface of clavicle. Contraction of this muscle clearly plays a significant role in elongation of the neck and in head control. The trapezius muscle is innervated by the accessory nerve (eleventh cranial nerve).

Summary

- The diaphragm is an exceptionally important muscle of inspiration, but many accessory muscles of inspiration and expiration also serve respiration.
- Generally, muscles of the thorax and neck that elevate the rib cage serve an accessory function for inspiration.

MUSCLES OF FORCED EXPIRATION

Active expiration requires muscles to act on the lungs indirectly to "squeeze" the air out of them. This is achieved in two ways. The front-to-back dimension of the rib cage is reduced when the rib cage is pulled down by the internal intercostal muscles, the innermost intercostal muscles, and the transversus thoracis muscles. The second means of reducing the volume of the thorax is by reducing the superior-inferior dimension. We can forcefully expire by contracting the muscles of the abdominal region which, in turn, squeeze the abdomen and force the viscera upward, reducing the size of the thorax. The abdominal muscles of expiration (see Figure 2–29) are very much like a cummerbund, wrapping the abdomen—front, side, and back—into a neat package.

The layers of abdominal muscles provide excellent support for the rib cage during lifting and other body movements. These movements virtually force immobilization of the thorax by inflating the lungs and closing off the vocal folds, and the abdominal muscles help to compress the viscera while simultaneously stabilizing the thorax.

Muscles of Thorax: Anterior-Lateral Thoracic Muscles

Internal Intercostal, Interosseous Portion. The *interosseous portion* of the *internal intercostal* muscles is a significant contributor to forced expiration. The internal

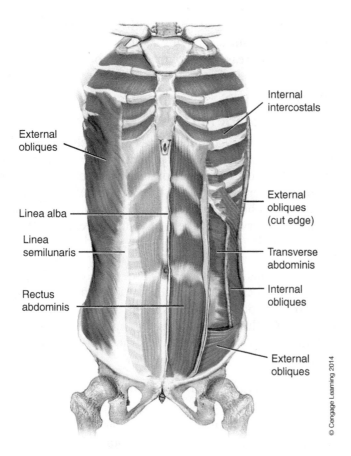

External
obliques

Internal
intercostals

Linea alba

External
obliques
(cut edge)

Linea
semilunaris

Transverse
abdominis

Rectus
abdominis

Internal
obliques

External
obliques

© Cengage Learning 2014

Figure 2–29. Accessory muscles
of expiration and landmarks of
the abdominal aponeurosis.

intercostal muscles are pervasive in the thorax, originating
on the superior margin of each rib and running up and
medially to insert into the inferior surface of the rib above.
They are absent in the posterior aspect of the rib cage near
the vertebral column. Because the external intercostal
muscles run at nearly right angles to the internals, these
two sets of muscles provide significant support for the rib
cage and protection of the ribs, as well as maintenance of
rib spacing.

The internal intercostal muscles also provide a mechanism for depressing the rib cage. As you can see from the
schematic of Figure 2–30, when the interosseous portion of
the internal intercostal contracts and shortens, the direction
of movement is down, and the expanded rib cage becomes
smaller. The internal intercostal muscles are innervated by
the intercostal nerves.

Transversus Thoracis. As the name implies, the *transversus
thoracis* ("transverse muscles of thorax") muscles are found
on the inner surface of the rib cage. The muscles originate

on the margin of the sternum, with fibers coursing to the inner chondral surface of ribs 2 through 6. Contraction of the muscles decreases the volume of the thoracic cavity. The thoracic intercostal nerves innervate the transversus thoracis (see Figure 2–30).

Posterior Thoracic Muscles

Subcostals. The *subcostal muscles* are widely variable but generally take a course parallel to the internal intercostal muscles and thus can serve expiration. The subcostals are on the inner posterior wall of the thorax. Unlike the intercostal muscles, the subcostals can span more than one rib. The subcostals are innervated by the intercostal nerves of the thorax.

Serratus Posterior Inferior. The *serratus posterior inferior* muscles originate on the spinous processes of T11, T12, and L1 through L3 and course up and laterally to insert into the lower margin of the lower five ribs. Contraction of these muscles pulls the rib cage down for expiration. The serratus posterior inferior is innervated by the intercostal and subcostal nerves.

Abdominal Muscles of Expiration

If you consider the human skeleton and imagine placing muscles in the region between the rib cage and the pelvis, you will realize that there are few places from which muscles can originate. To deal with this, nature has provided a tendinous

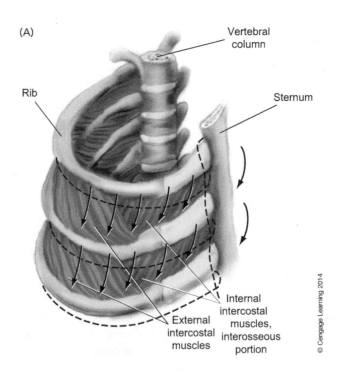

(A)

Vertebral column

Rib

Sternum

Internal intercostal muscles, interosseous portion

External intercostal muscles

© Cengage Learning 2014

Figure 2–30. (A) Effect of contraction of the interosseous portion of the internal intercostals is to pull the rib cage down, thereby decreasing the volume of the lungs. (B) Transversus thoracis and innermost intercostals pull the rib cage medially for expiration.   *(continues)*

(B)

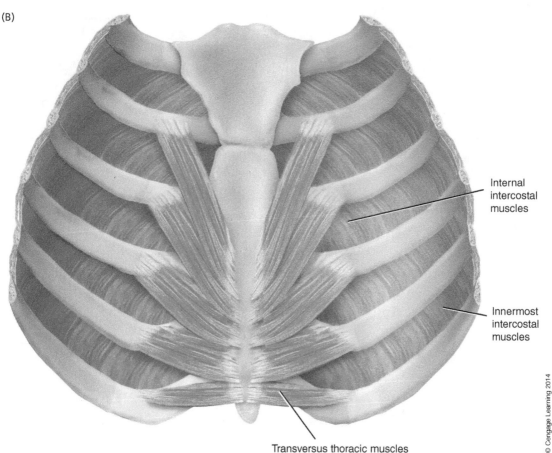

Internal
intercostal
muscles

Innermost
intercostal
muscles

Transversus thoracic muscles

© Cengage Learning 2014

Figure 2–30. continued

structure, the abdominal aponeurosis. Figure 2–31 shows
a schematic representation of the abdominal aponeurosis
from the front, as well as in the transverse section. The *linea
alba* ("white line") runs from the xiphoid process to the pubic symphysis, forming the midline structure for muscular
attachment. In the transverse view, you can see that as the
linea alba progresses laterally, and it differentiates into two
sheets of aponeurosis, between which is placed the rectus
abdominis. This aponeurotic wrapping comes back together
to form another band of tendon, the *linea semilunaris*. This
tendon once again divides, but this time into three sheets
of aponeurosis, which provide a way to attach three more
muscles to this structure.

In the posterior aspect, the fasciae join to form the *lum-
bodorsal fascia*. This structure connects the three abdominal
muscles (transversus abdominis, internal and external oblique
abdominis) with the vertebral column. The *external oblique
aponeurosis* communicates directly with the fascia covering
the rectus abdominis, forming a continuous layer of connective tissue from the linea alba to the external oblique muscle.

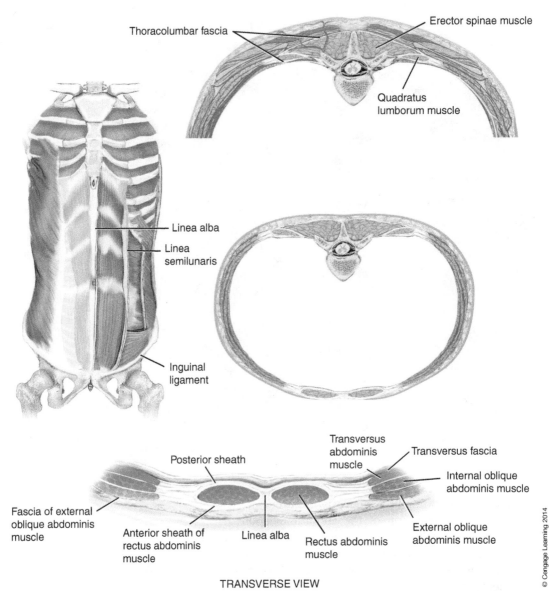

Figure 2–31. Schematic of abdominal aponeurosis as related to the abdominal muscles of expiration.

Anterolateral Abdominal Muscles. The abdominal muscles of expiration function by compression of the abdominal viscera.

Transversus Abdominis. The transversus abdominis (see Figure 2–31) runs laterally, originating in the posterior aspect at the vertebral column via the thoracolumbar fascia of the abdominal aponeurosis. Its anterior attachment is to the transversus abdominis aponeurosis, as well as to the inner surface of ribs 6 through 12. Its inferior-most attachment is at the pubis. Contraction of the transversus significantly reduces the volume of the abdomen. Innervation of the transversus abdominis is via the thoracic and lumbar nerves.

Internal Oblique Abdominis. The *internal oblique abdominis* is located between the external oblique abdominis and the transversus abdominis. As seen in Figure 2–31, this muscle fans out from its origin on the inguinal ligament and iliac crest to the cartilaginous portion of the lower ribs and the portion of the abdominal aponeurosis lateral to the rectus abdominis, and thus, by association, inserts into the linea alba. Contraction of the internal oblique abdominis assists in rotation of the trunk when unilaterally contracted or flexion of the trunk when bilaterally contracted. Innervation of the rectus abdominis is via the thoracic and lumbar nerves.

External Oblique Abdominis. The *external oblique abdominis* muscles are the most superficial of the abdominal muscles, as well as the largest of this group. These muscles originate along the osseous portion of the lower seven ribs and fan downward to insert into the iliac crest, inguinal ligament, and abdominal aponeurosis (lateral to rectus abdominis). Bilateral contraction of these muscles flexes the vertebral column, and unilateral contraction results in trunk rotation. These muscles receive innervation from the thoracoabdominal nerve arising from T7 through T11 and the subcostal nerve from T12.

Rectus Abdominis. The *rectus abdominis* muscles are the prominent midline muscles of the abdominal region, with inferior origin at the pubis (see Figure 2–31 and Figure 2–32). The superior attachment is at the xiphoid process of the sternum and the cartilage of the last true rib (rib 7) and the false ribs. These "rectangular" (i.e., rectus) muscles are manifest in a series of four or five segments connected (and separated) by tendinous slips known as tendinous intersections. Contraction draws the chest closer to the knees and compresses the abdominal contents. Innervation of the rectus abdominis is by means of the intercostal and subcostal nerves.

Posterior Abdominal Muscles

Quadratus Lumborum. As seen in Figure 2–31, the *quadratus lumborum* muscles are located in the dorsal aspect of the abdominal wall. These muscles originate along the iliac crest and fan up and into the transverse processes of the lumbar vertebrae and inferior border of the twelfth rib. Unilateral contraction of the quadratus lumborum assists lateral movement of the trunk, whereas bilateral contraction fixes the abdominal wall in support of abdominal compression. These muscles are innervated by the lowest thoracic nerve, T12, and the first four lumbar nerves.

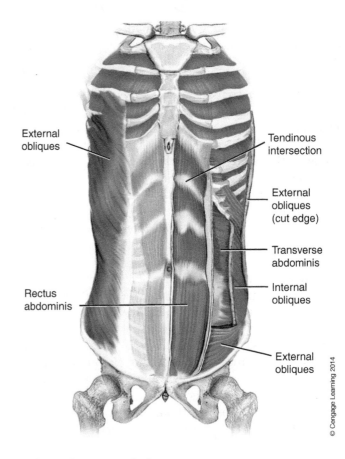

External
obliques

Tendinous
intersection

External
obliques
(cut edge)

Transverse
abdominis

Internal
obliques

Rectus
abdominis

External
obliques

© Cengage Learning 2014

Figure 2–32. Transversus
abdominis, rectus abdominis,
and external and internal
oblique abdominis muscles.

Muscles of Upper Limb

Latissimus Dorsi. The *latissimus dorsi* muscle (see
Figure 2–28) originates from the lumbar, sacral, and lower
thoracic vertebrae, with fibers rising fanlike to insert into
the humerus. Its primary role is in movement of the upper
extremity, but it clearly plays a role in chest stability, and perhaps expiration. With the arm immobilized, contraction of
the latissimus dorsi stabilizes the posterior abdominal wall,
performing a function similar to that of the quadratus lumborum. Innervation for this muscle arises from the posterior
branch of the brachial plexus.

Summary

- To inflate the lungs, you need to expand the cavity that
  holds them so that air can rush in.
- To do this, you can either increase the lung dimension
  fairly easily by contracting the diaphragm or you can
  elevate the rib cage with just a little bit more effort.
- Forced expiration reverses this process by pulling the
  thorax down and in and by forcing the diaphragm
  higher into the thorax.

PHYSIOLOGY OF RESPIRATION

Respiration requires muscular effort, and the degree to which an individual can control that musculature determines, in large part, the efficiency of respiration. Respiratory function (physiology) changes as we exercise, age, or suffer setbacks in health. Considering its importance in speech, it is no wonder that as the respiratory system goes, so goes communication. We are capable of both quiet and forced expiration.

The process of expiration eliminates the waste products of respiration. Attend to your own respiratory cycle to learn an important aspect of quiet expiration. Close your eyes while you breathe in and out ten times, quietly and in a relaxed manner. Pay particular attention to the area around your diaphragm, including your rib cage and your abdomen. What you experienced is the active contraction of the diaphragm, followed by a simple relaxing of the musculature. You actively contract to breathe in, and then simply let nature take its course for expiration. It is a little like blowing up a balloon, because the balloon will deflate as soon as you let go of it. The forces on the balloon that cause it to lose its air are among those that cause your lungs to deflate. The forces we need to talk about are elasticity and gravity.

Respiration is, above all, a biological function that is essential for life. Our bodies will always do what is necessary to keep us alive and well oxygenated, and that is essential information for a speech-language pathologist to know. As a simple example, a person with nasal congestion that makes it difficult to breathe through the nose will open up his or her mouth to increase respiratory flow, naturally, simply, and without voluntary effort. This may not be a very effective breathing pattern for speech (i.e., it can cause problems with dentition and even swallowing if it becomes a long-term requirement for a person, as in chronic nasal obstruction) but it is an effective pattern for survival!

The primary element that drives passive expiration is elasticity. There is elasticity in both the muscles and the lungs. Return to our earlier discussion of the elevation of the rib cage by the external intercostals and the accessory muscles of inspiration. When those muscles pull the rib cage up and out, the anterior cartilage comes under some twisting strain. As soon as the muscles stop pulling on the rib cage, it returns to its original shape thanks to the restoring forces of elastic cartilage, which cause the rib cage to drop back down to its resting state.

Recall that the lungs are highly elastic, porous tissue. They are sponge-like and when they are compressed (as in forced expiration), they tend to expand. Likewise, if you were

Aspiration

Aspiration refers to entry of liquid or solid materials into the lungs, but it can also refer to the removal of materials from the lungs (more commonly referred to as suctioning). Fluid or solids can enter the lungs as a result of some failure in muscular strength, coordination, sensation, or awareness.

Aspiration of foreign matter into the lungs is a very real danger in cases of neurological deficit, and the individual suffering from stroke or traumatic brain injury is particularly vulnerable. Sometimes a patient loses sensation in the laryngeal region, so that a protective cough or "clearing" response does not occur when food or liquid contacts the larynx. If a patient has muscular weakness, he or she might also demonstrate diminished or ineffective (nonproductive) cough and reduced elevation of the larynx during swallow.

Because the client with neurological deficit may not be aware of this problem or competent to seek help, it is wise to know the symptoms of aspiration. If the client's voice sounds wet or gurgly or if the client has a history of respiratory illnesses, the client is at risk for aspiration pneumonia. Likewise, the client may have a weak, breathy vocalization or cry, indicating laryngeal muscle weakness and the possibility of inadequate protective function.

to grab a sponge by its edges and stretch it, when you release it, the sponge would return to its original shape and size.

During early human development, the lungs completely fill the thorax so that they are not stretched to fit the relaxed rib cage. As the child develops, the rib cage grows at a faster rate than the lungs, and the pleural linings and increased negative intrapleural pressure provide a means for the lungs to be stretched out to fill that space.

The result of this stretching is greatly increased capacity and reserve in adults, but not in infants. Because the infant's thorax and lungs are equal in size, an infant must breathe two to three times as often as an adult for adequate respiration. The adult's lungs are stretched out and never completely compressed, so there is always a reserve of air in them that is not undergoing gas exchange.

Upon increasing the thorax size, the lungs expand just as if you had grabbed them and stretched them out. When the muscles expanding the rib cage relax, the lungs tend to return to their original shape and size. In addition, when you inhale and your abdomen protrudes, you are stretching the abdominal muscles. Relaxing the inspiratory process lets those muscles return to their original length; that is, the abdominal muscles tend to push your abdominal viscera back in and to force the diaphragm up.

The second force that supports passive expiration is gravity. When a person stands or sits erect, gravity is acting on the ribs to pull them back after they have been expanded through the effort of the accessory muscles of inspiration. Gravity also works in favor of maximizing your overall capacity because it pulls the abdominal viscera down, leaving more room for the lungs. We will talk about this more because body position becomes a significant issue in the efficiency of respiration.

Summary

- We are capable of quiet respiration as well as forced inspiration and expiration.
- Quiet inspiration uses the diaphragm and often the external intercostals, but forced inspiration uses many of the accessory muscles.
- Expiration can be passive, driven by the forces of elasticity and gravity.
- We also can use muscles that reduce the size of the thorax by compressing the abdomen or pulling the rib cage down, and this forces air out of the lungs beyond that which is expired in passive expiration.

Measurement of Respiration

The quantity of air processed through respiration is dictated primarily by bodily needs, and speech physiology operates within these limits. We will discuss respiration in terms of rate of air flow, volume and lung capacities, and pressure.

Respiratory flow, volumes, and capacities are measured with a spirometer (see Figure 2–33). The classic wet

spirometer: *Device that measures volume of air expelled or inspired.*

Protection Against Trauma

The lungs are obviously important for life function, and seem to be designed with damage control in mind. The two lungs are encased in separate pleural linings, so that if one lung is penetrated by an object (e.g., a lung is punctured by a broken rib), the other lung continues to function. Likewise, the segmented nature of lungs is a protective device. If a lung is punctured, the extremely rich vascular bed bleeds significantly and dangerously. The segmented nature of the lungs provides some protection against total lung failure. Bleeding in one segment is isolated to that segment, at least until the bronchial tree is filled with blood.

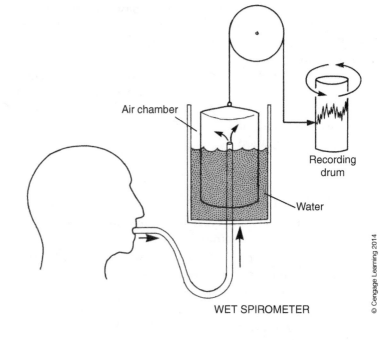

Air chamber

Recording
drum

Water

WET SPIROMETER

© Cengage Learning 2014

Figure 2–33. Wet spirometer is used to measure lung volumes. When the individual exhales into the tube, gas entering the air chamber displaces the water, causing the chamber to rise. These changes are charted on the recording drum.

manometer: *Device that measures pressure.*

spirometer involves a tube connected to a container that is open at the bottom. This container is placed inside another container that is full of water. To measure lung volume, an individual breathes into the tube, causing a volume of water to be displaced. The amount of water displaced gives an accurate estimate of the amount of air that was required to displace it.

The classic U-tube manometer is one means of measuring pressure, as shown in Figure 2–34. A subject is asked to place the tube in his or her mouth and to blow. The force of the subject's expiration is exerted on a column of water that is pushed down the tube, around the U-bend and up the other end of the tube. The more force the person uses, the higher the column rises. We can measure the effects of that force in inches or in centimeters of water (cm H_2O). For comparison, note that barometric pressure is often reported in millimeters of mercury (mm Hg), which measures how many millimeters of mercury were elevated by the pressure. Because water is considerably less dense than mercury, the same amount of pressure will elevate a column of water much higher than a similar column of mercury. For this reason we measure the rather small pressures of respiration with the water standard, although mechanical and electronic techniques are eliminating the water-filled tube.

Breathing requires that gas exchange be ongoing. The body has specific needs that must be met continually, so we will need to discuss respiration in terms of the rate of airflow into and out of the lungs (airflow is measured as cubic

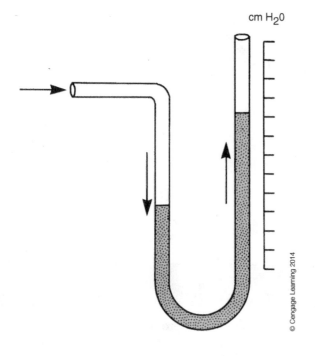

cm H$_2$0

© Cengage Learning 2014

Figure 2–34. U-tube manometer for measurement of respiratory pressure.

centimeters per second or minute). We also need to speak of the quantities or volumes involved in this gas exchange (measured in liters [L], milliliters [mL], cubic centimeters [cc], or on occasion, cubic inches).

Respiration for Life

The respiratory process is a direct function of the action of the diaphragm and muscles of respiration. As discussed earlier, contraction of muscles of inspiration causes expansion of the alveoli, resulting in a negative alveolar pressure and air being drawn into the lungs. Understanding the pressure changes in this process is critical.

Respiratory Cycle

A cycle of respiration is defined as one inspiration and one expiration. During *quiet respiration*, adults complete between 12 and 18 cycles of respiration per minute (see Figure 2–35). This quiet breathing pattern, known as quiet tidal respiration (because it can be visualized as a tidal flow of air into and out of the lungs) involves about 500 mL (0.5 liter) of air with each cycle. A quick calculation reveals that we process something in the order of 6000 to 8000 mL (6–8 liters) of air every minute. As work output increases, an adult increases his or her oxygen requirements up to a factor of 20.

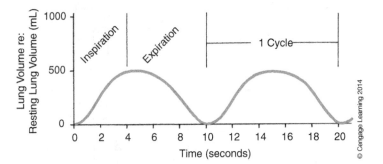

Figure 2–35. Volume display of two cycles of quiet respiration.

Emphysema

Emphysema is generally considered to be a product of a modern society that has not solved its pollution problems. Often the disease results from tobacco smoking, but it can arise from living in an industrial environment. Its progression is slow and may be arrested to some degree by altering the respiratory environment.

The mechanism for emphysema appears to be as follows. Recall that the bronchial passageway is richly infused with ciliated epithelial cells that beat continuously to remove contaminants from the respiratory tract. This continuous waste-removal process is seriously hampered by pollutants that, in the early stages of emphysema, destroy the epithelium.

The absence of ciliated epithelium greatly reduces the respiratory system's ability to clean and remove waste products, which allows deposition of pollutants in the alveoli. The alveoli undergo a significant morphological (form) change: The walls of the alveoli break down, and alveoli recombine so that clusters of alveoli become one sac. Although this change may seem benign, it has a devastating effect in that the surface area for gas exchange is greatly reduced as a result.

A second morphological change arises as a compensation to the first. The individual with emphysema is faced with an ongoing shortage of oxygen and is forced to attempt continually deeper inspirations to compensate; a characteristic "barrel chest" results from these efforts.

This second change causes a third pathological response. Recall that the lower margin of the rib cage marks the point of attachment of the diaphragm. Because the rib cage is flared out due to emphysema, contraction of the diaphragm (which pulls on the rib cage) causes the rib cage to pull down and in medially, which actually reduces the size of thorax rather than increases it.

The final change arising from this trilogy of tragedy is respiratory failure. The respiratory mechanism is highly compromised, leaving the individual susceptible to respiratory diseases such as pneumonia.

Pleurisy

Pleurisy is a condition in which the pleural linings of the thoracic cavity are inflamed. When the inflammation results in "dry pleurisy," the patient is experiencing extreme pain upon breathing because the lubricating quality of the intrapleural fluid has been lost. "Adhesions" may result, in which portions of the parietal pleurae adhere to the visceral pleurae. (The patient may experience "breaking up" of these adhesions for quite some time following his or her bout with pleurisy.) Pleurisy can be unilateral or bilateral and may result in movement of excessive fluid (potentially purulent) into the pleural space.

Developmental Processes of Respiration

The lungs undergo a great deal of prenatal development, as seen in Figure 2–36. By the time a healthy infant is born, the cartilaginous conducting airway is complete, although the number of alveoli will increase from about 25 million at birth to more than 300 million by 8 years of age. We retain that number throughout life. The conducting airways grow steadily in diameter and length until thorax growth is complete, although the thorax expands to a greater degree than the lungs. As the thorax expands, the lungs are stretched to fill the cavity, a fact that helps to explain two differences between adults and children. As mentioned earlier, adults breathe between 12 and 18 times per minute while at rest, but a newborn breathes an average of 40 to 70 cycles per minute. By 5 years, the child is down to about 25 breaths per minute (bpm), and that number drops to about 20 bpm at 15 years of age. The adult has a considerable volume of air that is never expelled, but the infant does not have this reserve. In essence, the thorax expands during growth and development and stretches the lungs beyond their natural volume (see Figure 2–37).

Accessory muscles of inspiration used to augment diminished respiratory support most typically include the anterior, middle, and posterior scalene muscles (to elevate the first and second ribs) and the sternocleidomastoid (to elevate the sternum and increase the anteroposterior dimension of the rib cage). You may have seen people with severe respiratory difficulties stretch their arms in front of them and hold onto the back of a chair to breathe: When they do this, they give the pectoralis major muscles something to work against, thus allowing these muscles to increase the anteroposterior dimension. You may have also seen these patients "shrugging," a sure sign that the trapezius muscle is in use to raise the rib cage.

breaths per minute (bpm): *The number of complete inhalations and exhalations performed in 1 minute.*

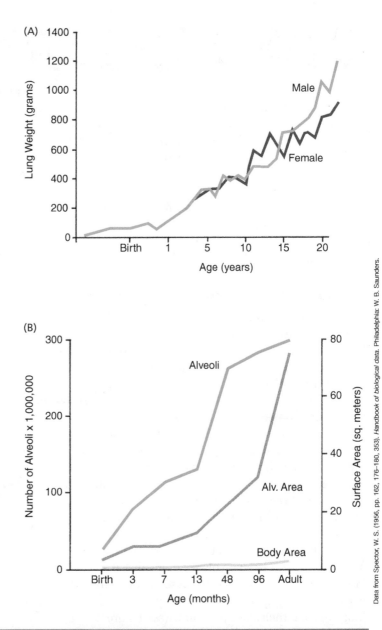

Figure 2–36. (A) Changes in lung weight as a function of age. Males and females are essentially equivalent in lung weight until puberty, at which time the increased thoracic cavity size of the male is reflected in larger lung weight. (B) Changes in lung tissue with age. The number of alveoli increases radically through the fourth year of life, and the total alveolar area stabilizes around puberty when the thorax approximates its volume.

Data from Spector, W. S. (1956, pp. 162, 176–180, 353). *Handbook of biological data.* Philadelphia: W. B. Saunders.

Clavicular Breathing

Clavicular breathing is a form of respiration in which a major source of thorax expansion is elevation of the rib cage via contraction of the accessory muscles of inspiration, most notably the sternocleidomastoid. Clavicular breathing often is an adaptive response by an individual to some previous or present pathological condition (e.g., chronic obstructive pulmonary disease) that prohibits other means to expand the thorax. Because elevation of the sternum results in only a small increase in thorax size, clavicular breathing is a less-than-perfect solution to the problem of respiration.

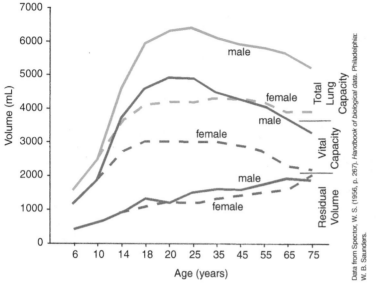

Data from Spector, W. S. (1956, p. 267). *Handbook of biological data.* Philadelphia: W. B. Saunders.

Figure 2–37. Vital capacity, total lung volume, and residual volume as a function of age.

As a result of this expansion, there is a volume of air in the adult lung that cannot be expelled (residual volume), and this volume helps to account for the reserve capacity of adults relative to infants. Infant lungs have yet to undergo the proliferation of the alveoli seen during childhood, and infants must breathe more frequently to meet their metabolic needs.

Volumes and Capacities

Respiration is the product of a number of forces and structures, and for us to make sense of them we need to define some volumes and capacities of the lungs. When we refer to volumes, we are partitioning off the respiratory system so that we can accurately estimate the amount of air each compartment can hold. Capacities are more functional units. Capacities refer to combinations of volumes that express physiological limits. Volumes are discrete, whereas capacities represent functional combinations of volumes.

Both volumes and capacities are measured in milliliters (mL, thousandths of a liter) or cubic centimeters (1 cc = 1 mL). To get an idea of what these volumes and capacities really amount to, look at a 2-liter soda bottle. One liter is 1000 mL, which is also 1000 cc. There are five volumes that we should consider. Refer to Figure 2–38 as we discuss them.

Tidal Volume. The volume of air that we breathe in during a respiratory cycle is referred to as tidal volume (TV). The average quiet tidal volume (tidal volume at rest) for adult males is around 600 cc, and for adult females it is approximately 450 cc. This works out to an average of 525 cc for adults, or approximately one quarter of the volume of a

volume: *In respiration, the displacement of air that represents specifically partitioned components of the respiratory system, measured in cubic centimeters or cubic inches.*

capacity: *Functional unit that is a combination of respiratory volumes, used to express physiological limits.*

milliliter (mL): *One thousandth of a liter.*

cubic centimeter (cc): *A milliliter or one thousandth of a liter.*

tidal volume (TV): *The volume of air exchanged during one cycle of respiration.*

quiet tidal volume: *Tidal volume at rest.*

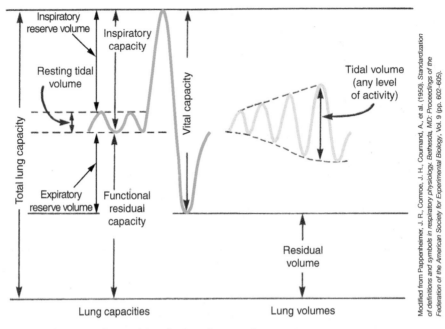

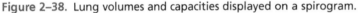

Figure 2–38. Lung volumes and capacities displayed on a spirogram.

Trunk Stability and Upper Body Mobility

Control of speech musculature depends in large part on the development of trunk control. If an infant fails to develop neck extension, he or she will not develop the ability to balance neck extensors and flexors. While the normal neck extension begins developing, the back muscles begin to come under control, again becoming dynamically opposed by anterior trunk muscles. Through this interplay of antagonist and agonist trunk muscles, the infant develops the ability to rotate the trunk, stabilize the hips, and elevate the head in preparation for speech. Once controlled, the infant can rotate his or her head, differentiate mandible movement from head movement, and differentiate tongue movement from mandible movement. All the while, the infant is developing the dynamic aspects of laryngeal control that permit the larynx to descend and the tongue to become controlled.

inspiratory reserve volume (IRV):
The volume of air that can be inhaled after a tidal inspiration (approximately 2475 cc for adults).

2-liter soda bottle every 5 seconds. You will breathe in the air in three of these bottles every minute. Tidal volume increases markedly as effort increases. You may wish to refer to Table 2–2.

Inspiratory Reserve Volume. The second volume of interest is **inspiratory reserve volume (IRV)**. Inspiratory reserve

Table 2–2. Typical Respiratory Volumes and Capacities in Adults

Volume/Capacity	Males* (cc)	Females** (cc)	Average (cc)
Resting tidal volume	600	450	525
Inspiratory reserve volume	3000	1950	2475
Expiratory reserve volume	1200	800	1000
Residual volume	1200	1000	1100
Vital capacity	4800	3200	4000
Functional residual capacity	2400	1800	2200
Inspiratory capacity	3600	2400	3000
Total lung capacity	6000	4200	5100

Note: Volumes and capacities vary as a function of body size, gender, age, and body height. These volumes represent approximate values for healthy adults between 20 and 30 years of age. Vital capacity is estimated by accounting for age (in years) and height (in cm) as follows:

*Males: VC in mL $= (27.63 - (0.112 \times$ age in yr$)) \times$ ht. in cm.

**Females: VC in mL $= (21.78 - (0.101 \times$ age in yr$)) \times$ ht. in cm.

Source: Data from Baldwin, Cournand, and Richards (1948) as cited in Kao, F. F. (1972, p. 39). *An Introduction to Respiratory Physiology,* Amsterdam: Excerpta Medica; and Peters, R. M. (1969, p. 49). *The Mechanical Basis of Respiration,* Boston: Little, Brown.

volume is the volume that can be inhaled after a tidal inspiration. It is the volume of air that is in reserve for use beyond the volume you would breathe in tidally, averaging 2475 cc for adults.

Expiratory Reserve Volume. The parallel volume for expiration is the **expiratory reserve volume (ERV)**. Expiratory reserve volume is the amount of air that can be expired following passive, tidal expiration, amounting to about 1000 cc (1.0 liter). This volume is referred to as resting lung volume (RLV) also because it is the volume of air in the resting lungs after a passive exhalation.

Residual Volume. The third volume of interest is **residual volume (RV)**. Residual volume is the amount of air that cannot be expelled after a maximum exhalation. No matter how forcefully you exhale, there is a volume of air (about 1.1 liters) that cannot be eliminated. This volume exists because the lungs are stretched as a result of the relatively expanded thorax. By the way, this does not mean we do not use that air, but rather that it is a volume that is not eliminated during expiration.

expiratory reserve volume (ERV): *The volume of air that can be expired following passive, tidal expiration (approximately 1000 cc for adults).*

residual volume (RV): *The volume of air in the lungs after a maximum exhalation (approximately 1100 cc in adults).*

dead air space: *The space, representing the conductive passageway of the respiratory system, that contains a volume of air that never undergoes gas exchange (approximately 150 cc in adults).*

Dead Air Space. The air in the conducting passageways cannot be involved in gas exchange because there are no alveoli there. The volume that cannot undergo gas exchange in the lungs is dead air space, and an adult has a volume of about 150 cc. The volume associated with dead air is included in residual volume because both are volumes associated with air that cannot be expelled.

The volumes can be combined in a number of ways to characterize physiological needs. Four capacities are useful combinations of air volumes: vital, functional residual, total lung, and inspiratory capacities.

vital capacity (VC): *The combination of inspiratory reserve volume, expiratory reserve volume, and tidal volume, representing the capacity of air available for speech (approximately 4000 cc in adults).*

Vital Capacity. Of the capacities, vital capacity (VC) is the one most often cited in speech and hearing literature because it represents the capacity of air available for speech. Vital capacity is the combination of inspiratory reserve volume, expiratory reserve volume, and tidal volume. That is, vital capacity represents the total volume of air that can be inspired after a maximal expiration. VC = IRV + ERV + TV, and this calculation shows that VC is approximately 4000 cc in the average adult.

functional residual capacity (FRC): *The volume of air in the thorax after a passive exhalation (approximately 2100 cc in adults).*

Functional Residual Capacity. Functional residual capacity (FRC) is the volume of air in the body after a passive exhalation (FRC = ERV + RV). In the average adult, this comes to approximately 2100 cc.

total lung capacity (TLC): *The total volume of the respiratory system that can undergo gas exchange, equaling the sum of tidal volume, inspiratory reserve volume, expiratory reserve volume, and residual volume (approximately 5100 cc in adults).*

Total Lung Capacity. Total lung capacity (TLC) is the sum of all the volumes (TLC = TV + IRV + ERV + RV), which comes to approximately 5100 cc. Note that TLC is different from vital capacity. Vital capacity represents that volume of air that is involved in a maximal respiratory cycle, whereas total lung capacity includes the residual volume. Residual volume serves as a buffer in respiration because it does not immediately interact with the environment.

inspiratory capacity (IC): *The maximum inspiratory volume possible after tidal expiration (approximately 3000 cc in adults).*

Inspiratory Capacity. Inspiratory capacity (IC) is the maximum inspiratory volume possible after tidal expiration (IC = TV + IRV). This refers to the capacity of the lungs for inspiration and represents a volume of approximately 3000 cc in the adult.

Summary

- The volumes of respiration indicate arbitrary partitioning of the respiratory system and include tidal volume (the volume inspired and expired in a cycle of respiration), inspiratory reserve volume (air inspired beyond tidal inspiration), expiratory reserve volume (air expired beyond tidal expiration), residual volume (air that remains in the lungs after maximal expiration), and dead air, which cannot undergo gas exchange.

- Vital capacity is the volume of air that can be inspired after a maximal expiration.
- Functional residual capacity is the air that remains in the body after passive exhalation.
- Total lung capacity represents the sum of all lung volumes.
- Inspiratory capacity is the volume of air that can be inspired from resting lung volume.

Pressures of the Respiratory System

There are five specific pressures for nonspeech and speech: alveolar, intrapleural, subglottal, intraoral, and atmospheric (see Figure 2–39). The atmosphere in which we live exerts

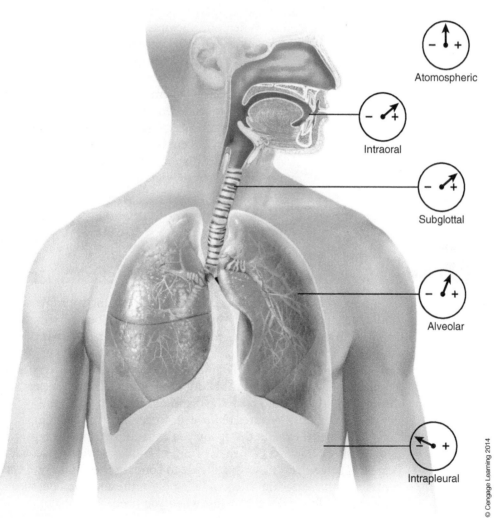

Figure 2–39. Pressures of respiration.

atmospheric pressure (P$_{atm}$):
*Pressure generated as a result
of the weight of atmospheric
gases.*

intraoral (mouth) pressure (P$_m$):
Pressure in the oral cavity.

subglottal pressure (P$_s$): *Pressure
beneath the level of the vocal
folds.*

**alveolar, or pulmonary, pressure
(P$_{al}$):** *Pressure in the alveolus.*

intrapleural pressure (P$_{pl}$):
*Pressure between the visceral
and parietal pleurae.*

a sizable pressure on the surface of the earth (760 mm Hg; that is, sufficient pressure to elevate a column of mercury 760 mm against gravity). **Atmospheric pressure (P$_{atm}$)** is actually our reference in discussions of the respiratory system, and so we will treat it as a constant zero against which to compare respiratory pressures. **Intraoral,** or **mouth, pressure (P$_m$)** is the pressure in the mouth that can be measured, while **subglottal pressure (P$_s$)** is the pressure below the vocal folds. We can assume that subglottal and intraoral pressures are equal to alveolar pressure during normal respiration with open vocal folds. As we progress more deeply into the lungs, we can estimate **alveolar,** or **pulmonary pressure (P$_{al}$)**, the pressure in the individual alveolus. If we were to measure the pressure in the space between parietal and visceral pleurae, we would refer to it as pleural, or **intrapleural, pressure (P$_{pl}$)**. Intrapleural pressure is negative throughout respiration. Recall that the lungs, inner thorax, and diaphragm are wrapped in a continuous sheet of pleural lining. When one attempts to separate the visceral from parietal pleurae, a negative pressure ensues.

These pressure measurements are all relative to atmospheric pressure. When we refer to alveolar pressure as being, for instance, $+3$ cm H_2O, it means that, through muscular effort, we have generated $+3$ cm H_2O pressure above and beyond atmospheric pressure (if atmospheric pressure is 1033 cm H_2O, then alveolar pressure would be 1036 cm H_2O). When the diaphragm is pulled down for tidal inspiration, Boyle's law predicts that alveolar pressure will drop

"Getting the Wind Knocked Out of You"

Why does a blow to the abdomen result in your losing your breath? Logic would dictate that you would lose your breath from being hit in the chest.

Try to recall what happened the last time you had the wind knocked out of you. First, something hit you in the abdominal region or you fell and landed on your stomach. Remember that forced expiration depends in large part on contraction of the abdominal muscles which, in turn, causes the abdominal viscera to push the diaphragm up and pull the thorax down. Both of these gestures remove air forcefully from the lungs.

This doesn't explain the agony you experience trying to regain respiratory control, however. When large muscles are passively stretched, a reflex is triggered that causes the muscle to contract involuntarily. This contraction increases the effect of being hit in the abdomen because it causes you to forcefully exhale just when you needed to inhale!

(relative to atmospheric pressure), and it does. In quiet tidal inspiration, alveolar pressure drops to approximately −2 cm H_2O until equalized with atmospheric pressure by inspiratory flow. Likewise, during expiration the pressure at the alveolar level becomes positive with reference to the atmosphere, increasing to +2 cm H_2O during quiet tidal breathing.

Figure 2–40 is a schematic of the alveolar pressures, intrapleural pressures, and change in lung volume during quiet tidal breathing. This figure shows the alveolar pressure associated with a cycle of respiration and illustrates what we have been talking about. We have placed markers on it so that we can discuss how this whole system of pressures and flows works together.

Look at the curve labeled lung volume; it shows the periodic function that represents tidal respiration. Point A represents the peak of that inspiration, and the lungs have about 500 cc of air in them. Point B represents the end of the expiratory cycle, when our subject has relaxed the forces of inspiration and the lungs have passively evacuated down to resting lung volume. At the bottom of the figure, point C represents the electromyographic activity recorded from the diaphragm as it contracted. Putting these two traces together, you can see that as the diaphragm contracts the volume increases to a maximum at the point where the diaphragmatic contraction is complete.

Let us examine the airflow component. As the diaphragm contracts, there is a fairly steady flow of air into the lungs (measured in mL/second), indicated by point D. When the inspiratory effort is completed (represented by the termination of the diaphragm activity and the volume peak at A), the flow of air into the lungs ends. That is, when the diaphragm stops contracting, air stops flowing. As air leaves the lungs, the airflow becomes negative at point E (which simply means that the air is flowing in a different direction). Alveolar pressure goes positive (+2 cm H_2O) during expiration. To summarize, when the diaphragm contracts, airflow begins and is fairly steady throughout the inspiratory cycle. When the diaphragm stops contracting, the air begins to flow out of the lungs.

This is a good time to examine the pressures driving this process. If you recall that contraction of the diaphragm causes the alveolar pressure to drop, the point marked F will make sense. When the diaphragm is contracted (C), pressure deep in the lungs drops. At this point, alveolar pressure reaches its maximum negativity during this tidal respiration (−2 cm H_2O relative to atmospheric pressure), because the negative pressure is responsible for airflow into the lungs. Looking at point G will explain why that pressure drops. You will recall that intrapleural pressure is constantly

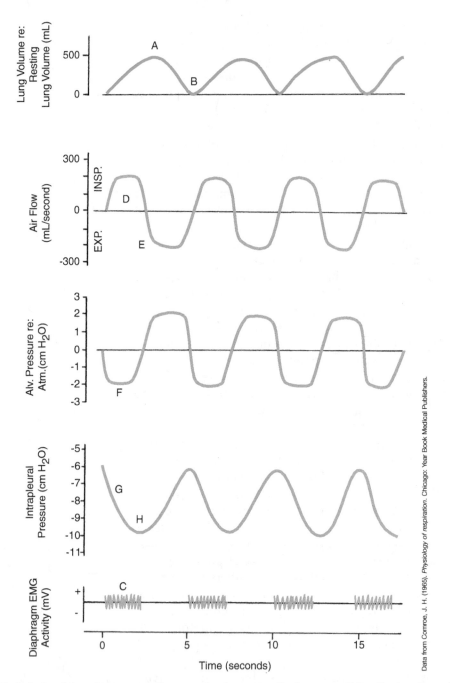

Figure 2–40. Relationships of pressures, flows, and volumes to diaphragm activity. Contraction of the diaphragm causes a drop in intrapleural and alveolar pressure, which results in an increase in airflow and lung volume.

negative relative to atmospheric pressure, and the lungs are in a state of continued expansion in the thoracic cavity. This is reflected in the fact that the highest pressure on the intrapleural plot is negative (-6 cm H_2O).

When the diaphragm contracts, the intrapleural pressure becomes even more negative as the diaphragm attempts to pull the diaphragmatic pleurae away from the visceral pleurae. During the entire period of contraction of the diaphragm, the pressure continues to drop: The diaphragm is pulling farther away from its resting point, and the pressure between the pleurae increases proportionately. As the diaphragm reaches the end of its contraction, intrapleural pressure reaches a maximum negativity (point H), which reverses upon relaxation of the diaphragm. When the diaphragm contracts, the volume (space) between the two pleural linings increases; as Boyle's law predicts, the pressure drops.

Depression of the diaphragm for quiet tidal inspiration results in an intrapleural pressure of approximately -10 cm H_2O, but relaxing the diaphragm during quiet expiration does not return the pressure to atmospheric level, but rather returns it to a constant rest pressure of -6 cm H_2O. In the average, healthy individual, intrapleural pressure remains negative at all times, becoming increasingly negative as muscles of inspiration act on the lungs.

The fact that this intrapleural pressure remains negative underscores two important notions. First, the lungs are in a state of continual expansion because the thorax is larger than the lungs that fill it. Second, the lungs are never completely deflated under normal circumstances. During inspiration and expiration, two more pressures are of interest to us. Subglottal pressure is the pressure beneath the level of the vocal folds (*glottis* refers to the space between the vocal folds). Above the vocal folds the respiratory pressure in the oral cavity is referred to as intraoral pressure. When the vocal folds are open, intraoral pressure, subglottal pressure, and alveolar pressure are the same.

The pressure beneath and above the vocal folds is directly related to what is happening in the lungs, as long as the vocal folds are open for air passage. If the lungs are drawing air in, the pressure at both of these locations is negative. If the lungs are in expiration, the pressure is relatively positive. Things get more difficult when the vocal folds are closed.

When we close vocal folds for phonation (voicing), we place a significant blockage in the flow of air through the upper respiratory pathway. Closing the vocal folds causes an immediate increase in the subglottal air pressure as the lungs continue expiration. At the same time, closing the vocal folds causes the intraoral pressure to drop to near atmospheric level, resulting in a large difference in pressure between the

supraglottal: *The region above the vocal folds.*

supraglottal (above vocal folds) and subglottal regions. If this increased pressure exceeds 3 to 5 cm H_2O, the vocal folds will be blown open and voicing will begin. This turns out to be a critical pressure in itself because it marks the minimal requirement of respiration for speech.

You can now view these critical pressures as a system: We are continually playing the respiratory system against the relatively stable atmospheric pressure. Contraction of the diaphragm and muscles of inspiration decreases the intrapleural pressure markedly, which, in turn, expands the lungs. When the lungs expand, alveolar pressure drops relative to

Use of Abdominal Muscles for Childbirth and Other Biological Functions

Nature has a way of getting the most use out of structures, and the abdominal muscles are a great example. Clearly, we use the abdominal muscles to force air out of the lungs, but they serve several other worthwhile (even vital) functions. The act of vomiting requires evacuation of the gastric contents, and to do so necessitates forceful action from the abdominal muscles.

A less obvious function has to do with thoracic fixation. For the muscles of the upper body to gain maximum benefit, they need to pull against a relatively rigid structure. The thorax can be made rigid by inhaling and then capturing the respiratory charge by closing off the vocal folds. To demonstrate this process, take a very deep breath and hold it. To do this, you must close off the folds.

This thoracic fixing gives leverage for lifting (notice that you "grunt" when you lift because some air is escaping past the vocal folds, having been compressed by your muscular effort), but it also gives leverage in the other direction. Defecation requires compression of the abdomen and increase in abdominal pressure, and that process also demands thoracic fixation for efficiency.

Another not immediately obvious use for abdominal muscle contraction is childbirth. Although you may not have experienced this directly, you are probably familiar with midwives, nurses, or partners whose job it was to remind the mother-to-be to "breathe." It shouldn't surprise you to realize that the mother has not forgotten this basic biological process, but rather she has an overwhelming, deep biological urge to "push." Besides providing supportive encouragement, the person who is cheerleading is doing so to synchronize breathing with contractions and to keep the mother from closing the vocal folds (you can't breathe through closed folds) because if she does, she will start pushing the baby to its new home before the time has come (Creasy, 1997).

atmospheric pressure, causing air to enter the lungs. Relaxing the muscles of inspiration permits the natural recoil of the lungs and cartilage to draw the chest back to its original position, and the relaxed diaphragm again returns to its relatively elevated position in the thorax. When this happens, intrapleural pressure increases (but still stays negative), alveolar pressure becomes positive relative to atmospheric pressure, and air leaves the lungs.

Summary

- Volumes and pressures vary as a direct function of the forces acting on the respiratory system.
- With the vocal folds open, oral pressure, subglottal pressure, and alveolar pressure are roughly equivalent.
- Intrapleural pressure remains constantly negative, increasing in negativity during inspiration.
- These pressures are all measured relative to atmospheric pressure.
- During inspiration, expansion of the thorax decreases the already negative intrapleural pressure, and the increased lung volume results in a negative alveolar pressure.
- Air from outside the body flows into the lungs when the pressure in the lungs is negative relative to the atmosphere.
- During expiration, this pressure differential is reversed, with air escaping the lungs to equalize the positive alveolar pressure with the relatively negative atmospheric pressure.

Pressures Generated by Tissue

At this point, we should address the forces of expiration more deeply. Expiration capitalizes on elasticity and gravity to reclaim some of the energy expended during inspiration. When muscles of inspiration contract, they stretch tissue and the cartilage of the ribs, and they distend the abdomen.

These restoring forces actually generate pressures themselves. Elastic forces govern how much effort is required to inhale. This relationship is described in the curve of Figure 2–41.

The dashed line on this figure is the relaxation point, the point at which no pressure is generated because all parts of the system are at equilibrium. The dashed relaxation point of zero pressure represents about 38% of vital capacity. When you relax entirely with open airway, the lungs still have 38% of the total exchangeable volume left, and this could be forcefully exhaled. Said another way, from this point you can actively inhale 62% of your vital capacity.

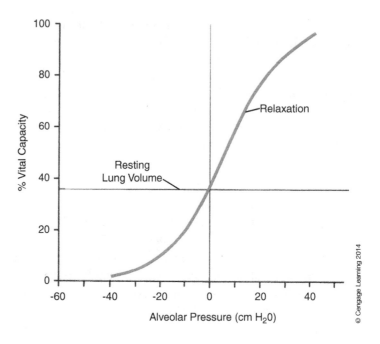

Figure 2–41. Relaxation pressure curve representing pressures generated by the passive forces of the respiratory system.

Summary

- The process of contracting musculature deforms the cartilage and connective tissue, and recoil forces will drive the respiratory system back to equilibrium after inspiration or expiration.

- Relaxing the musculature after inspiration results in a positive alveolar pressure that decreases as volume approaches resting lung volume.

- When the pressure is measured following forced expiration, a negative relaxation pressure is found, increasing to equity at resting lung volume.

Effects of Posture on Respiration

Body posture is a significant contributor to efficiency of respiration, and any condition that compromises posture also compromises respiration (see Figure 2–42). As the body is shifted from an erect, sitting position to a supine posture, the relationship between the physical structures of respiration and gravity changes. In the sitting posture, gravity is pulling the abdominal viscera down (supporting inspiration), as well as pulling the rib cage down (supporting expiration). When the body is in the supine position, gravity is pulling the abdominal viscera toward the spine. The result of this is spread of the viscera toward the thorax and further distention of the diaphragm into the thoracic cavity. When a body is supine, gravity supports neither expiration nor

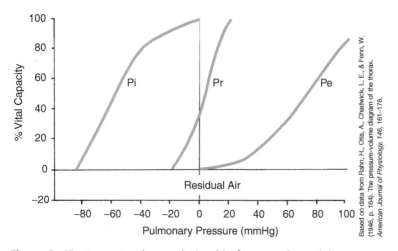

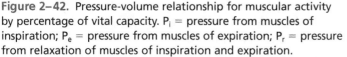

Figure 2–42. Pressure-volume relationship for muscular activity by percentage of vital capacity. P_i = pressure from muscles of inspiration; P_e = pressure from muscles of expiration; P_r = pressure from relaxation of muscles of inspiration and expiration.

inspiration: Muscles of inspiration must elevate both abdomen and rib cage against gravity.

Although vital capacity is not affected, the ability to completely inflate the lungs is. Because of the shift in viscera and effects of gravity on the rib cage, the lung volume is significantly reduced from approximately 38% of vital capacity in the sitting position to 20% when supine.

You may have already realized the danger this poses to a person whose illness requires that he or she stay in bed for long periods. Pneumonia is a major complication of conditions that immobilize a person.

Summary

- Posture and body position play important roles in volumes for respiration.
- When the body is reclining, the abdominal contents shift rostrally as a result of the forces of gravity.
- Aside from reducing the resting lung volume, the force of gravity on the abdomen increases the effort required for inspiration when supine.

Pressures of Speech

The respiratory system operates at two levels of pressure virtually simultaneously. The first level is the relatively constant supply of subglottal pressure required to drive the vocal folds. To produce sustained voicing of a given intensity, this pressure is relatively constant. As we will see, the minimum driving pressure to make the vocal folds move would elevate a column of water between 3 and 5 cm (3–5 cm H_2O), with conversational speech requiring between 7 and 10 cm H_2O. Loud speech requires a concomitant increase in pressure.

The second level of pressure requires microcontrol. Even as we maintain the constant pressure needed for phonation, we are also quite capable of rapidly and briefly changing the pressure for linguistic purposes such as syllable stress. With quick bursts of pressure (and laryngeal adjustments), we can have rapid and brief increases in vocal intensity and vocal pitch. To maintain that constant pressure for speech, we must first charge the system. During normal respiration, inhalation takes up approximately 40% of the cycle and expiration takes up about 60% (see Figure 2–43).

In fact, the respiratory cycle for speech is markedly different. You need a long, drawn-out expiration to produce long utterances, and you need a very short inspiration to maintain the smooth flow of communication. When you

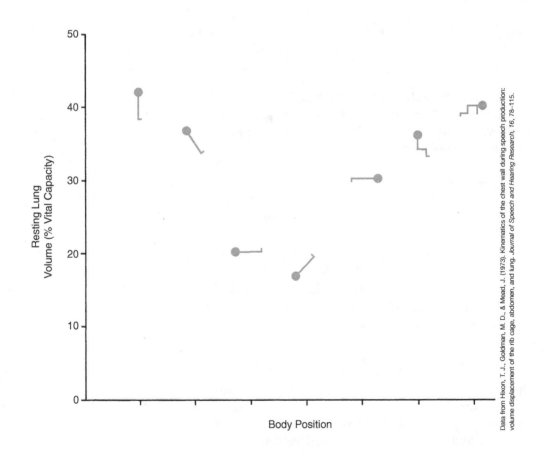

Data from Hixon, T. J., Goldman, M. D., & Mead, J. (1973). Kinematics of the chest wall during speech production: volume displacement of the rib cage, abdomen, and lung. *Journal of Speech and Hearing Research, 16*, 78–115.

Figure 2–43. Vital capacity changes resulting from postural adjustment.

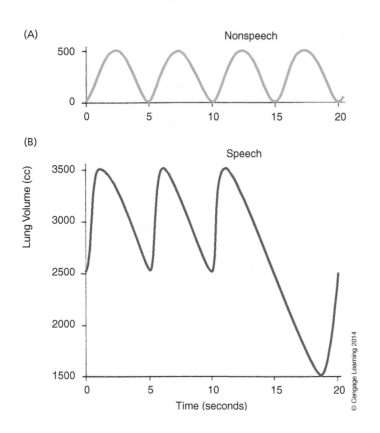

Figure 2–44. Modification of respiratory cycle during speech compared with nonspeech respiratory cycle. (A) This trace represents quiet tidal respiration, with volume related to resting lung volume. (B) This trace is related to total lung capacity. The speaker rapidly inhales a markedly larger volume than during quiet tidal inspiration and then slowly exhales the air during speech. Note that inspiration occurs with the same timing in both speech and nonspeech, but that the expiratory phase is proportionately longer during speech. In the final portion of the trace, the speaker is called on to speak on expiratory reserve volume.

breathe in for speech, you spend only 10% of the respiratory cycle on inspiration and about 90% breathing out. This does not change the amount of air we breathe in and out. We still breathe exactly the volume we need for our metabolic processes (too much and we take in too much oxygen, or hyperventilate; too little and we take in too little oxygen and become hypoxic) (see Figure 2–44).

Instead of letting the air out through total relaxation when we speak, we let the air out slowly, using muscles to restrain the airflow. If you remember that the lungs are attempting to empty as a result of their being stretched for inspiration, then you might realize that if you were to hold that inspiration position you would impede the outflow of air. This process is called **checking action**. That is, you "check" (impede) the flow of air out of your inflated lungs by means of the muscles that got it there in the first place—the muscles of inspiration.

There is an expiratory parallel to checking action, and that is the process of speaking on expiratory reserve. What happens when we get down to that resting lung volume point of 38% during speech? If we have more to say before we inhale, we have to enlist the muscles of expiration to push beyond that resting lung volume.

checking action: *Using the muscles of inspiration to impede the outflow of air during expiration.*

Summary

- During speech we modify our respiratory activities to balance bodily needs and communication needs.
- During respiration for speech we spend markedly less time in inspiration than in expiration, thus capitalizing on the positive pressures generated.
- We also meter out that respiratory charge through checking action, using the muscles of inspiration to restrain expiration.
- We use our muscles of expiration to capitalize on the expiratory reserve volume for speech.
- Even as we maintain this relatively constant subglottal pressure through muscles of inspiration and expiration, we also use those muscles to produce small surges in pressure for syllable stress during speech.

Muscular Activity during Respiration

Electromyography: *is the process of measuring and recording the electrical activity associated with muscular contraction.*

Electromyography is the process of measuring and recording the electrical activity associated with muscular contraction. For many years we assumed that muscles of inspiration became entrained sequentially as a person breathed increasingly deeper, beginning with the diaphragm, and then including the external intercostals (Draper, Ladefoged, and Whitteridge, 1959). Hixon and Weismer (1995) re-examined some of those assumptions and clarified our understanding, so we now know that the interaction of these respiratory muscles is much more complex than earlier portrayals led us to believe. For instance, we originally thought that the abdominal muscles were activated only in deep expiration, and we now know that they are active during all of speech production. Examination of Figure 2–44 also reinforces the concepts we have been discussing throughout the chapter on respiration about muscular activity. Although it doesn't show the activity of individual muscles during respiration, you can see the effects of those muscles: During inspiration the diaphragm and external intercostal activity will dominate, although you should realize that even the abdominal muscles will have activity to support the postures associated with inspiration. As depth of inspiration increases, we can expect increasing involvement of the muscles of inspiration. Likewise, expiration will be dominated by the abdominal musculature, whether for speech or nonspeech function.

As the speaker continues to speak beyond resting lung volume, he or she is using expiratory reserve and must exert the muscles of forced expiration to capitalize on that reserve. As the speaker reaches deeper and deeper into expiratory reserve, the muscles of expiration will increasingly be called into duty. The musculature is recruited as needed to develop increasingly greater abdominal pressure (and, subsequently, alveolar pressure). To plumb the depths of the respiratory system, increasingly more muscular activity of the expiratory muscles is needed.

CHAPTER SUMMARY

Respiration is the process of gas exchange between an organism and its environment. The rib cage, made up of the vertebral column and ribs, houses the lungs, which are the primary organs of respiration. By means of the cartilaginous trachea and bronchial tree, air is brought into the lungs for gas exchange within the minute alveolar sacs. Oxygen enters the blood, and carbon dioxide is removed, to be expired.

Air is drawn into the lungs through muscular effort. The diaphragm, placed between the thorax and abdomen, contracts during inspiration. The lungs expand when the diaphragm contracts, drawn by pleurae linked through surface tension and negative pressure. When lungs expand, the air pressure in the lungs becomes negative with respect to the outside atmospheric pressure, and Boyle's law dictates that air will flow from the region of higher pressure to fill the lungs. Accessory muscles provide added expansion of the rib cage for further inspiration. Expiration can occur passively, through the forces of elasticity and gravity acting on the ribs and rib cage. It also can be forced, by use of muscles of the abdomen and those that depress the rib cage to evacuate the lungs.

Respiration requires the balance of pressures. Decreased alveolar pressure is the product of expansion of the thorax. When the thorax expands, the pressure between the pleurae decreases as the thorax and diaphragm are pulled away from the lungs. The force of the distended lungs increases the negative intrapleural pressure, and the expansion causes a drop in alveolar pressure as well. The relatively lower alveolar pressure represents an imbalance between pressures of the lungs and the atmosphere, and air will enter the lungs to equalize the imbalance. Expiration requires reduction in thorax size, which results in a positive pressure within the alveoli, with air escaping through the oral and nasal cavities. The intrapleural pressure becomes less negative during expiration, but it never reaches atmospheric pressure.

Several volumes and capacities can be identified in the respiratory system. Tidal volume is the volume inspired and expired in a cycle of respiration, and inspiratory reserve volume is the air inspired beyond tidal inspiration. Expiratory reserve volume is air expired beyond tidal expiration, and residual volume is air that remains in the lungs after maximal expiration. Dead air space contains air that cannot undergo gas exchange. Vital capacity is the volume of air that can be inspired after a maximal expiration, and functional residual capacity is the air that remains in the body after passive exhalation. Inspiratory capacity is the volume that can be inspired from resting lung volume. Total lung capacity is the sum of all lung volumes.

For speech we must work within the confines of pressures and volumes required for life. We alter the respiratory cycle to capitalize on expiration time and restrain that expiration through checking action. We also generate pressure through contraction of the muscles of expiration when the lung volume is less than resting lung volume. With these manipulations we maintain a respiratory rate to match our metabolic needs, and even use the accessory muscles of inspiration and expiration to generate small bursts of pressure for syllabic stress.

STUDY QUESTIONS

1. _____ is defined as force distributed over area.

2. _____ pressure causes air to enter the container until the pressure is equalized.

3. How many of each of the following vertebrae are there?

_____ cervical vertebrae

_____ thoracic vertebrae

_____ lumbar vertebrae

_____ sacral vertebrae

_____ coccygeal vertebrae (fused)

4. On the accompanying figure identify the indicated landmarks.

A. _____ process

B. _____ process

C. _____ (structure)

D. _____ facet

E. _____ facet

F. _____ facet

G. _____ foramen

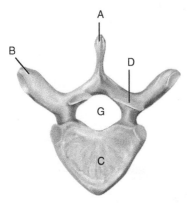
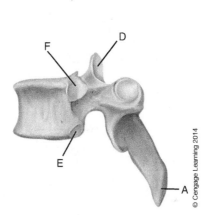

5. The _____ passes through the vertebral foramen.

6. On the following figure identify the indicated landmarks.

A. _____ (bone)

B. _____ (bone)

C. _____ (bone)

D. _____

E. _____

F. _____

G. _____

H. _____ (bone)

I. _____ (bone)

J. _____

K. _____

L. _____

M. _____

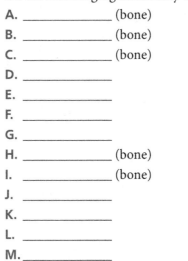

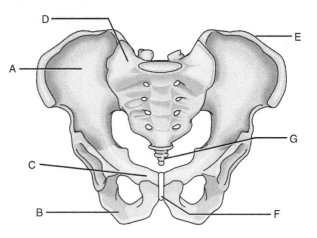

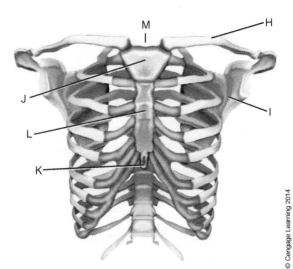

7. On the accompanying figure please identify the indicated landmarks.

A. _____

B. _____

C. _____

D. _____

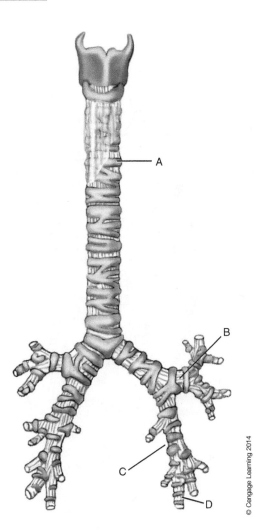

© Cengage Learning 2014

8. On the following figure identify the muscles and indicated structures.

A. _____

B. _____

C. _____

D. _____

E. _____

F. _____ ligament

G. _____

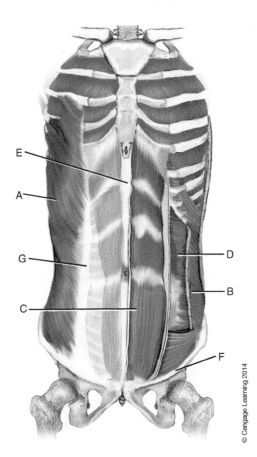

9. On the accompanying figure identify the indicated muscles.

A. _____

B. _____

C. _____

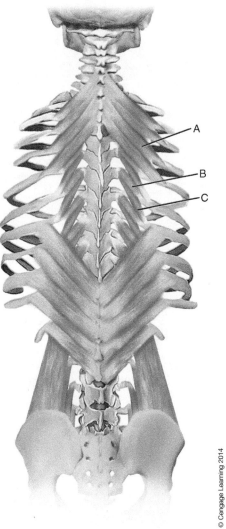

10. Identify the muscles indicated in the accompanying figure.

   A. _____

   B. _____

   C. _____

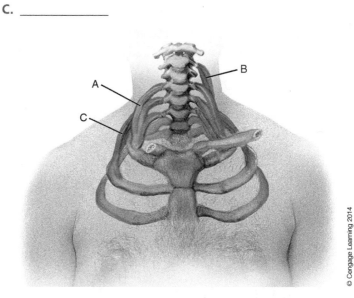

11. Identify the muscles and portions of muscles indicated in the accompanying figure.

   A. _____

   B. _____ head

   C. _____ head

   D. _____

   E. _____

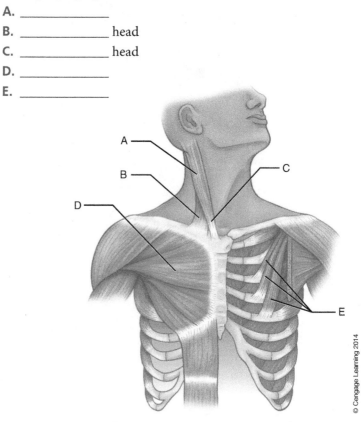

12. _____ Contraction of the diaphragm increases the dimension of the thorax.

13. _____ Contraction of the accessory muscles of inspiration increases the dimension of the thorax.

14. _____ Contraction of the muscles of expiration decreases the volume of the thorax.

15. _____ are the two forces involved in passive expiration.

16. Identify the following described volumes and capacities.

 A. _____ volume: The volume of air that we breathe in during a respiratory cycle.

 B. _____ volume: The volume that can be inhaled after a tidal inspiration.

 C. _____ volume: The volume that can be exhaled after a tidal expiration.

 D. _____ volume: The volume that remains in the lungs after a maximal exhalation.

 E. _____ capacity: The combination of inspiratory reserve volume, expiratory reserve volume, and tidal volume.

 F. _____ capacity: The volume of air in the body after a passive exhalation.

 G. _____ capacity: The sum of all the volumes.

17. _____ is the volume of air that cannot undergo gas exchange.

18. _____ pressure is the air pressure in the oral cavity.

19. _____ pressure is the air pressure below the vocal folds.

20. _____ pressure is the pressure in the alveolus.

21. _____ pressure is the pressure between the visceral and parietal pleural membranes.

22. When the diaphragm contracts, pressure in the alveolus _____ (increases/decreases).

23. When air pressure in the lungs is lower than that of the atmosphere, air will _____ (enter/leave) the lungs.

24. When the body is reclining, the resting lung volume _____ (increases/decreases).

25. _____ is the term that describes use of the muscles of inspiration to impede the outward flow of air during speech.

26. Emphysema results in a breakdown of the alveolar wall, resulting in enlargement of alveolar clusters and consequent enlargement of the thorax known as "barrel chest." The result of this is that the diaphragm is pulled down at rest. Discuss the implications of the muscular action of inspiration and expiration on this altered system.

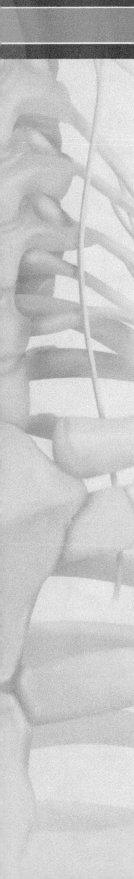

REFERENCES

Agostoni, E., & Mead, J. (1964). Statics of the respiratory system. In W. Fenn & H. Rahn (Eds.), *Handbook of physiology, respiration* (Vol. 1, Sect. 3). Washington, DC: American Physiological Society.

Araujo, J. A., Barajas, B, Kleinman, M., et al. (2008). Ambient particulate pollutants in the ultrafine range promote early atherosclerosis and systemic oxidative stress. *Circulation Research, 102*(5), 589–596; published online before print, January 17, 2008, 0.1161/CIRCRESAHA.107.164970.

Arnott, W. M. (1973). *Disorders of the respiratory system.* Oxford, England: Blackwell Scientific.

Baken, R., & Cavallo, S. (1981). Prephonatory chest wall posturing. *Folia Phoniatrica, 33,* 193–202.

Baken, R., Cavallo, S., & Weissman, K. (1979). Chest wall movements prior to phonation. *Journal of Speech and Hearing Research, 22,* 862–872.

Baken, R., & Orlikoff, R. F. (1999). *Clinical measurement of speech and voice* (2nd ed.). San Diego: Singular Publishing Group.

Basmajian, J. V. (1975). *Grant's method of anatomy.* Baltimore: Williams & Wilkins.

Bateman, H. E., & Mason, R. M. (1984). *Applied anatomy and physiology of the speech and hearing mechanism.* Springfield, IL: Charles C. Thomas.

Beck, E. W. (1982). *Mosby's atlas of functional human anatomy.* St. Louis: Mosby.

Bergman, R., Thompson, S., & Afifi, A. (1984). *A catalog of human variation.* Baltimore: Urban & Schwarzenberg.

Bly, L. (1994). *Motor skills acquisition in the first year.* Tucson, AZ: Therapy Skill Builders.

Burrows, B., Knudson, R. J., & Kettel, L. J. (1975). *Respiratory insufficiency.* Chicago: Year Book Medical Publishers.

Campbell, E. (1958). An electromyographic examination of the role of the intercostal muscles in breathing in man. *Journal of Physiology, 129,* 12–26.

Campbell, E., Agostoni, E., & Davis, J. (1970). *The respiratory muscles, mechanics and neural control.* Philadelphia: W. B. Saunders.

Chusid, J. G. (1985). *Correlative neuroanatomy and functional neurology* (17th ed.). Los Altos, CA: Lange Medical Publications.

Comroe, J. H. (1974). *Physiology of respiration.* Chicago: Year Book Medical Publishers.

Creasy, R. K. (1997). *Management of labor and delivery.* Malden, MA: Blackwell Science.

Des Jardins, T. (1984). *Clinical Manifestation of Respiratory Disease.* Chicago, IL: Year Book Medical Publishers.

Des Jardins, T., & Burton, G. G. (2001). *Clinical manifestation and assessment of respiratory disease.* St. Louis: Mosby.

Draper, M., Ladefoged, P., & Whitteridge, D. (1959). Respiratory muscles in speech. *Journal of Speech and Hearing Research, 2,* 16–27.

Ganong, W. F. (2003). *Review of medical physiology* (21st ed.). New York: McGraw-Hill/Appleton & Lange.

Gordon, M. S. (1972). *Animal physiology: Principles and adaptations.* New York: Macmillan.

Gosling, J. A., Harris, P. F., Humpherson, J. R., Whitmore, I., & Willan, P. L.T. (1985). *Atlas of human anatomy.* Philadelphia: J. B. Lippincott.

Gray, H., Bannister, L. H., Berry, M. M., & Williams, P. L. (Eds.). (1995). *Gray's anatomy.* London: Churchill Livingstone.

Grobler, N. J. (1977). *Textbook of clinical anatomy* (Vol. 1). Amsterdam: Elsevier Scientific.

Hixon, T. J. (1973). Respiratory function in speech. In F. D. Minifie, T. J. Hixon, & F. Williams (Eds.), *Normal aspects of speech, hearing, and language* (pp. 73–126). Englewood Cliffs, NJ: Prentice-Hall.

Hixon, T. J. (2006). Rib torque does not assist resting tidal expiration or most conversational speech expiration. *Journal of Speech, Language and Hearing Research, 49,* 213–214.

Hixon, T. J., Goldman, M. D., & Mead, J. (1973). Kinematics of the chest wall during speech production: Volume displacement of the rib cage, abdomen, and lung. *Journal of Speech and Hearing Research, 16,* 78–115.

Hixon, T., & Weismer, G. (1995). Perspectives on the Edinburgh study of speech breathing. *Journal of Speech and Hearing Research, 38,* 42–60.

Hlastala, M. P., & Berger, A. J. (1996). *Physiology of respiration.* New York: Oxford University Press.

Hoit, J. D., & Hixon, T. J. (1987). Age and speech breathing. *Journal of Speech and Hearing Research, 30,* 351–366.

Kahane, J. (1982). Anatomy and physiology of the organs of the peripheral speech mechanism. In N. Lass, L. McReynolds, J. Northern, & D. Yoder (Eds.), *Speech, language, and hearing. Vol. 1: Normal processes* (pp. 109–155). Philadelphia: W. B. Saunders.

Kao, F. F. (1972). *An introduction to respiratory physiology.* Amsterdam: Exerpta Medica.

Kaplan, H. (1960). *Anatomy and physiology of speech.* New York: McGraw-Hill.

Kent, R. D. (1997). *The speech sciences.* Clifton Park, NY: Delmar Cengage Learning.

Konno, K., & Mead, J. (1968). Measurement of the separate volume changes of rib cage and abdomen during breathing. *Journal of Applied Physiology, 22,* 407–422.

Kuehn, D. P., Lemme, M. L., & Baumgartner, J. M. (1989). *Neural bases of speech, hearing, and language.* Boston: Little, Brown.

Langley, M. B., & Lombardino, L. J. (1991). *Neurodevelopmental strategies for managing communication disorders in children with severe motor dysfunction.* Austin: Pro-Ed.

Lass, N., McReynolds, L., Northern, J., & Yoder, D. (Eds.) (1982). *Speech, language, and hearing. Vol. I: Normal processes.* Philadelphia: W. B. Saunders.

Lee, D. H. K. (1972). *Environmental factors in respiratory disease.* New York: Academic Press.

Logemann, J. (1998). *Evaluation and treatment of swallowing disorders* (2nd ed.). Austin: Pro-Ed.

MacKay, L. E., Chapman, P. E., & Morgan, A. S. (1997). *Maximizing brain injury recovery.* Gaithersburg, MD: Aspen.

McMinn, R. M. H., Hutchings, R. T., & Logan, B. M. (1994). *Color atlas of head and neck anatomy.* London: Mosby-Wolfe.

McReynolds, L., Northern, J., & Yoder, D. (Eds.). *Speech, language, and hearing. Vol. I: Normal processes.* Philadelphia: W. B. Saunders.

Miller, A. D., Bianchi, A. L., & Bishop, B. P. (1997). *Neural control of the respiratory muscles.* Boca Raton, FL: CRC Press.

Mohr, J. P. (1989). *Manual of clinical problems in neurology.* Boston: Little, Brown.

Moser, K. M., & Spragg, R. G. (1982). *Respiratory emergencies.* St. Louis: Mosby.

Murray, J. F. (1976). *The normal lung. The basis for diagnosis and treatment of pulmonary disease.* Philadelphia: W. B. Saunders.

Netter, F. H. (1983a). *The CIBA collection of medical illustrations. Vol. 1. Nervous system: Part I. Anatomy and physiology.* West Caldwell, NJ: CIBA Pharmaceutical Company.

Netter, F. H. (1983b). *The CIBA collection of medical illustrations. Vol. 1. Nervous system: Part II. Neurologic and neuromuscular disorders.* West Caldwell, NJ: CIBA Pharmaceutical Company.

Netter, F. H. (1997). *Atlas of human anatomy.* Los Angeles: Icon Learning Systems.

Pace, W. R. (1970). *Pulmonary physiology.* Philadelphia: F. A. Davis.

Pappenheimer, J. R., Comroe, J. H., Cournand, A., et al. (1950). *Standardization of definitions and symbols in respiratory physiology. Bethesda, MD: Proceedings of the Federation of the American Society for Experimental Biology,* Vol. 9 (pp. 602–605).

Peters, R. M. (1969). *The mechanical basis of respiration.* Boston: Little, Brown.

Rahn, H., Otis, A., Chadwick, L. E., & Fenn, W. (1946). The pressure–volume diagram of the thorax and lung. *American Journal of Physiology, 146,* 161–178.

Rohen, J. W., Yokochi, C., Lutjen-Drecoll, E., & Romrell, L. J. (2002). *Color atlas of anatomy* (5th ed.). Philadelphia: Williams & Wilkins.

Rosse, C., Gaddum-Rosse, P., & Rosse, G. (1997). *Hollinshead's textbook of anatomy.* Philadelphia: Lippincott-Raven.

Scott, J. R., Disaia, P. J., Hammond, C. B., & Spellacy, W. N. (1994). *Danforth's obstetrics and gynecology* (7th ed.). Philadelphia: J. B. Lippincott.

Snell, R. S. (1978). *Gross anatomy dissector.* Boston: Little, Brown.

Spector, W. S. (1956). *Handbook of biological data.* Philadelphia: W. B. Saunders.

Taylor, A. (1960). The contribution of the intercostal muscles to the effort of respiration in man. *Journal of Physiology, 151,* 390.

Tokizane, T., Kawamata, K., & Tokizane, H. (1952). Electromyographic studies on the human respiratory muscles. *Japan Journal of Physiology, 2,* 232.

Twietmeyer, A., & McCracken, T. D., (1992). *Coloring guide to regional human anatomy* (2nd ed.). Philadelphia: Lea & Febiger.

Zemlin, W. R. (1998). *Speech and hearing science: Anatomy and physiology* (4th ed.). Needham Heights, MA: Allyn & Bacon.

3

Anatomy and Physiology of Phonation

OUTLINE

C. Structure of the vocal folds
  1. Vocal ligament
  2. Aditus
  3. Glottis
D. Structure of the larynx
  1. Cricoid cartilage
  2. Thyroid cartilage
  3. Arytenoid cartilage
  4. Corniculate cartilage
  5. Epiglottis
  6. Cuneiform cartilages
  7. Hyoid bone
E. Movement of the cartilages
  1. Cricothyroid joint
  2. Cricoarytenoid joint
F. Laryngeal musculature
  1. Intrinsic laryngeal muscles
    a. Adductors
      1) Lateral cricoarytenoid
      2) Transverse arytenoid
      3) Oblique arytenoid
    b. Abductor: Posterior cricoarytenoid muscle
    c. Glottal tensors
      1) Cricothyroid muscle
      2) Thyrovocalis muscle
    d. Relaxer: thyromuscularis muscle
  2. Extrinsic laryngeal muscles
    a. Hyoid and laryngeal elevators
      1) Digastricus anterior and posterior
      2) Stylohyoid muscle
      3) Mylohyoid muscle
      4) Geniohyoid muscle
      5) Hyoglossus muscle
      6) Genioglossus muscle
      7) Thyropharyngeus and cricopharyngeus muscles
    b. Hyoid and laryngeal depressors
      1) Sternohyoid muscle
      2) Omohyoid muscle
      3) Sternothyroid muscle
      4) Thyrohyoid muscle

III. **Physiology of Phonation**
A. Nonspeech laryngeal function
  1. Protective function of the larynx
  2. Coughing
B. Laryngeal function for speech
  1. Attack
    a. Simultaneous attack

INTRODUCTION TO PHONATION

The larynx is a critically important structure for survival in that it provides a way to protect the airway from foreign bodies. It sits at the entryway to the trachea, and consists of cartilages and muscles that can quickly and effectively seal off that airway, both voluntarily and reflexively. The larynx is an exquisite sphincter in that the vocal folds are capable of a very strong and rapid clamping of the airway in response to threat of intrusion by foreign objects. As evidence of this primary function, there are three pairs of laryngeal muscles directly responsible for either **approximating** (bringing folds into contact) or tensing the vocal folds, but only one pair of muscles is responsible for opening them. The vocal folds are "wired" to close immediately on stimulation by outside agents, such as food or liquids, a response followed quickly by a rapid and forceful exhalation. This combination of gestures stops intrusion by foreign matter and rapidly expels that matter away from the airway's opening.

approximation: *When referring to vocal folds, making contact.*

The larynx has other important functions as well. Because the vocal folds provide an excellent seal to the respiratory system, they permit you to hold your breath for such activities as swimming.

Holding your breath also serves other functions. Lifting heavy objects requires you to "fix" your thorax by inhaling and clamping your laryngeal sphincter (vocal folds). This gives the muscles of the upper body a solid framework with which to work. You might remember from Chapter 2 that tightly clamping the vocal folds plays an important role in the labor of childbirth.

Spoken communication uses both voiceless and voiced sounds, and this chapter is concerned with the critical distinction between the two. *Phonation* refers to the quasi-periodic vibration of the vocal folds for production of speech voicing. Voiceless or devoiced sounds (voiceless phonemes) are produced without use of the **vocal folds** (for example, the /s/ or /f/ sounds). Voiced sounds like /z/ and /v/, are produced by action of the vocal folds. Just as we referred to respiration as the source of energy for speech, phonation is the source of voice for speech. Respiration is the energy source that permits phonation, and without respiration there would be no voicing.

vocal folds (vocal cords): *The vibrating component of the larynx used to produce sound.*

The vocal folds, or vocal cords, are located in the airstream at the upper end of the trachea. As the airstream passes between the vocal folds, they may be made to vibrate, much as a flag flaps in the wind. We call this vibration "phonation."

MECHANISMS OF PHONATION

Vocal folds are bands of tissue that can be set into vibration. The larynx is the cartilaginous structure that houses vocal folds. The paired vocal folds are situated on both sides of the larynx so that they actually intrude into the airstream, as you can see in Figure 3–1. In the view from above, you can see

(A)

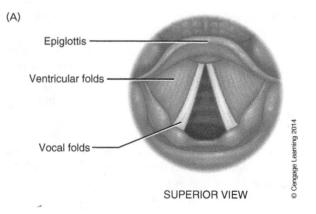

Epiglottis

Ventricular folds

Vocal folds

SUPERIOR VIEW

© Cengage Learning 2014

Figure 3–1. (A) Vocal folds viewed from above. *(continues)*

(B)

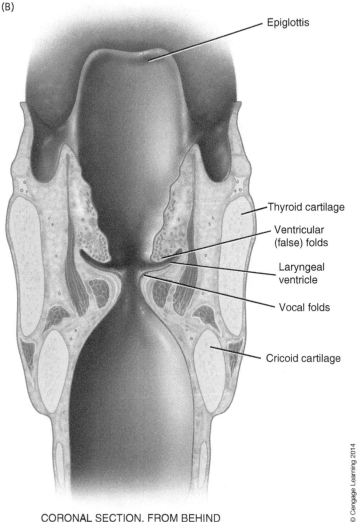

Epiglottis

Thyroid cartilage

Ventricular (false) folds

Laryngeal ventricle

Vocal folds

Cricoid cartilage

CORONAL SECTION, FROM BEHIND

© Cengage Learning 2014

Figure 3–1. continued
(B) View of larynx from behind, showing constriction of laryngeal space caused by the vocal folds.

that the vocal folds are bands of tissue that are visible from a point immediately behind your tongue (shown in front of the epiglottis) looking down toward the lungs. Looking from behind in coronal section, you can see that the vocal folds also constrict the airway, a critical concept for phonation.

You will remember from our discussion of respiratory physiology that any constriction of the airway greatly increases airway turbulence. The vocal folds are a source of turbulence in the vocal tract. Without them, air would pass relatively unimpeded out of the lungs and into the oral cavity.

Daniel Bernoulli, a seventeenth-century Swiss scientist, recognized the effects of constricting a tube during fluid flow. The Bernoulli effect states that given a constant volume flow of air or fluid, at a point of constriction there will be a decrease in air pressure and an increase in velocity of the flow. If you put a constriction in a tube, air will flow faster

Bernoulli effect (principle): *Given a constant volume flow of air or liquid, at a point of constriction there will be a decrease in air or liquid pressure perpendicular to the flow and an increase in velocity of flow.*

as it detours around the constriction and the pressure on the wall at the point of constriction will be lower than that of the surrounding area. Let us further examine this statement.

Airflow Increase

If you have placed your thumb over a garden hose, you know that the rate of water flow increases as a result of that constriction. Likewise, if you have been white-water rafting, you will immediately recognize that the white water comes from constriction in the flow of the river, in the form of boulders. As the water flows through the constriction, the rate of flow increases, giving you a thrill as you speed uncontrollably toward your fate.

Air Pressure Drop

To get an intuitive feel for the pressure drop, think about the flow in terms of molecules of air. Look at Figure 3–2. We have drawn it so you can count the number of molecules of air

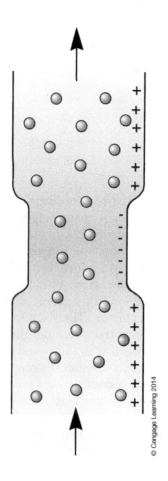

Figure 3–2. Rate of airflow through the tube increases at the point of constriction, and air pressure decreases at that point.

© Cengage Learning 2014

in the tube relative to the tube's length. In the unconstricted regions, you can count 10 molecules of air. Where the tube is narrower, there are fewer air molecules because there is less space for them to occupy, so there are only 5 in that area. Where the constriction ends, you once again see 10 molecules.

When air is forced into a narrow tube, that volume of air has to squeeze into a smaller space. Because each unit mass of air becomes longer and narrower, it covers a longer stretch of the tube's walls. The pressure exerted by this mass, although the same in an overall sense, is now distributed over more of the wall. The result is that each atom of the wall feels less force from the air molecules, and the narrow part of the tube is more likely to collapse. This effect occurs only when the air is forced to move; air without forced movement will sooner or later equalize its pressure everywhere. If you remember that pressure is force exerted on an area ($P = F/A$), a drop in pressure makes perfect sense.

The Bernoulli Effect in Everyday Life

The next time you go flying in an airplane, feel free to thank Daniel Bernoulli for the flight. While the thrust of the engines has a very large contribution to keeping the plane aloft, the configuration of the wings is critical to keeping you aloft so that you can arrive at your destination. If you viewed a wing in cross section from the end you would note that the front of the wing is fatter, while the back is tapered, giving a more stream-lined shape. This configuration causes the air on the upper surface of the wing to move a little faster than that of the underbelly of the wing, which corresponds to a reduction in air pressure *above* the wing. This low pressure above "sucks" the airplane up into the sky as airflow increases, so that the net result is an airplane that rises! (This is why wings are treated for ice in winter: Ice changes the aerodynamics of the wing, destabilizing the difference between upper and lower surfaces, greatly compromising the lift that can be gained.)

For those of you who prefer fly balls to flying, realize that the pitcher in a baseball game is capitalizing on the Bernoulli effect as well. To throw a curve ball, the pitcher ensures that the ball begins its flight with the smooth surface toward the front and that the seam on the ball rotates to the side of the ball sometime during its brief flight. The seam acts as a constriction; the pressure on the seam side is lower than that on the opposite smooth side, and the ball is "sucked" toward the seam (there are other processes involved, but we'll ignore them here). At least one pitcher has demonstrated the ability to "weave" the ball through a series of fence posts by putting just the right spin on the ball. For an excellent discussion of this effect, see Adair (1995).

The vocal folds are made up of muscle and epithelial tissue. Because these are soft tissues, the folds are capable of moving when sufficient force is exerted on them. In Figure 3–3A the vocal folds are closed. In Figure 3–3B the air pressure generated by the respiratory system is beginning to force the vocal folds open, but there is no transglottal flow because the folds are still making full contact. By part D the vocal folds have been blown open. Because the vocal folds are elastic, they tend to return to the point of equilibrium, which is the point of rest. They cannot return to equilibrium, however, as long as the air pressure is so great that they are kept apart. When they are apart, however, there is a drop in pressure at the point of constriction (the Bernoulli effect), and we already know that if there is a drop in pressure, something is going to move to equalize that pressure.

In parts E, F, and G you can see the result of the negative pressure. The vocal folds are being sucked back toward the midline (E) as a result of the negative pressure and tissue

Figure 3–3. One cycle of vocal fold vibration seen through a frontal section. (A) Air pressure beneath the vocal folds rises from respiratory flow. (B) Air pressure causes the vocal folds to separate in the inferior. (C) Superior aspect of vocal folds begins to open. (D) Vocal folds are blown open, flow between the folds increases, and pressure at the folds decreases. (E) Decreased pressure and elastic quality of vocal folds causes folds to move back toward midline. (F) Vocal folds make contact inferiorly. (G) The cycle of vibration is completed.

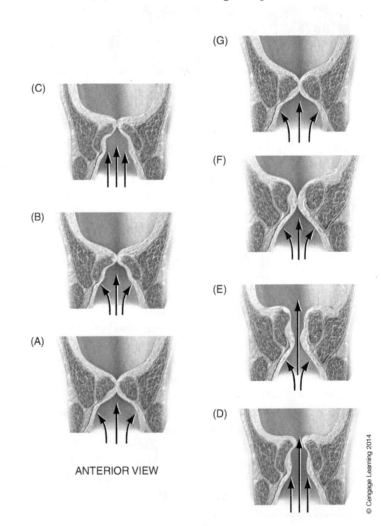

ANTERIOR VIEW

© Cengage Learning 2014

elasticity. Parts F and G show the folds again making contact, with airflow completely halted. The vocal folds are, in essence, sucked back to midline by the pressure drop at the constriction. When the vocal folds are pulled back toward midline by their tissue-restoring forces, they completely block the flow of air for an instant as they make contact. When they are in contact, air has stopped flowing briefly, and therefore the negative pressure related to flow is gone also. Instead, there is the force of respiratory charge beneath the folds ready to blow them apart once again. By the way, the minimum subglottal pressure that will blow the vocal folds apart to sustain phonation is approximately 3 to 5 cm H_2O, although much larger subglottal pressures are required for louder speech.

What you hear as voicing is the product of the repeated opening and closing of the vocal folds. The motion of the tissue and airflow disturb the molecules of air, causing the phenomenon we call sound.

The act of bringing the vocal folds together for phonation is **adduction**, and the process of drawing the vocal folds apart to terminate phonation is **abduction**. As we will see, both of these movements use specific muscles, but the actual vibration of the vocal folds is the product of airflow interacting with the tissue in absence of repetitive muscular contraction.

adduction: *The process of moving two structures closer together.*

abduction: *The process of moving two structures farther apart.*

Summary

- Phonation, or voicing, is the product of vibrating vocal folds in the larynx.
- The vocal folds vibrate as air flows past them; the Bernoulli phenomenon and tissue elasticity help maintain phonation.
- The Bernoulli principle states that given a constant volume flow of air or fluid, at a point of constriction there will be a decrease in air pressure perpendicular to the flow and an increase in velocity of the flow.
- The interaction of subglottal pressure, tissue elasticity, and constriction of the airflow caused by the vocal folds produces sustained phonation as long as pressure, flow, and vocal fold approximation are maintained.

A TOUR OF THE PHONATORY MECHANISM

This is a good opportunity to walk you through the vocal mechanism. We will get into details soon enough, but for now let us look at the larger picture.

Framework of the Larynx

The larynx is a structure made of muscle and cartilage located at the superior (upper) end of the trachea. It comprises three unpaired and three paired cartilages bound by ligaments and lined with mucous membrane.

In Figure 3–4 you can see the relation between the trachea and larynx. The *cricoid cartilage* is a complete ring resting atop the trachea and is the most inferior of the laryngeal cartilages. The *thyroid cartilage* is the largest of the laryngeal cartilages, articulating with the cricoid cartilage below by means of paired processes that let it rock forward and backward at that joint. With this configuration, the paired *arytenoid cartilages* ride on the high-backed upper surface of the cricoid cartilage, forming the posterior point of attachment for the vocal folds. The *corniculate cartilages* ride on the superior surface of each arytenoid. The inner surface of the thyroid cartilage provides the anterior point of attachment for the vocal folds.

The thyroid cartilage articulates with the hyoid bone by means of a pair of superior processes. Medial to the hyoid bone and thyroid cartilage is the *epiglottis*, a leaf-shaped cartilage.

process: *Protrusion of an anatomical structure.*

Summary

- The larynx is a musculo-cartilaginous structure located at the upper end of the trachea that comprises the cricoid, thyroid, and epiglottis cartilages, as well as the paired arytenoid, corniculate, and cuneiform cartilages.
- The thyroid and cricoid cartilages articulate by means of the cricothyroid joint, which lets the two cartilages come closer together in front.
- The arytenoid and cricoid cartilages also articulate with a joint that permits a wide range of arytenoid motion.
- The corniculate cartilages rest on the upper surface of the arytenoids, and the cuneiform cartilages reside in the aryepiglottic folds.

Inner Larynx

The vocal folds are bands of mucous membrane, connective tissue, and muscle that are slung between the arytenoid cartilages and the thyroid cartilage so that they can be moved into and out of the airstream. Muscles attached to the arytenoids perform both adductory and abductory functions.

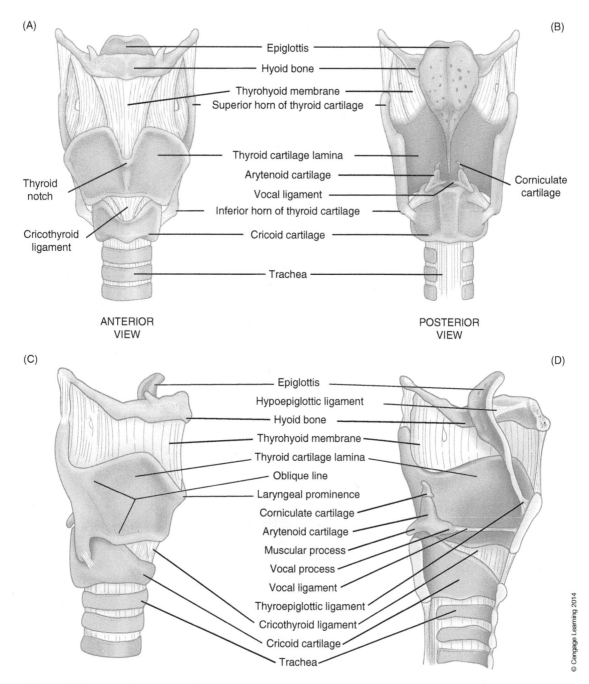

Figure 3–4. Larynx in anterior (A) and posterior (B) views (upper). (C) Lateral view of larynx. (D) View of relationship of cricoid and arytenoid cartilages, as seen in larynx that has been cut in sagittal section at midline. *(continues)*

(E)

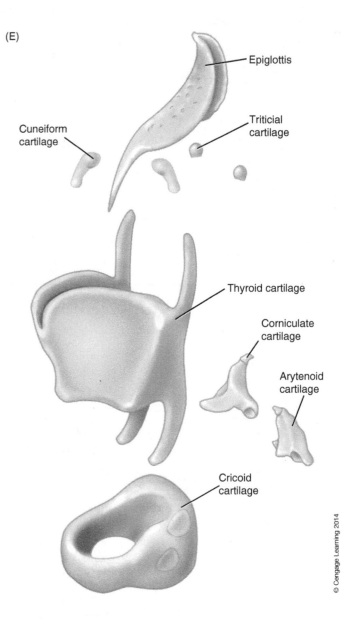

Epiglottis

Triticial cartilage

Cuneiform cartilage

Thyroid cartilage

Corniculate cartilage

Arytenoid cartilage

Cricoid cartilage

© Cengage Learning 2014

Figure 3–4. continued
(E) Exploded view of
disarticulated laryngeal
cartilages.

Laryngeal Membranes

The cavity of the larynx is a constricted tube with a smooth
and reasonably aerodynamic surface (see Figure 3–5). The
thyrohyoid membrane stretches across the space between the
greater cornu of hyoid and the lateral thyroid cartilage.

Intrinsic ligaments connect the cartilages of the larynx
and form the support structure for the cavity of the larynx,
as well as that of the vocal folds themselves. The *fibroelastic
membrane* of the larynx is composed of the upper quadrangular membranes and *aryepiglottic folds,* the lower *conus
elasticus,* and the *vocal ligament,* which is actually the upward free extension of the conus elasticus.

Laryngectomy

People who undergo laryngectomy (surgical removal of the larynx) lose the structures necessary to produce sound. The larynx is removed and the oral cavity is sealed off from the trachea and lower respiratory passageway as a safeguard because the protective function of the larynx is also lost. Laryngectomees (individuals who have undergone laryngectomy) must alter their activities because they now breathe through a tracheostoma, an opening placed in the trachea through a surgical procedure known as a tracheostomy.

Loss of the ability to phonate is but one of the difficulties facing the laryngectomee. They have difficulty with expectoration (elimination of phlegm from respiratory passageway) and coughing, and are no longer able to enjoy swimming or other activities that would expose the stoma to water or pollutants. The air entering the person's lungs is no longer humidified or filtered by the upper respiratory passageway, and a filter must be kept over the stoma to prevent introduction of foreign objects. The flavor of foods is greatly reduced because the person no longer breathes through the nose, and our perception of food relies heavily on the sense of smell. Depending on pre- and postoperative treatment, laryngectomees may also experience extreme dryness of oral tissues arising from damage to salivary glands from radiation therapy.

If you will look at the profile of the larynx in Figure 3–6, you will appreciate some of the relationships among the structures. The **aditus** is the entry to the larynx from the pharynx above. View A of Figure 3–7 is looking through the aditus into the vestibule. You can see two "bumps" under the aryepiglottic folds that are caused by the cuneiform cartilages embedded in the folds. The second set of prominences posterior to the first two are from the *corniculate cartilages* on the arytenoids.

aditus: *The entrance of the larynx.*

The vestibule is the cavity between the entry to the larynx, or aditus, and the **ventricular**, or vestibular, folds. The ventricular folds are known also as the false vocal folds because they are not used for phonation. The space between the margins of the false vocal folds and the true vocal folds below is the *laryngeal ventricle*, or laryngeal sinus, and the anterior extension of this space is the *laryngeal saccule*. The saccule, or pouch, is endowed with more than 60 mucous glands that secrete lubricating mucus into the laryngeal cavity. These sacs are actually endowed with muscle to squeeze the mucus out for lubrication.

ventricular: *Referring to cavities or passageways to structures.*

The **glottis** is the space between the vocal folds, inferior to the ventricle and superior to the conus elasticus. This is the most important laryngeal space for speech because

glottis: *The space between the vocal folds.*

(A)

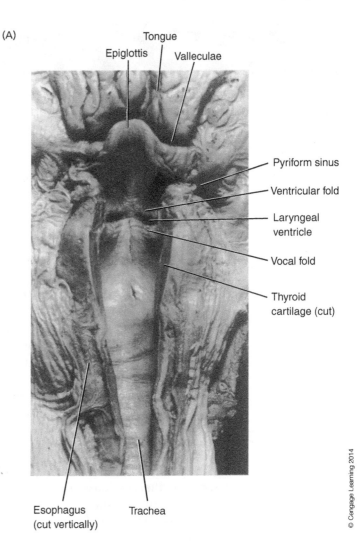

Figure 3–5. (A) Cavity of
the larynx with landmarks.
(continues)

Esophagus   Trachea
(cut vertically)

© Cengage Learning 2014

anterior commissure of glottis:
*The anterior-most region
of the glottis.*

posterior commissure of glottis:
*The posterior-most region
of the glottis.*

it is defined by the variable sphincter that permits voicing. In adults at rest, the length of the glottis is approximately 20 mm from the **anterior commissure** (anterior-most opening) to the **posterior commissure** (between the arytenoid cartilages). The glottis area is variable, depending on the moment-to-moment configuration of the vocal folds. At rest, the posterior glottis is approximately 8 mm wide, and this dimension doubles during forced respiration.

At the margins of the glottis are the vocal folds and the arytenoid cartilage. The anterior three fifths of the vocal margin is made up of the soft tissue of the vocal folds. (You might see this referred to as the membranous glottis because some anatomists define the glottis as the entire vocal mechanism.) In adult males the free margin of the vocal folds is approximately 15 mm long, and in females it is approximately 12 mm. This free margin of the vocal folds is the vibrating element that provides voice. The posterior

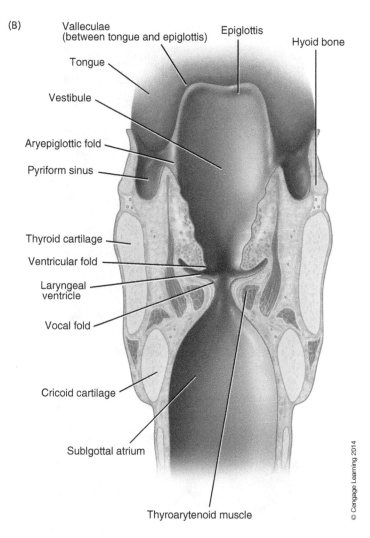

(B)

Valleculae
(between tongue and epiglottis)

Epiglottis

Hyoid bone

Tongue

Vestibule

Aryepiglottic fold

Pyriform sinus

Thyroid cartilage

Ventricular fold

Laryngeal
ventricle

Vocal fold

Cricoid cartilage

Sublgottal atrium

Thyroarytenoid muscle

© Cengage Learning 2014

Figure 3–5. continued
(B) Drawing of cavity of
larynx, as viewed from behind
through coronal section.

two fifths of the vocal folds is the cartilage of the arytenoids.
(This is often referred to as the cartilaginous glottis.) This
portion of the vocal folds is between 4 mm and 8 mm long,
depending on sex and body size.

The cover-body theory of phonation (Titze, 1994) helps
to explain the complex vibration that occurs from vocal fold
vibration. The vocal folds are composed of five layers of tissue. The most superficial layer is a protective layer of squamous epithelium, which combines with a basement layer to
connect it with the next layer. This layer gives the vocal folds
a "glistening" appearance when viewed using a laryngoscope. The next layer is called the superficial lamina propria
and is highly elastic. Deep to that is the intermediate lamina
propria, and finally the deep lamina propria. The layers of
the lamina propria provide great strength to the vocal folds,
and the intermediate and deep layers make up the vocal ligament. The final layer of the vocal folds is the thyroarytenoid
muscle itself (thyrovocalis + thyromuscularis).

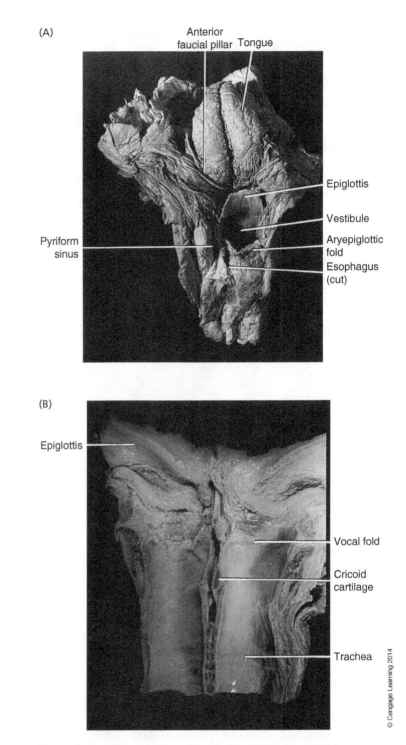

(A)

Anterior
faucial pillar Tongue

Epiglottis

Vestibule

Aryepiglottic
fold

Esophagus
(cut)

Pyriform
sinus

(B)

Epiglottis

Vocal fold

Cricoid
cartilage

Trachea

© Cengage Learning 2014

Figure 3–6. (A) Larynx seen from behind and above. (B) Larynx that has been cut sagittally and the sides reflected, revealing the two halves of the larynx. *(continues)*

(C)

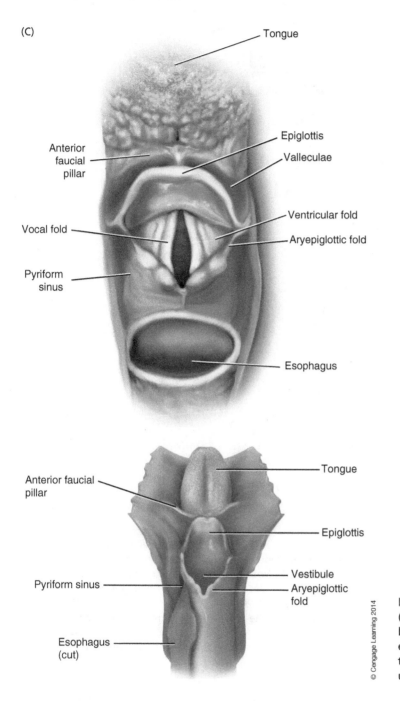

Figure 3–6. continued (C) Drawing of larynx showing landmarks. Note that the esophagus is closed when the airway is open and unprotected.

© Cengage Learning 2014

Summary

- The cavity of the larynx is a constricted tube with a smooth surface.
- Sheets and cords of ligaments connect the cartilages, and smooth mucous membrane covers the medial-most surface of the larynx.

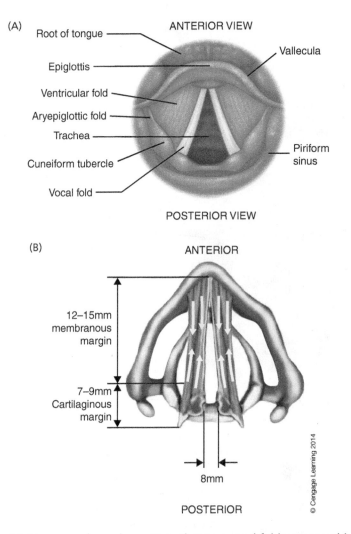

(A)

ANTERIOR VIEW

Root of tongue

Vallecula

Epiglottis

Ventricular fold

Aryepiglottic fold

Trachea

Cuneiform tubercle

Piriform sinus

Vocal fold

POSTERIOR VIEW

(B)

ANTERIOR

12–15mm membranous margin

7–9mm Cartilaginous margin

8mm

POSTERIOR

© Cengage Learning 2014

Figure 3–7. (A) Vocal folds as seen from above. Note that true vocal folds appear white upon examination as a result of the superficial layer of squamous epithelial tissue. Seen immediately superior to the true vocal folds are the ventricular or false folds. Note the corniculate and cuneiform tubercles. These prominences arise from the presence of the corniculate and cuneiform cartilages deep in the aryepiglottic folds. (B) Same view of vocal folds, but with the membranous lining and supportive muscle of lanrynx removed, to reveal only cartilages and the thyroarytenoid muscle (thyrovocalis and thyromuscularis). The membranous margin of the vocal folds is approximately 12 to 15 mm long in adults and the cartilaginous margin is approximately 7 to 9 mm long. The space between the vocal folds (glottis) at rest is approximately 8 mm.

- The fibroelastic membrane is composed of the upper quadrangular membranes and aryepiglottic folds, the lower conus elasticus, and the vocal ligament, which is actually the upward free extension of the conus elasticus.
- The aryepiglottic folds course from the side of the epiglottis to the arytenoid apex.
- The vocal ligament is made of elastin. The aditus is the entryway of the larynx, marking the entry to the vestibule.

- The ventricular and vocal folds are separated by the laryngeal ventricle.
- The glottis is the variable space between the vocal folds.

STRUCTURAL ELEMENTS OF THE LARYNX

Cricoid Cartilage

As the most inferior cartilage of the larynx, the cricoid cartilage is the approximate diameter of the trachea. It is higher in the back than in the front. There are several important landmarks on the cricoid. The low, anterior cricoid arch provides clearance for the vocal folds that will pass over that point, and the posterior elevation provides the point of articulation of the arytenoid cartilages. On the lateral surfaces of the cricoid are articular facets, or "faces," marking the point of articulation of the inferior horns of the thyroid cartilage (see Figure 3–8).

Thyroid Cartilage

The unpaired thyroid cartilage is the largest laryngeal cartilage. As you can see in Figure 3–9, the thyroid has a prominent anterior surface made up of two plates called the *thyroid laminae*, joined midline at the *thyroid angle*. At the superior-most point of that angle is the *thyroid notch*. On the lateral superficial aspect of the thyroid laminae you can see the *oblique line*. This marks the point of attachment for two of the muscles we will talk about shortly.

The posterior aspect of the thyroid is open, and it is characterized by two prominent sets of cornua, or horns. The *inferior cornua* project downward to articulate with the cricoid cartilage, and the *superior cornua* project upward to articulate with the hyoid. Some individuals have a small *triticial cartilage* (*cartilago triticea*) between the superior cornua of the thyroid cartilage and the hyoid bone.

Arytenoid and Corniculate Cartilages

The paired arytenoid cartilages are among the most important parts of the larynx for phonation. They reside on the superior surface of the cricoid cartilage and provide the mechanical structure that permits onset and offset of voicing. To aid visualization, the form of the arytenoid can be likened to

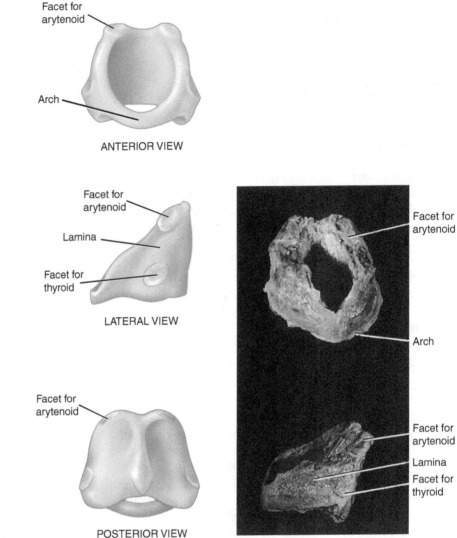

Facet for arytenoid

Arch

ANTERIOR VIEW

Facet for arytenoid

Lamina

Facet for thyroid

LATERAL VIEW

Facet for arytenoid

POSTERIOR VIEW

Facet for arytenoid

Arch

Facet for arytenoid

Lamina

Facet for thyroid

© Cengage Learning 2014

Figure 3–8.
Cricoid cartilage and landmarks.

a pyramid (see Figure 3–10). Each cartilage has two processes and four surfaces.

The apex is the superior portion of the arytenoid cartilage, and above it is the corniculate cartilage. The inferior surface of the arytenoid cartilage is termed the base, and its concave surface is the point of articulation with the convex arytenoid facet of the cricoid cartilage. There are two processes on each arytenoid. The *vocal process* projects toward the thyroid notch, where the vocal folds attach in the anterior. The *muscular process* forms the lateral outcropping of the arytenoid pyramid and is the point of attachment for muscles that adduct and abduct the vocal folds.

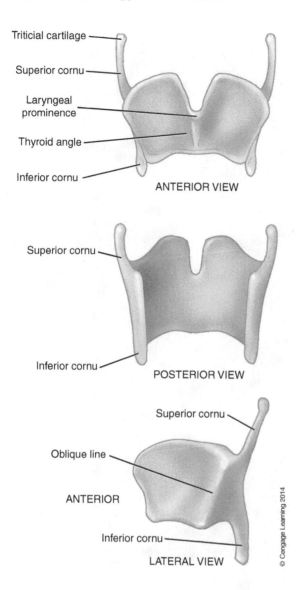

Figure 3–9. Thyroid cartilage and landmarks. *(continues)*

Epiglottis

The unpaired epiglottis is a leaflike structure that arises from the inner surface of the angle of the thyroid cartilage just below the notch, attached there by the *thyroepiglottic ligament*. The sides of the epiglottis are joined with the arytenoid cartilages via the aryepiglottic folds, which are the product of the membranous lining draping over muscle and connective tissue.

The epiglottis projects upward beyond the larynx and above the hyoid bone. It is attached to the root of the tongue by the median *glosso-epiglottic fold* and the paired lateral glosso-epiglottic folds. This juncture produces the valleculae, important landmarks in swallowing deficit.

valleculae: *Pair of small indentations between the tongue and epiglottis.*

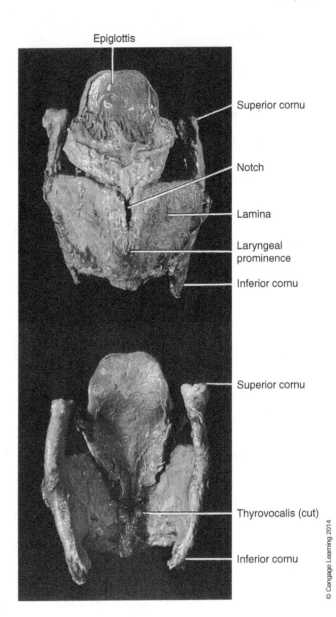

Epiglottis
Superior cornu
Notch
Lamina
Laryngeal prominence
Inferior cornu
Superior cornu
Thyrovocalis (cut)
Inferior cornu

© Cengage Learning 2014

Figure 3–9. continued

fossa: *Indentation or cavity.*

pharyngeal recesses: *Valleculae and piriform sinuses.*

During swallowing, food passes over the epiglottis, and from there laterally to the *piriform* (also pyriform) *sinuses*, which are small fossae, or indentations, between the aryepiglottic folds medially and the mucous lining of the thyroid cartilage. Together the piriform sinuses and valleculae are called the pharyngeal recesses (see Figure 3–7).

Cuneiform Cartilages

The cuneiform cartilages are small cartilages embedded in the aryepiglottic folds. They are situated above and anterior to the corniculate cartilages, and they cause a small bulge on

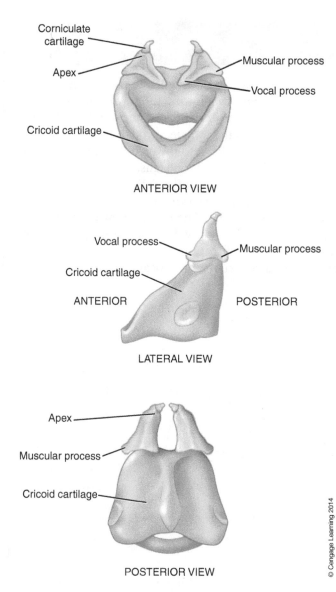

Corniculate cartilage

Apex

Muscular process

Vocal process

Cricoid cartilage

ANTERIOR VIEW

Vocal process

Muscular process

Cricoid cartilage

ANTERIOR

POSTERIOR

LATERAL VIEW

Apex

Muscular process

Cricoid cartilage

POSTERIOR VIEW

© Cengage Learning 2014

Figure 3–10. Arytenoid cartilages articulated with cricoid cartilage.

the surface of the membrane that looks white under illumination. These cartilages apparently provide support for the membranous laryngeal covering.

Hyoid Bone

The *hyoid bone* is the union between the tongue and the laryngeal structure. This unpaired small bone articulates loosely with the superior cornu of the thyroid cartilage, and it has the distinction of being the only bone of the body that is not attached to other bone (see Figure 3–11).

The front of the **corpus** of the hyoid bone is convex and the inner surface is concave. The corpus is the point of attachment for six muscles (mylohyoid, sternohyoid,

corpus: *Body.*

Valleculae and Swallowing

The valleculae are "little valleys," formed by the membrane between the tongue and epiglottis. During normal swallowing the larynx elevates and the epiglottis folds down to protect the airway from food and liquid. The food and liquid pass over the back of the tongue, through the valleculae, on either side of the base of the epiglottis, into the piriform sinuses lateral to the laryngeal aditus, and finally into the esophagus.

When swallowing is compromised, as in the deficit caused by cerebrovascular accident (CVA, or stroke), the larynx may not elevate properly, and food can accumulate in the valleculae. The resultant malodorous breath in a neurologically compromised individual may be a significant indicator of a dangerous swallowing dysfunction; if the epiglottis is not covering the airway, there is a good chance that the vocal folds are not doing their job in protecting the lungs.

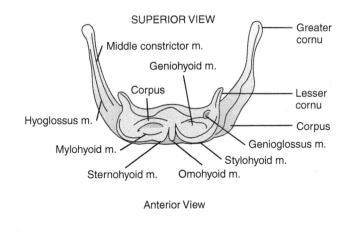

SUPERIOR VIEW

Greater cornu

Middle constrictor m.

Geniohyoid m.

Corpus

Lesser cornu

Hyoglossus m.

Corpus

Mylohyoid m.

Genioglossus m.

Stylohyoid m.

Sternohyoid m.   Omohyoid m.

Anterior View

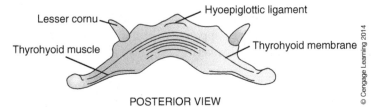

Lesser cornu

Hyoepiglottic ligament

Thyrohyoid muscle

Thyrohyoid membrane

POSTERIOR VIEW

© Cengage Learning 2014

Figure 3–11. Hyoid bone seen from above and behind. Points of attachment of muscles and membranes are indicated in parentheses.

cornu: *Horn.*

omohyoid, stylohyoid, genioglossus, and geniohyoid). The greater **cornu** is on the lateral surface of the corpus, projecting posteriorly. At the junction of the corpus and greater cornu, you can see the *lesser cornu*. Three additional muscles (hypoglossus, middle constrictor, and thyrohyoid) are attached to these two structures.

MOVEMENT OF THE CARTILAGES

The *cricothyroid* and *cricoarytenoid joints* are the only functionally mobile points of the larynx. The cricothyroid joint is the junction of the cricoid cartilage and inferior cornu of the thyroid cartilage. These joints permit the cricoid and thyroid to rotate and glide relative to each other. As seen in Figure 3–12, rotation at the cricothyroid joint permits the thyroid cartilage to rock down in front, and the joint also permits the thyroid to glide forward and backward slightly relative to the cricoid. This joint will provide the major adjustment for change in vocal pitch.

The cricoarytenoid joint is the articulation formed between the cricoid and arytenoid cartilages. These joints permit rocking, gliding, and minimal rotation. The arytenoid facet of the cricoid is a convex, oblong surface, and the axis of motion is around a line projecting back along the superior surface of the arytenoid and converging at a point above the arytenoid (see Figure 3–13). This rocking action folds the two vocal processes toward each other, permitting the

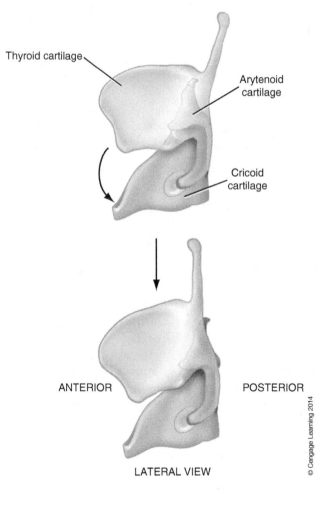

Thyroid cartilage

Arytenoid cartilage

Cricoid cartilage

ANTERIOR   POSTERIOR

LATERAL VIEW

© Cengage Learning 2014

Figure 3–12. Movement of the cricoid and thyroid cartilages about the cricothyroid joint. When the cricoid and thyroid move toward each other in front the arytenoid cartilage moves farther away from the thyroid cartilage, tensing the vocal folds.

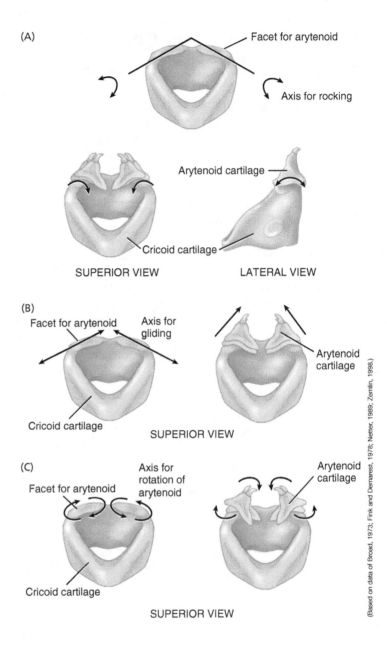

Figure 3–13. The articular facet for the arytenoid cartilage permits rocking, gliding, and rotation. (A) The shape of the articular facet of the arytenoid cartilage promotes inward rocking of the arytenoid cartilage and vocal folds (arced arrows). (B) The long axis of the facet permits limited anterior-posterior gliding (bidirectional arrows). (C) The arytenoids can also rotate, although this does not appear to be a functional gesture for adduction (circling arrows).

(Based on data of Broad, 1973; Fink and Demarest, 1978; Netter, 1989; Zemlin, 1998.)

vocal folds to make contact. The arytenoids are also capable of gliding on the long axis of the facet, facilitating changes in vocal fold length. The arytenoids may rotate upon a vertical axis drawn through the apex of the arytenoid, but this motion appears to be limited to extremes of abduction (Fink & Demarest, 1978). The combination of these gestures provides the mechanism for vocal fold approximation and abduction.

Your understanding of the movement of these cartilages in relation to each other will provide a valuable backdrop to understanding laryngeal physiology.

Vocal Fold Hydration

The vocal folds are extremely sensitive to the internal and external environments. Although the effects of smoking and other pollutants are known to irritate the tissues of the vocal folds, the internal environment appears to have an impact as well.

When the vocal folds are subject to abuse, problems such as contact ulcers and vocal nodules may occur. Hydration therapy is a frequent prescription to counteract the problems of irritated tissue. Dry tissue does not heal as well as moist tissue, so the patient will be told to spray the throat, drink fluids, or even take medications to promote water retention. This type of therapy makes more than medical sense. Verdolini, Titze, and Fennell (1994) found that the effort of phonation increases as individuals become dehydrated and decreases when they are hydrated beyond normal levels. Indeed, the airflow required to produce the same phonation is greatly increased by a poorly lubricated larynx. In addition, the vocal folds vibrate much more periodically (that is, they have greatly reduced perturbation, or cycle-by-cycle variation) when lubricated (Fukida et al., 1988). When the relative periodicity of the vocal folds decreases, the voice is hoarse.

Palpation of the Larynx

To palpate the larynx, first identify the prominent thyroid notch, or "Adam's apple." Once you have found it, place your index finger on the notch and your thumb and second finger on either side. Your thumb and second finger should feel a fairly flat surface, the thyroid lamina. Now bring your index finger straight down a little bit, and you will feel the prominent thyroid angle. Bring your finger back up to the top of the notch; the hard region contacting your fingernail is the corpus of the hyoid bone. In some people this is very hard to differentiate from the thyroid.

Palpate lateral to the notch on the superior surface and you will feel the superior cornu of thyroid. With a little discomfort you may feel the articulation of the hyoid and thyroid. If you draw your finger down the angle again, you can find the lower margin of the thyroid and feel the cricoid beneath. By carefully placing your thumb at the junction of the cricoid and thyroid, you can hum up and down the scale and feel the thyroid and cricoid moving closer together and farther apart as you do this. You will also feel the entire larynx elevate as you reach the upper end of your range. Finally, draw your finger down to find the lower margin of the cricoid, marking the beginning of the trachea. Palpate the tracheal rings.

Summary

- The laryngeal cartilages have a number of important landmarks to which muscles are attached.
- The cricoid cartilage is shaped like a signet ring, higher in back.
- The arytenoid cartilages ride on the superior surface of the cricoid, with the cricoarytenoid joint permitting rotation, rocking, and gliding.
- The corniculate cartilages attach to the upper margin of the arytenoids.
- The thyroid cartilage has two prominent laminae, superior and inferior horns, and a prominent thyroid notch.
- The hyoid bone attaches to the superior cornu of thyroid, and the cricoid cartilage attaches to the inferior horn via the cricothyroid joint.
- The epiglottis attaches to the tongue and thyroid cartilage, dropping down to cover the larynx during swallowing.
- The cuneiform cartilages are embedded in the aryepiglottic folds.

LARYNGEAL MUSCULATURE

intrinsic laryngeal muscles:
Muscles with both origin and insertion in the larynx.

extrinsic laryngeal muscles:
Muscles with one attachment in the larynx and one attachment outside the larynx.

As summarized in Table 3–1, muscles of the larynx are categorized either as intrinsic laryngeal muscles, which have both origin and insertion on laryngeal cartilages, or extrinsic laryngeal muscles, which have one attachment on a laryngeal cartilage and the other attachment on a non-laryngeal structure. The intrinsic muscles assume responsibility for opening, closing, tensing, and relaxing the vocal folds, and the extrinsic muscles make major adjustments of the larynx.

Intrinsic Laryngeal Muscles

Adductors

The *lateral cricoarytenoid muscle* attaches to the cricoid and the muscular process of the arytenoid, causing the muscular process to move forward and medially (see Figure 3–14). The origin of the lateral cricoarytenoid muscle is the superior-lateral surface of the cricoid cartilage. The muscle courses up and back to insert into the muscular process of the arytenoid cartilage. When it is contracted, the muscular process is drawn forward, which rocks the arytenoid inward and downward, adducting the vocal folds.

Table 3–1. Muscles Associated with Laryngeal Function

Intrinsic Muscles of Larynx
  Adductors
    Lateral cricoarytenoid
    Transverse arytenoid
    Oblique arytenoid
  Abductor
    Posterior cricoarytenoid
  Tensors
    Thyrovocalis (medial thyroarytenoid)
    Cricothyroid, pars recta, and pars oblique
  Relaxers
    Thyromuscularis (lateral thyroarytenoid)

Suprahyoid and Infrahyoid Muscles
  Hyoid and Laryngeal Elevators
    Stylohyoid
    Mylohyoid
    Geniohyoid
    Genioglossus
    Hyoglossus
    Inferior pharyngeal constrictor
    Digastricus anterior and posterior
  Hyoid and Laryngeal Depressors
    Sternothyroid
    Sternohyoid
    Omohyoid
    Thyrohyoid

The *transverse arytenoid muscle* also might be called the transverse interarytenoid muscle. This muscle spans the posterior surface of both arytenoid cartilages. Its function is to pull the two arytenoids closer together and to approximate the vocal folds. Motor innervation of the transverse arytenoid muscles is by means of the inferior branch of the recurrent laryngeal nerve arising from the vagus nerve, or tenth cranial nerve.

The *oblique arytenoid muscles* are immediately superficial to the transverse arytenoid muscles, and they perform a similar function. They take their origins at the posterior base of the muscular processes to course obliquely up to the apex of the opposite arytenoid. This course results in a characteristic X arrangement of the muscles as well as in the ability of these muscles to pull the apex medially. The result

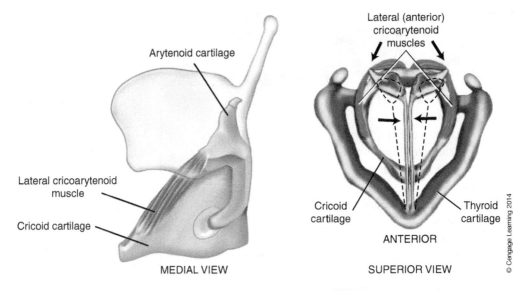

Arytenoid cartilage

Lateral (anterior)
cricoarytenoid
muscles

Lateral cricoarytenoid
muscle

Cricoid cartilage

Cricoid
cartilage

Thyroid
cartilage

ANTERIOR

MEDIAL VIEW

SUPERIOR VIEW

© Cengage Learning 2014

Figure 3–14. Course and effect of lateral cricoarytenoid muscle. The figure on the right shows that contraction of the lateral cricoarytenoid muscle pulls the muscular process forward, adducting the vocal folds (seen from above).

of this action is to promote adduction, enforce medial compression, and rock the arytenoid (and vocal folds) down and in. Innervation of the oblique arytenoid muscles is the same innervation of the transverse arytenoid muscles.

Abductor

The *posterior cricoarytenoid muscle* is the sole abductor of the vocal folds. As you can see in Figure 3–15, the posterior cricoarytenoid muscle originates on the posterior cricoid lamina. Fibers project up and out to insert into the posterior aspect of the muscular process of the arytenoid cartilage. The posterior cricoarytenoid muscles are direct antagonists to the lateral cricoarytenoids (see Figures 3–15 and 3–16).

Contraction of this muscle pulls the muscular process medially and back, rocking the arytenoid cartilage out on its axis and abducting the vocal folds. The posterior cricoarytenoid is innervated by the recurrent laryngeal nerve, a branch of the vagus nerve.

Glottal Tensors

The primary tensor of the vocal folds, the cricothyroid muscle, achieves its function by rocking the thyroid cartilage forward relative to the cricoid cartilage. The *cricothyroid muscle* is composed of two heads, the pars recta and pars oblique, as seen in Figure 3–17. The pars recta courses up and out to insert into the lower surface of the thyroid lamina. The pars oblique arises from the cricoid cartilage lateral to the pars

(A)

(B)

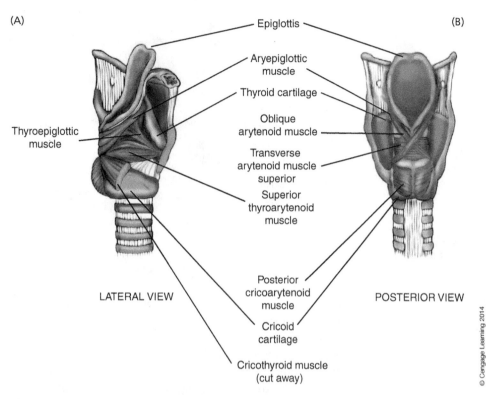

Epiglottis

Aryepiglottic
muscle

Thyroid cartilage

Oblique
arytenoid muscle

Transverse
arytenoid muscle
superior

Superior
thyroarytenoid
muscle

Thyroepiglottic
muscle

LATERAL VIEW

POSTERIOR VIEW

Posterior
cricoarytenoid
muscle

Cricoid
cartilage

Cricothyroid muscle
(cut away)

© Cengage Learning 2014

Figure 3–15. (A) Schematic illustrating relationship among posterior cricoarytenoid, lateral cricoarytenoid, superior thyroarytenoid, and aryepiglottic muscles. (B) Schematic of posterior cricoarytenoid muscle and transverse and oblique arytenoid muscles. Contraction of the transverse and oblique arytenoid muscles pulls the arytenoids closer together, thereby supporting adduction. Contraction of the posterior cricoarytenoid muscle pulls the muscular process medially and back, abducting the vocal folds.

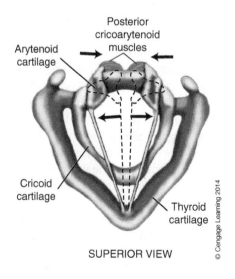

Posterior
cricoarytenoid
muscles

Arytenoid
cartilage

Cricoid
cartilage

Thyroid
cartilage

SUPERIOR VIEW

© Cengage Learning 2014

Figure 3–16. Superior view of action of the posterior cricoarytenoid muscle.

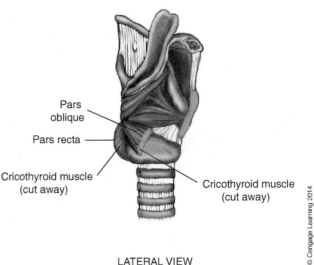

Pars oblique

Pars recta

Cricothyroid muscle (cut away)

Cricothyroid muscle (cut away)

© Cengage Learning 2014

Figure 3–17. Cricothyroid muscle, pars recta, and pars oblique.

LATERAL VIEW

recta, coursing obliquely up to insert at the juncture of the thyroid laminae and inferior horns.

Contraction of the pars recta rocks the thyroid cartilage downward, rotating on the cricothyroid joint. (Remember that the points of attachment of the vocal folds are the inner margin of the thyroid cartilage and arytenoid cartilages and that the arytenoid cartilages are well attached to the posterior cricoid cartilage.) Rocking the thyroid cartilage forward stretches the vocal folds. That is, rocking the thyroid and cricoid closer together in front makes the posterior cricoid more distant from the thyroid. The cricothyroid is innervated by the external branch of the *superior laryngeal nerve* of the vagus nerve. This branch courses lateral to the inferior pharyngeal constrictor to terminate on the cricothyroid muscle.

The *thyrovocalis muscle* is actually the medial muscle of the vocal folds. Contraction of the thyrovocalis tenses the vocal folds, especially when contracted in concert with the cricothyroid (see Figure 3–18). The thyrovocalis (abbreviated *vocalis*) originates from the inner surface of thyroid cartilage near the thyroid notch and inserts into the lateral surface of the arytenoid vocal process. Contraction of this muscle will draw the thyroid and cricoid cartilages farther apart in front, making this muscle a functional antagonist of the cricothyroid muscle (which draws the anterior cricoid and anterior thyroid closer together). This antagonistic function has earned the thyrovocalis classification as a glottal tensor. The thyrovocalis is innervated by the recurrent laryngeal nerve, a branch of the vagus nerve.

Innervation of all intrinsic muscles of the larynx is by means of the *vagus nerve*. The *recurrent laryngeal nerve* (RLN) is so named because of its course. The left RLN "re-courses" beneath the aorta, after which it ascends to innervate the larynx. The right RLN courses under the subclavian artery before ascending to the larynx.

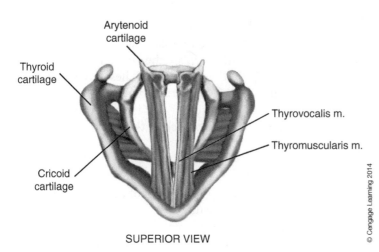

Arytenoid
cartilage

Thyroid
cartilage

Thyrovocalis m.

Thyromuscularis m.

Cricoid
cartilage

SUPERIOR VIEW

© Cengage Learning 2014

Figure 3–18. The thyromuscularis muscle is the lateral muscular component of the vocal folds; the thyrovocalis is the medial-most muscle of the vocal folds. Together they are often referred to as thyroarytenoid muscle.

Referral in Voice Therapy

The phonatory mechanism is extremely sensitive, and vocal variations can indicate a broad range of problems. We must always refer an individual to a physician when we identify vocal dysfunction, even if we are fairly certain that the problem is behavioral. When a client comes to us with a hoarse voice, we may find that the person is abusing his or her phonatory mechanism by spending too much time in loud, smoky settings that require raising the voice to speak. What we don't know from this information is whether there is some vocal pathological condition, perhaps secondary to the same behavioral conditions, that is developing on the vocal folds. Although we suspect vocal nodules, the client could be showing early signs of laryngeal cancer.

In a similar vein, a client who comes to us with a voice that is progressively weaker during the day and for whom muscular effort of any sort is extremely difficult as the day wears on should be referred to a neurologist. *Myasthenia gravis* is a myoneural disease that results in a complex of speech disorders including progressive weakening of phonation, progressive degeneration of articulatory function, and progressive hypernasality, all arising from use of the speech mechanism over the course of a day or even over a briefer time. The condition is quite treatable, but often the speech-language pathologist is the first to recognize the signs because the client sees it primarily as a speech problem. If you identify these signs in a patient, bring this to the attention to your supervising speech-language pathologist, who could assess further.

Laryngeal Relaxer

The *thyromuscularis muscles* (or simply, *muscularis*) are immediately lateral to each thyrovocalis. The thyromuscularis originates on the inner surface of the thyroid cartilage, near the notch and lateral to the origin of the thyrovocalis. It runs back to insert into the arytenoid cartilage at the muscular process and base. Contraction of the medial fibers of the thyromuscularis relaxes the vocal folds. These fibers pull the arytenoids toward the thyroid cartilage without influencing medial rocking. The thyromuscularis is innervated by the recurrent laryngeal nerve, a branch of the vagus.

Summary of Intrinsic Muscle Activity

The drawing in Figure 3–19 may help you to visualize the actions of phonation. Intrinsic muscles of the larynx include the thyrovocalis, thyromuscularis, cricothyroid, lateral and posterior cricoarytenoid, transverse arytenoid and oblique interarytenoid muscle, and superior thyroarytenoid muscles. The thyrovocalis and thyromuscularis muscles make up the muscular portion of the vocal folds. The cricothyroid pulls the anterior cricoid and anterior thyroid closer together, thereby stretching the vocal folds. The lateral cricoarytenoid adducts the vocal folds by rotating and rocking the arytenoids medially, while the posterior cricoarytenoid muscle abducts the vocal folds. The oblique and transverse arytenoid muscles pull the arytenoids closer together, assisting adduction. The superior thyroarytenoid muscle is a variable muscle that may or may not be present. If present, it would be positioned to relax the vocal folds.

Adduction and abduction of the vocal folds is achieved by coordinated effort of many of the larynx's intrinsic muscles. The lateral cricoarytenoid muscle is responsible for rocking

Vocal Hyperfunction

The range of phonatory "misbehavior" is broad and deep. The larynx is an exquisite structure of delicate tissues evolved for use as a protective mechanism. When we use it as a phonatory source, we capitalize on its flexibility. When we overuse the mechanism, we can get into trouble. Here are a few of the problems that occur from laryngeal misuse.

Vocal nodules arise from excessively loud phonation or excessively forceful adduction (shouting or screaming). Contact ulcers apparently develop from excessive force on the posterior aspect of the vocal folds, applied by attempting to force the vocal folds into a lower vocal range and higher vocal intensity.

The addition of toxins to your laryngeal environment can cause trouble as well. Alcohol consumption can irritate the vocal folds, as can cigarette and cigar smoke (primary or secondary smoke). Likewise, excessively dry air can irritate the vocal folds, leading to laryngitis. Esophageal reflux can also cause laryngeal irritation.

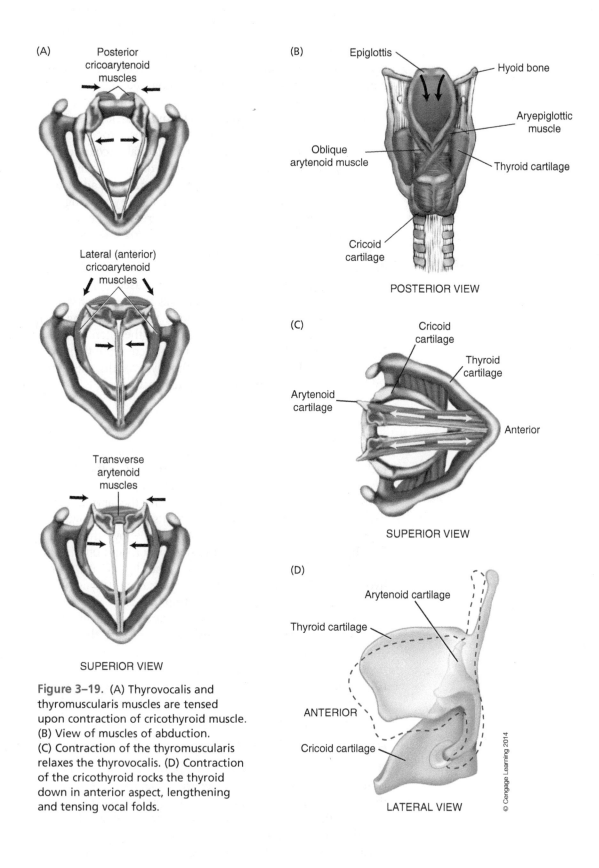

Figure 3–19. (A) Thyrovocalis and thyromuscularis muscles are tensed upon contraction of cricothyroid muscle. (B) View of muscles of abduction. (C) Contraction of the thyromuscularis relaxes the thyrovocalis. (D) Contraction of the cricothyroid rocks the thyroid down in anterior aspect, lengthening and tensing vocal folds.

153

the arytenoid cartilage on its axis, causing the vocal folds to tip in and slightly down. This action is directly opposed by contraction of the posterior cricoarytenoid muscle, which will rock the arytenoid (and vocal folds) out on that same axis. Contraction of the transverse arytenoid muscle draws the posterior surfaces of the two arytenoids closer together, but it is most effective as an adductor if the lateral cricoarytenoid muscle is contracted as well. Contraction of the oblique arytenoid helps the vocal folds dip downward as they are adducted.

Changing vocal pitch is accomplished by altering the mass and tension of the vocal folds. Increasing the tension on the vocal folds stretches them and thereby reduces the mass per unit length. Stretching the vocal folds does not decrease the mass of the muscle, but it does spread them over the length of the muscle. Both increased tension and reduced mass per unit length increases frequency of vibration of the vocal folds, causing pitch to rise; relaxing the vocal folds causes the frequency and thus the pitch to drop. Note that when the cricothyroid is contracted, the thyrovocalis stretches. If you also contract the thyrovocalis, the vocal folds become more tense and the pitch increases.

Extrinsic Laryngeal Muscles

The extrinsic musculature consists of muscles with one attachment to a laryngeal cartilage. These include the sternothyroid, thyrohyoid, and thyropharyngeus muscles. A number of muscles attached to the hyoid also move the larynx: infrahyoid muscles run from the hyoid to a structure below, and suprahyoid muscles attach to a structure above the hyoid. Infrahyoid muscles consist of the sternohyoid and omohyoid muscles; the suprahyoid muscles are the digastricus, stylohyoid, mylohyoid, geniohyoid, genioglossus, and hyoglossus muscles. They are often called the strap muscles.

A more meaningful categorization is based on function relative to the larynx. Muscles that elevate the hyoid and larynx are laryngeal elevators (digastricus, stylohyoid, mylohyoid, geniohyoid, genioglossus, hyoglossus, and thyropharyngeus muscles) and muscles that depress the larynx and hyoid are laryngeal depressors (sternohyoid, omohyoid, thyrohyoid, and sternothyroid muscles).

Hyoid and Laryngeal Elevators

Digastricus. As seen in Figure 3–20, the *digastricus muscle* is actually composed of two separate "bellies" (the belly is the central portion of a muscle). The anterior and posterior bellies of the digastricus muscle converge at the hyoid bone, and their paired contraction elevates the hyoid. The digastricus anterior muscle originates on the inner surface of

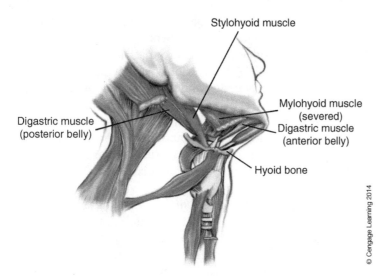

Stylohyoid muscle

Mylohyoid muscle (severed)

Digastric muscle (anterior belly)

Digastric muscle (posterior belly)

Hyoid bone

© Cengage Learning 2014

Figure 3–20. Schematic of digastricus, stylohyoid, and mylohyoid muscles.

the mandible at the digastricus fossa, courses medially and down to the level of the hyoid, and joins the posterior digastricus by means of an intermediate tendon. The posterior digastricus originates on the mastoid process of the temporal bone, behind and beneath the ear. The intermediate tendon passes through and separates the fibers of another muscle, the stylohyoid, as it inserts into the hyoid at the juncture of the hyoid corpus and greater cornu.

Contraction of the anterior component draws the hyoid up and forward, whereas contraction of the posterior belly draws the hyoid up and back. Simultaneous contraction results in hyoid elevation without anterior or posterior movement.

Muscles attached to the mandible, such as the digastricus, also may be depressors of the mandible. That is, the digastricus could help to pull the mandible down if the musculature below the hyoid were to fix it in place. The anterior belly is innervated by the mandibular branch of the trigeminal nerve (cranial nerve V) via the mylohyoid branch of the inferior alveolar nerve. The posterior belly is supplied by the digastric branch of the facial nerve, or cranial nerve VII.

Stylohyoid Muscle. The *stylohyoid muscle* originates on the prominent styloid process of the temporal bone, a point medial to the mastoid process (see Figure 3–20). The course of this muscle is medially down, so that it crosses the path of the posterior digastricus and inserts into the corpus hyoid. Contraction of the stylohyoid elevates and retracts the hyoid bone. The stylohyoid is innervated by the motor branch of the facial nerves (cranial nerve VII).

Mylohyoid Muscle. The *mylohyoid muscle* originates on the underside of the mandible and courses to the corpus hyoid. The mylohyoid is fanlike, originating along the lateral aspects of the inner mandible on a prominence known as the mylohyoid line. The anterior fibers converge at the *median fibrous raphe* (ridge), a structure that runs from the mandible to the hyoid. The posterior fibers course directly to the hyoid. The fibers of mylohyoid form the floor of the oral cavity. The relationship between digastricus and mylohyoid can be seen in Figure 3–21. The mylohyoid elevates the hyoid and projects it forward, or alternately depresses the mandible. Mylohyoid is innervated by the alveolar nerve, arising from the trigeminal nerve, mandibular branch.

Geniohyoid Muscle. The *geniohyoid muscle* is superior to the mylohyoid, originating at the mental spines projecting in a course parallel to the anterior belly of the digastricus from the inner mandibular surface (see Figure 3–21). Fibers of this narrow muscle course back and down to insert into the hyoid bone at the corpus. When contracted, the geniohyoid elevates the hyoid and draws it forward. It may depress the mandible also if the hyoid is fixed. The geniohyoid is innervated by the hypoglossal nerve (cranial nerve XII).

Hyoglossus Muscle. The *hyoglossus* is a lateral muscle that arises from the entire superior surface of the greater cornu of hyoid and courses up into the side of the tongue. The point of insertion in the tongue is near that of the styloglossus, a muscle we will discuss in Chapter 4, which covers the articulators. The muscle takes on a quadrilateral appearance

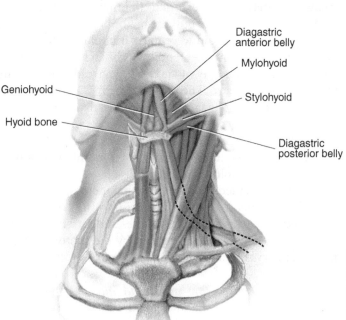

Figure 3–21. Schematic of the relationships among geniohyoid, mylohyoid, digastricus, and stylohyoid muscles.

© Cengage Learning 2014

and is a lingual depressor or hyoid elevator. The hyoglossus muscle is innervated by the motor branch of the hypoglossal nerve.

Genioglossus Muscle. Although the *genioglossus muscle* is more appropriately considered a muscle of the tongue, it definitely is a hyoid elevator. The genioglossus originates on the inner surface of the mandible at the symphysis and courses up, back, and down into the tongue and anterior surface of the hyoid corpus. The genioglossus muscle is innervated by the motor branch of the hypoglossal nerve.

Thyropharyngeus and Cricopharyngeus Muscles of the Inferior Constrictor. The *thyropharyngeus* and *cricopharyngeus muscles* comprise the inferior pharyngeal constrictor. The cricopharyngeus is the sphincter muscle at the orifice of the esophagus, and the thyropharyngeus is involved in propelling food through the pharynx. Its attachment to the cricoid and thyroid provides an opportunity for laryngeal elevation.

The thyropharyngeus arises from the posterior pharyngeal raphe, coursing down fanlike and laterally to the thyroid lamina and inferior cornu. Contraction of this muscle promotes elevation of the larynx while constricting the pharynx. The inferior constrictors are innervated by branches from the vagus nerve and the recurrent laryngeal nerves off the vagus.

Hyoid and Laryngeal Depressors

Laryngeal depressors depress and stabilize the larynx via attachment to the hyoid, but also stabilize the tongue by serving as antagonists to the laryngeal elevators.

Sternohyoid Muscle. As the name implies, the *sternohyoid* runs from sternum to hyoid. It originates from the posterior-superior region of the manubrium sterni, as well as from the medial end of the clavicle (see Figure 3–22). It courses superiorly to insert into the inferior margin of the hyoid corpus. Contraction of the sternohyoid depresses the hyoid. The sternohyoid is innervated by the *ansa cervicalis* (*ansa* = loop; i.e., cervical loop), arising from spinal nerves C1 through C3.

Omohyoid Muscle. The *omohyoid* is a muscle with two bellies. The *superior belly* terminates on the side of the hyoid corpus, while the *inferior belly* has its origin on the upper border of the scapula. The bellies are joined at an intermediate tendon. As you can see from Figure 3–22, the omohyoid passes deep to the sternocleidomastoid that, along with the deep cervical fascia, restrains the muscle to retain that characteristic "dogleg" configuration. When contracted, the omohyoid depresses the hyoid bone and larynx.

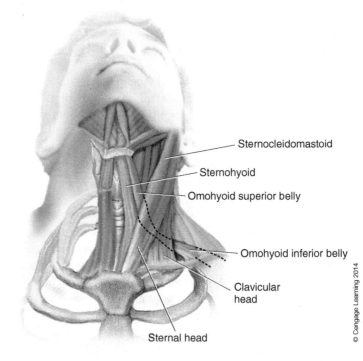

Sternocleidomastoid

Sternohyoid

Omohyoid superior belly

Omohyoid inferior belly

Clavicular head

Sternal head

© Cengage Learning 2014

Figure 3–22. Schematic of the relationships among omohyoid, sternocleidomastoid, and sternohyoid muscles.

The superior belly is innervated by the superior ramus of the ansa cervicalis arising from spinal nerve C1, whereas the inferior belly is innervated by the main ansa cervicalis, arising from spinal nerves C2 and C3.

Sternothyroid Muscle. As shown in Figure 3–23, contraction of the *sternothyroid muscle* depresses the thyroid cartilage. It originates at the manubrium sterni and first costal cartilage, coursing up and out to insert into the oblique line of the thyroid cartilage. The sternothyroid is innervated by fibers from spinal nerves C1 and C2, which pass in the hypoglossal nerve (cranial nerve XII).

Thyrohyoid Muscle. The *thyrohyoid muscle* courses from the oblique line of the thyroid cartilage to the inferior margin of the greater cornu of hyoid bone. The thyrohyoid muscle either depresses the hyoid or raises the larynx (see Figure 3–23). It is innervated by the fibers of spinal nerve C1, which course with the hypoglossal nerves.

Summary

- The extrinsic muscles of the larynx are the sternothyroid, thyrohyoid, and thyropharyngeus muscles.
- The digastricus anterior and posterior muscles together elevate the hyoid, whereas the stylohyoid retracts it.

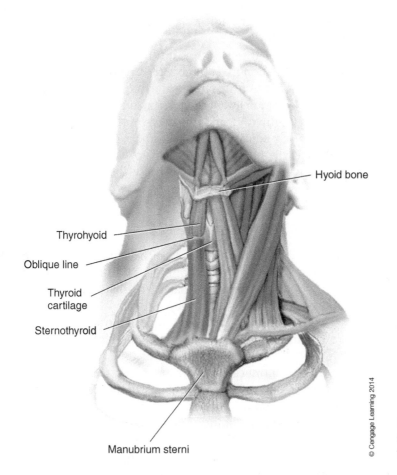

Hyoid bone

Thyrohyoid

Oblique line

Thyroid
cartilage

Sternothyroid

Manubrium sterni

© Cengage Learning 2014

Figure 3–23. The
sternothyroid and
thyrohyoid muscles.

- The mylohyoid and hyoglossus muscles elevate the hyoid, and the geniohyoid elevates the hyoid and draws it forward.
- The thyropharyngeus and cricopharyngeus muscles elevate the larynx, and the sternohyoid, sternothyroid, thyrohyoid, and omohyoid muscles depress the larynx.

Interaction of Musculature

The larynx is virtually suspended from a broad sling of muscles, referred to collectively as the hyoid sling muscles, which must work in concert to achieve the complex motions required for speech and nonspeech functions. Movement of the larynx and its cartilages requires both gross and fine adjustments. It appears that the gross movements associated with laryngeal elevation and depression provide stability for the fine adjustments of phonatory control. The suprahyoid and infrahyoid muscles raise and lower the larynx, changing the vocal tract length, but the intrinsic laryngeal muscles are responsible for the fine adjustments associated with phonation control.

The musculature works as a unit. The simple gesture of laryngeal elevation must be countered with the controlled antagonistic action of the laryngeal depressors. Elevation of the tongue tends to elevate the larynx and increase the tension of the cricothyroid, and this must be countered through intrinsic muscle adjustment to keep the articulatory system from driving the phonatory mechanism. It is time to move to physiology of phonation to see how these components work together.

Mechanics of Vibration

You may be familiar with the notion that things are capable of vibrating. When a physical body is set into vibration, it tends to continue vibrating (that is, oscillating), and that vibration tends to continue at the same rate.

Let us examine why a body tends to oscillate. If you have a guitar or other stringed instrument, pluck one of the strings. As you listen to the twang of the string, you will notice that it continues vibrating for quite a while before finally quieting down. The tone remains about the same pitch throughout the audible portion of its vibration.

The process of vibration is determined by a lawful interplay among the elastic restoring forces of a material; the stiffness of the material; and inertia, a quality of its mass. Elasticity is the property of a material that causes it to return to its original shape after being displaced. Stiffness refers to the strength of the forces held within a given material that restore it to its original shape on being distended. Inertia is the property of mass that dictates that a body in motion tends to stay in motion. If we discuss the vibration of the guitar string in detail, the interaction of these elements may become clearer. Look at Figure 3–24A as we discuss this.

In the first frame of the figure, the guitar string is at its resting point; all forces are balanced. Next, the string is being displaced by someone's finger; a displacing force is distending the string. Next, the string has been released and is moving toward its starting point. This is a direct result of the restoring forces of the elastic material. The elastic qualities of the material from which the string is made and the stiffness of that material determine the efficiency with which the string returns. (If you tried this with a very inelastic material, such as a bar of lead or a slab of roast beef, would it return?)

In the next part of the figure, when the string reaches it original position, it is moving too fast to stop and sails on by it, even though it is the point of equilibrium. Just as when you push someone in a swing, the swing does not simply

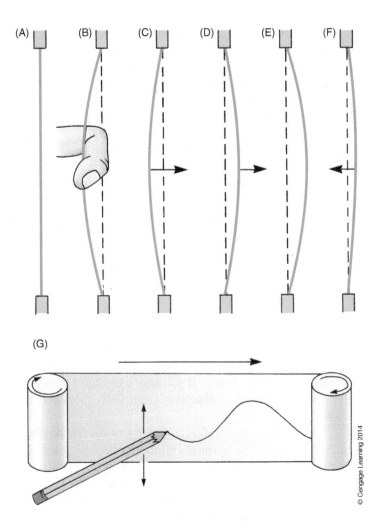

Figure 3–24. A guitar string illustrates oscillation. (A) The string is at rest. (B) A finger forces the string into displacement. (C) The string is released and its elastic elements cause it to return toward the rest position. (D) The string overshoots the rest position because of its inertia. (E) The string reaches the extreme point of its excursion past the rest position. (F) Elastic forces in the string cause the string to return toward the rest position. (G) Periodic motion of a vibrating body graphically recorded.

© Cengage Learning 2014

return to the point of rest and stop, but rather overshoots that point. The reason the string travels past the point of rest is that it has mass. It takes energy to move mass and it takes energy to stop it once it has started moving. The string will not only return to its original resting position because of elastic restoring forces, but it will fly past that position because of the inertia associated with moving the mass of the object. In the last part of this vibration, the string eventually stops moving because it is now being distended in the opposite direction. The energy you expended in the first distension has now been translated into an opposite distortion as a result of inertia. In the final panel, the string can now begin its return trip toward the starting point, but it will once again overshoot that point because of inertia.

If you had set a pencil into vibration instead of a string and we had moved a sheet of paper in front of it as it vibrated, it might have drawn a picture something like Figure 3–24B, which depicts the periodic motion of a vibrating body. This picture is a graphic representation of the vibration of that object. The drawing represents a waveform, which is the representation of displacement of a body over time, and displays what the pencil or string was doing as it vibrated.

This waveform is periodic. When we say that vibration is periodic, we mean that it repeats itself in a predictable fashion. If it took the pencil 1/100 (0.01) of a second to move from the first point of distension back to that point again, it will take 0.01 second to repeat that cycle if it is vibrating periodically.

Moving from one point in the vibratory pattern to the same point again defines one cycle of vibration, and the time it takes to pass through one cycle of vibration is referred to as the period. In our example, the period of vibration was 1/100 second, or 0.01 second. Frequency refers to how often something occurs, as in the frequency with which you shop for groceries (e.g., two times per month). The frequency of vibration is how often a cycle of vibration repeats itself, which in our example is 100 times per second. Frequency and period are the inverse of each other, and that relationship may be stated as $f = 1/T$ or $T = 1/f$. That is, frequency (f) equals 1 divided by period T (time). For our example, frequency = 1/0.01 second. If you take a moment with your calculator, you will find that this calculation gives a result of 100.

Because frequency refers to the repetition rate of vibration, we speak of it in terms of number of cycles per second. The pencil vibrated with a frequency of 100 cycles per second, but cycles per second is known as Hertz (Hz), after Heinrich Hertz. When we set the pencil into vibration, it vibrated with a period of 0.01 second and a frequency of 100 Hz.

We said that a body's frequency of vibration is governed by its elasticity, stiffness, and mass. If you had added a large weight to the guitar string, it would have vibrated slower. As mass increases, frequency of vibration decreases.

If you were to make the string stiffer, it would vibrate more rapidly. Increased stiffness would drive the string to return to its point of equilibrium faster, increasing the frequency of vibration.

PHYSIOLOGY OF PHONATION

Discussion of the function of the larynx and vocal folds revolves around the movable components and the results of that movement. We will concentrate on the nonspeech functions initially, which will help examine speech and vocal function. Speech-language pathologists and assistants use their knowledge of these nonspeech functions in the treatment of voice disorders, so you will need to be very familiar with these functions.

Laryngeal Stability

Laryngeal stability is the key to laryngeal control, and this stability is gained through development of the infrahyoid and suprahyoid musculature. You can think of the larynx as a box connected to a flexible tube on the lower end (trachea) and loosely attached above. This "box" has liberal movement in the vertical dimension and some horizontal movement as well, but there must be a great deal of control in contraction of all of this musculature for this arrangement to work.

The larynx is intimately linked, via the hyoid bone, to the tongue so that movement of the tongue is translated to the larynx. During development, the infant begins to gain control of neck musculature as early as 4 weeks, as seen in the ability to elevate the neck while prone. This ability to extend the previously flexed neck heralds the beginning of oral motor control because the ability to balance neck extension and flexion permits the child to control the gross movement of the head. During this stage, the larynx is quite elevated, so much so that you can easily see the superior tip of the epiglottis behind the tongue of a 2-year-old. In the early stages, the elevated larynx facilitates the anterior tongue protrusion required in infancy for nursing.

As the child develops, the larynx descends, starting a process of muscular differentiation between the tongue and the larynx. In the "nursing" position of the tongue, laryngeal stability is not very important. As the child begins to eat solid food, the ability to move food around in the oral cavity is quite important. Now the child will develop the ability to move the tongue and larynx independently, permitting a much wider set of oral gestures. With this differentiation comes the control needed for accurate speech production. For more information on head and neck control in children with motor dysfunction, you may wish to examine Jones-Owens (1991), and Bly (1994) provides more detail about the development of muscle control.

Nonspeech Laryngeal Function

The protective function of the larynx is its most important role because failure to prohibit entry of foreign objects into the lungs is life-threatening. This function is fulfilled through the cough and other associated reflexive gestures. Coughing is a response by the tissue of the respiratory passageway to an irritant or foreign object, mediated by the visceral afferent (sensory) portion of the vagus nerve innervating the bronchial mucosa. Coughing is a violent and broadly predictable behavior, which includes deep inhalation through widely abducted vocal folds, followed by tensing and tight adduction of the vocal folds and elevation

cough: *Forceful expiration of air following tight adduction of the vocal folds, for the purpose of expelling foreign matter from the airway.*

of the larynx. The axis of movement of the arytenoids guarantees that, as they are rocked for adduction, they also are directed somewhat downward, providing more force in opposition to expiration. Significant positive subglottal pressure for the cough comes from tissue recoil and muscles of expiration. The high pressure of forced expiration blows the vocal folds apart.

The aerodynamic benefit of the cough is that the person coughing generates a maximal flow of air through the passageway to expel the irritating object. The negative side of the cough is the force required for its production. Chronic irritation of the respiratory system leads to vocal abuse in the form of repeated coughing. The "near cousin" of the cough is throat clearing. It is not as violent as the full cough, but is nonetheless stressful.

So far we have dealt primarily with laryngeal functions focused on tight adduction of the vocal folds, but abduction has its place as well. Abduction dilates the larynx,

paralysis: *Loss of voluntary motor function due to lesion in the nervous system.*

paresis: *Weakness arising from lesion in the nervous system.*

sign: *Measurable or objective component of illness or condition.*

Vocal Fold Paralysis

Paralysis refers to loss of voluntary motor function, whereas **paresis** refers to weakness. Either occurs from damage to the neurons supplying the muscle.

Vocal fold paralysis takes several forms, depending on the nerve damage. If only one side of the recurrent laryngeal nerve is damaged, the result is unilateral vocal fold paralysis. Bilateral vocal fold paralysis results from bilateral lower motor neuron damage.

If the result of damage is adductor paralysis, the vocal folds remain in the abducted position. In unilateral paralysis, one vocal fold is still capable of motion. Phonation can still occur, but production will be markedly breathy. Bilateral adductor paralysis results in virtually complete loss of phonation. If the superior laryngeal nerve is involved, the individual loses the ability to alter vocal pitch because the cricothyroid is innervated by this nerve.

There are several causes of vocal fold paralysis, but the most common causes are damage to the nerve during thyroid surgery and blunt trauma, often from the steering wheel of an automobile. Cerebrovascular accidents (CVA: hemorrhage or other condition causing loss of blood supply to the brain) may damage upper or lower motor neurons, resulting in paralysis, and a host of neurodegenerative diseases can weaken or paralyze the vocal folds. Paralysis may also occur as a result of aneurysm of the aortic arch. An aneurysm is a focal "ballooning" of a blood vessel caused by a weakness in the wall. When the aneurysm balloons out, it compresses the recurrent laryngeal nerve, causing paresis or paralysis. A phonatory **sign** (objective evidence of phonatory deficit) is not to be taken lightly.

an important function for respiration during physical exertion. Oxygen use increases significantly during work and exertion. During normal quiet respiration, an adult's vocal folds are abducted to a width of about 8 mm. During forced respiration, the need for air causes you to dilate, or open, the respiratory tract as widely as possible, doubling that width.

Summary

- We use the larynx and associated structures for many nonspeech functions, including coughing, throat clearing, abdominal fixation, and increasing airflow.
- These functions serve important biological needs, and understanding them provides background for useful clinical intervention techniques.

Laryngeal Function for Speech

Phonation is an extremely important component of the speech signal. To accomplish phonation, we must adduct the vocal folds to begin phonation (attack), hold the vocal folds in a fixed position in the airstream to sustain phonation, and abduct the vocal folds to terminate phonation (see Figure 3–25).

Attack

Attack is the process of bringing vocal folds together to begin phonation. There are three basic types of attack. When we initiate phonation using **simultaneous vocal attack**, we coordinate adduction and onset of respiration so that they occur simultaneously. The vocal folds reach the critical degree of adduction at the same time that the respiratory flow is adequate to support phonation. You are using simultaneous attack when you say the word "zany," for example, because to start the flow of air before voicing would add the unvoiced /s/ to the beginning of the word.

simultaneous vocal attack: *Phonation initiated through simultaneous vocal folds adduction and expiration.*

Breathy vocal attack involves starting airflow before adducting the vocal folds. This occurs frequently during running speech, as in the sentence "Harry is my friend."

breathy vocal attack: *Phonation by initiating expiration before adduction of the vocal folds.*

The third type of attack is **glottal attack**, in which adduction of the vocal folds occurs prior to the airflow, much like a cough. Try this. Bring your vocal folds together (be gentle!) as if to cough, but instead of opening your vocal folds as you push air through the folds, keep them adducted and say /a/. That was a glottal attack. You use a glottal attack when saying any word beginning with a vowel, such as "onion."

glottal attack: *Phonatory onset that occurs with the adduction of the vocal folds before onset of expiration.*

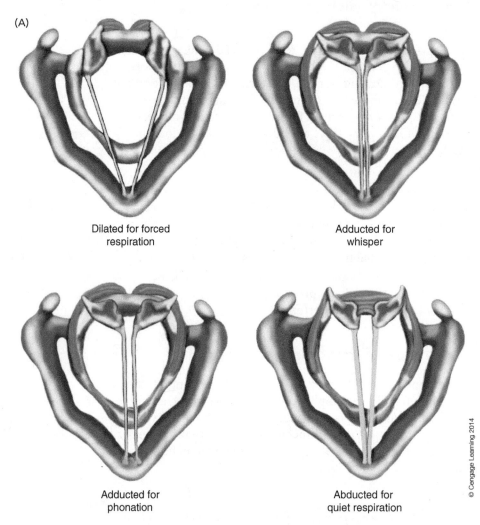

(A)

Dilated for forced
respiration

Adducted for
whisper

Adducted for
phonation

Abducted for
quiet respiration

© Cengage Learning 2014

Figure 3–25. Laryngeal postures for various functions. (A) During adduction for phonation the vocal folds are approximated. For quiet respiration the folds are moderately abducted, but for forced respiration they are widely separated. Adduction for whisper involves bringing the folds close together but retaining an open space between the arytenoid cartilages. *(continues)*

Ventricular Phonation

The false, or ventricular, vocal folds are technically unable to vibrate for voice, but in some instances clients may use them for this purpose. Boone (1999) cites instances in which clients use ventricular phonation as an adaptive response to severe vocal fold dysfunction, such as growths on the folds. Apparently the client forces the lateral superior walls closely together during the adductory gesture, permitting the folds to make contact and vibrate.

The ventricular folds are thick, and the phonation heard is deep and often raspy. The false folds may hypertrophy (increase in size), facilitating ventricular phonation.

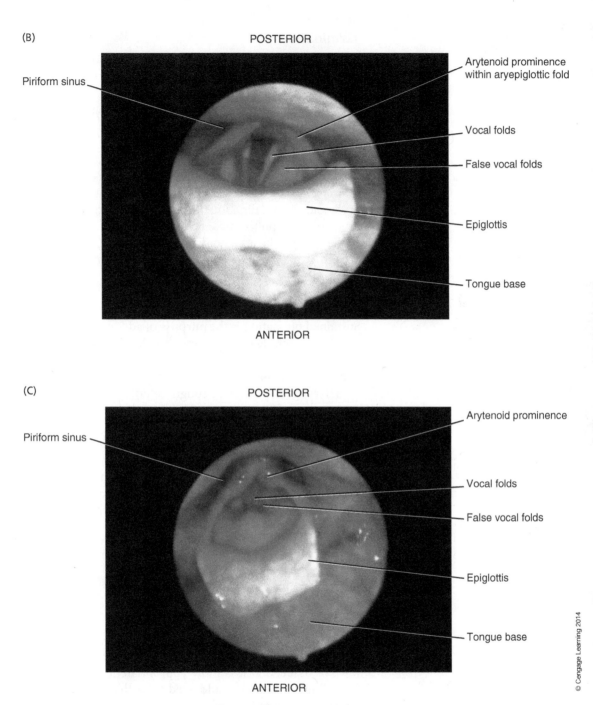

Figure 3–25. continued (B) Fiberoptic endoscopic view of superior larynx with abducted vocal folds. (C) Fiberoptic endoscopic view of superior larynx with adducted vocal folds.

Termination

Termination of phonation requires that we abduct the vocal folds. We pull the vocal folds out of the airstream far enough to reduce the turbulence, and the vocal folds stop vibrating. As with attack, we terminate phonation many times during running speech to accommodate voiced and voiceless speech sounds.

Adduction is a constant in all types of attack. The arytenoid cartilages are capable of moving in three dimensions—*rotating, rocking,* and *gliding.* It appears that the primary arytenoid gesture for adduction is inward rocking. When the arytenoids are pulled medially on the convex arytenoid facet of the cricoid, the arytenoids will rock down. These motions are the product of the lateral cricoarytenoid muscle and the lateral portion of the thyromuscularis.

Sustained Phonation

Sustained phonation is the purpose of adduction and abduction for speech. Let us examine this closely. Vocal attack requires muscular action, as does termination of phonation. In contrast, sustaining phonation simply requires maintenance of a laryngeal posture through tonic (sustained tensing) contraction of musculature. This is a very important point. The vibration of the vocal folds is achieved by placing and holding the vocal folds in the airstream so that their physical qualities interact with the airflow, causing vibration. The vocal folds are held in place during sustained phonation. Vibration of the vocal folds is *not* the product of repeated adduction and abduction of the vocal folds.

Fundamental Frequency Generation

Figure 3–26 shows the vocal folds from the sides and from above. In the vertical mode of phonation, the vocal folds open from inferior to superior (bottom to top), and they also close from inferior to superior. The folds are an undulating wave of tissue, and it is more appropriate to think of air as "bubbling" through the adducted folds than of them opening and closing as if hinged.

The second mode of vibration of the vocal folds is in the anterior-posterior dimension. The vocal folds tend to open from posterior to anterior, but that closure at the end of a cycle is made by contact of the medial edge of the vocal fold, but with the posterior closing last.

The primary frequency of vibration of the vocal folds is the **fundamental frequency**. This is the number of cycles the vocal folds go through per second, and it is audible.

fundamental frequency: *The lowest component of a harmonic series. In phonation, the lowest frequency of the voiced source.*

Vocal Fold Nodules

Vocal fold nodules are aggregates of tissue arising from abuse. This condition makes up a large share of the voice disorder cases seen by school clinicians. Common forms of vocal abuse are yelling, screaming, cheerleading, or "barking" commands (e.g., by a drill sergeant). The result of this abuse is a sequence of events that can lead to permanent change in the vocal fold tissue. You are probably familiar with laryngitis, which is hoarseness, often with loss of voice (aphonia). The laryngeal effect is swelling (edema) of the delicate vocal fold tissue so that it is difficult to make the folds vibrate. In fact, they are often bowed so badly that expiratory flow will pass between them, even as phonation occurs; we refer to this as a breathy voice.

Vocal abuse typically leads to soreness, which is a message from your body to stop doing what made the vocal folds hurt in the first place. Continued abuse results in growth of a protective layer of epithelium, which is callus-like and not a very effective oscillator. If the vocal hyperfunction continues, the hardened tissue will increase in size until a nodule may be found on one (unilateral) or both (bilateral) vocal folds. The site of abuse is usually at the juncture of the anterior and middle thirds of the vocal folds because this is the point of greatest impact during phonation. Although untreated vocal nodules may eventually have to be removed surgically, voice therapy to reverse the vocal behavior driving the phenomenon is always appropriate. If the vocal hyperfunction is not eliminated, the vocal nodules will return after surgery. Surgery may be avoided if therapy is initiated soon enough.

aphonia: *Loss of voicing.*

The movement of the vocal folds in air produces an audible disturbance known as sound. That sound is transmitted through the air as a wave, with molecules compressed by movement of the vocal folds.

Besides the fundamental frequency, the vocal folds produce an extremely rich set of harmonics, which are whole-number multiples of the fundamental. These harmonics provide important acoustical information for identification of voiced phonemes.

Because the vocal folds offer resistance to airflow, the minimum driving pressure of the vocal folds in modal phonation is approximately 3 to 5 cm H_2O subglottal pressure. If pressure is lower than this, the folds will not be blown apart. This is clinically important because a client who cannot generate pressure of 3 to 5 cm H_2O and sustain it for 5 seconds cannot use the vocal folds for speech. (See Figure 3–27 for an illustration of a simple clinical manometer.)

Figure 3–26. Graphic representation of vertical and transverse phase relationships during one glottal cycle. Note that generally the vocal folds open from inferior to superior and also close from inferior to superior. Simultaneously, the glottis grows generally from posterior to anterior, but the vocal folds close from anterior to posterior.

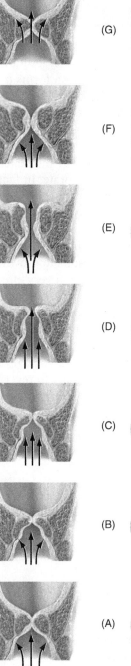

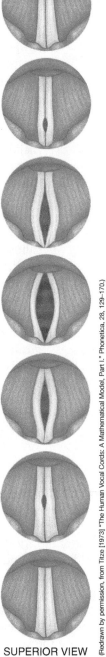

(G)

(F)

(E)

(D)

(C)

(B)

(A)

A. ANTERIOR VIEW

SUPERIOR VIEW

(Redrawn by permission, from Titze [1973] "The Human Vocal Cords: A Mathematical Model, Part I." Phonetica, 28, 129–170.)

Sustained and Maximum Phonation

Physical systems, such as those encompassing the mechanisms of speech, are rarely employed at maximum output and stress. For instance, we generally don't breathe in maximally or speak using our entire vital capacity, although we are capable of doing so. When clinicians wish to examine whether there is a deficit in a system, one useful technique is to ask the client to perform a test of maximal output for a given parameter. In respiration, such tests would be examination of vital capacity, inspiratory reserve, and expiratory reserve.

This useful concept may be extended to voicing. If you ask a client to sustain a vowel for as long as he or she can, you are testing not only how well the vocal folds function but also the vital capacity and checking action of the person under examination. If the respiratory system is intact, an average adult female between the ages of 17 and 41 years will be able to sustain the /a/ vowel for approximately 15 seconds, and the male will be able to sustain that vowel for 23 seconds. This function changes with age, increasing through the second decade of life. Generally you can expect the phonation time to increase from about 10 seconds at 6 years, but you may be interested in looking at the norms by age as summarized by Kent, Kent, and Rosenbek (1987). By the way, did you wonder why males are able to phonate a little longer than females? If you blamed it on larger vital capacity, you were right.

Another phonation-related task involves maximum duration of the sustained sibilants, /s/ and /z/. Boone (1999) states that individuals are able to sustain these phonemes for approximately the same durations, but that physical change to the vocal folds (such as vocal nodules) will cause a significant reduction in the duration of the voiced /z/. Males again produce longer fricatives (e.g., /s/), and the duration increases with age. Clinicians calculate the ratio of s:z duration to aid their decisions. If the two durations are the same, the value is 1.0, and as the /z/ duration drops, the ratio increases. Although the ratio undergoes continual examination for its clinical utility, many studies have substantiated the use of this clinical tool.

Related to these tasks is your client's ability to sustain respiration for phonation. Figure 3–27 shows a portable manometer, which is an extremely affordable means of giving your client feedback about whether he or she is generating sufficient subglottal pressure to drive the vocal folds into vibration. Generally, a client who can sustain 3 to 5 cm H_2O for 5 seconds has adequate respiratory support for phonation.

Vocal Register

The *mode of vibration* of the vocal folds during sustained phonation refers to the pattern of activity that the vocal folds undergo during a cycle of vibration. Moving from one point in the vibratory pattern to the same point again defines one cycle of vibration, and within one cycle, the vocal folds undergo

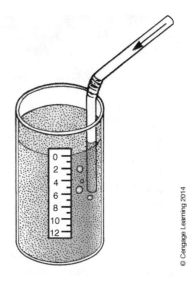

Figure 3–27. A useful clinical tool described by Hixon, Hawley, and Wilson (1982), this portable manometer gives the client feedback concerning respiratory ability and provides the clinician with a measure of function.

© Cengage Learning 2014

some very significant changes, and these variations in vibratory pattern in large part differentiate vocal registers. A number of *modes* or *vocal registers* have been differentiated perceptually.

The three registers most commonly referred to are modal register, glottal fry or pulse register, and falsetto. We will be also interested in whispered speech, although it is not a phonatory pattern since the vocal folds do not vibrate.

modal register: *The mode of vibration used for daily speaking.*

Modal Register. The first register, known as the modal register, or modal phonation, refers to the pattern of phonation used most often. This pattern is the most important one for the speech-language pathologist and the speech-language pathology assistant, and it is the most efficient.

glottal fry: *A low-frequency mode of vibration characterized by syncopated rhythm and generated by low subglottal air pressure.*

Glottal Fry. The second register is known as glottal fry, but is known also as pulse register. What "fry" and "pulse" allude to is the crackly, "popcorn" quality of this voice. Perceptually, this voice is extremely low in pitch and sounds rough, almost like eggs frying in a pan.

Glottal fry is the product of a complex glottal configuration, and it occurs in frequencies ranging as low as 30 Hz, up to 80 or 90 Hz. This mode of vibration requires low subglottal pressure to sustain it (on the order of 2 cm H_2O), and tension of the vocalis is significantly reduced relative to modal vibration so that the vibrating margin is flaccid and thick. The lateral portion of the vocal folds is tensed, producing strong medial compression with short, thick vocal folds and low subglottal pressure. If either vocalis tension or subglottal pressure is increased, the popcorn-like perception of this mode of vibration is lost.

In glottal fry, the vocal folds take on a secondary, syncopated mode of vibration, with a secondary beat for every cycle of the fundamental frequency. In addition to this syncopation, the vocal folds spend up to 90% of the cycle in approximation.

Puberphonia

During normal development, children undergo a great deal of change during puberty, the time in a person's life when he or she becomes capable of reproduction. Puberty occurs between the ages of 13 and 15 years for boys and between 9 and 16 years for girls and is characterized by rapid muscle development and significant gains in height and weight. The thyroid cartilage and thyroarytenoid are not left out of development. They grow rapidly during this time, although the larynges of boys grow considerably more than those of girls.

The result of this spurt of laryngeal growth is that the person (typically a boy) has periods of voice change (mutation) in which his voice "breaks down" in pitch as he is speaking. This is, of course, a normal result of the changing tissue and the young man's attempt to control it for phonation, but it is nonetheless disturbing. *Puberphonia* refers to the maintenance of the childhood pitch despite having passed through the developmental stage of puberty. It likely represents an attempt to hold something constant during the roller-coaster ride of puberty, but the result is a significant mismatch between the large body of the developing teenaged boy and the high-pitched voice of the prepubescent child. Typically, the young man is speaking in falsetto but is aware of the "lower" voice. To help the individual alter habitual pitch therapy performed over the summer vacation, in absence of peer pressures associated with school, is quite effective.

Falsetto. The third and highest register of phonation, the falsetto, also is characterized by a vibratory pattern that varies from modal production. In falsetto, the vocal folds lengthen and become extremely thin and "reedlike." When set into vibration, they tend to vibrate along the tensed, bowed margins, in contrast to the complex pattern seen in other modes of phonation. Compared with modal phonation, the vocal folds make contact only briefly, and the degree of movement (amplitude of excursion) is reduced. The posterior portion of the vocal folds tends to be damped, so that the length of the vibrating surface is decreased to a narrow opening. Contrast this to elevated pitch in modal phonation, which involves lengthening the vocal folds.

The perception of falsetto is one of an extremely "thin," high-pitched vocal production. The difference between falsetto and modal vibration is not simply one of the frequencies of vibration (in the 300–600 Hz range). Although it is true that falsetto is the highest register, the modal and falsetto registers overlap.

Whispering. Whispering is not really a phonatory mode, because no voicing occurs. This does not mean that there are no laryngeal adjustments, but rather that they do not

falsetto: *Phonation is high in frequency, which is produced by significant increase in laryngeal tension that results in thinned vocal fold margins.*

whispered speech: *Speech produced without vocal fold vibration by causing air to pass along the edges of the tensed vocal folds, thus producing a friction sound source.*

produce vibration in the vocal folds. Prove this to yourself. In respiration the vocal folds are abducted, but for whispering they must be partially adducted and tensed to develop turbulence in the airstream, and that turbulence is the noise you use to make speech.

The interplay of the elasticity and mass of the vocal folds leads them to vibrate in a periodic fashion. *Intensity* refers to the relative power or pressure of an acoustic signal, measured in decibels (abbreviated dB). In phonation, we may refer to the intensity of voice as vocal intensity. Intensity is a direct function of the amount of pressure exerted by the sound wave (as opposed to air pressure generated by the respiratory system). As molecules vibrate from movement of the vocal folds, the movement of molecules exerts an extremely small but measurable force over an area, and that is defined as pressure. The larger the excursion of the vibrating body, the greater the intensity of the signal produced because air will be displaced with greater force. The next two sections deal with frequency and intensity of vocal fold vibration.

Summary

- We must adduct the vocal folds to initiate phonation, and this may take several forms, including breathy, simultaneous, and glottal attacks.
- Termination of phonation requires abduction of the vocal folds, a process that must occur with the transition of voiced to voiceless speech sounds.
- Sustained phonation can take several forms, depending on the laryngeal configuration.
- Fundamental frequency is the measure of how fast the vocal folds vibrate.
- Falsetto occupies the upper range of laryngeal function, while glottal fry is found in the lower range.
- Vocal fold vibration varies among phonatory modes, and the differences are governed by laryngeal tension, medial compression, and subglottal pressure.

FREQUENCY, PITCH, AND PITCH CHANGE

pitch: *The perceptual correlate of frequency of vibration.*

Pitch is the perceptual correlate of frequency and is closely related to frequency: As frequency increases, pitch increases, and as frequency decreases, so does pitch.

oscillation: *Repeated vibration of a body at the same frequency.*

The vocal folds are made up of mass and elastic elements that promote **oscillation**, or repeated vibration, at the same frequency, and as long as mass and elasticity

Prosody and Neuromuscular Disorder

The prosodic element of speech can be a window on speech physiology in neuropathology. **Prosody** is the combination of changes in fundamental frequency and vocal intensity that produces linguistically relevant intonation and stress characteristics, such as emphasizing the word *he* in the sentence "He went to town." When the neuromuscular system is compromised, prosody may be affected. When muscle tone increases (**hypertonus**) due to spasticity, the individual may demonstrate prosody characterized by even and equal stress with inappropriately high vocal intensity on each syllable or word. It is as if each syllable is forced out, the uttered sentence has an essentially flat intonation contour.

When an individual has ataxic signs from cerebellar damage, she will have disrupted prosody from the discoordination of respiratory, phonatory, and articulatory systems. Speech syllable timing will be defective, and control of phonatory elements will be seriously deficient.

In many of the hyperkinetic dysarthrias the element of speech control is over-ridden by movements of speech structures that are involuntary and uncontrollable. In these cases, prosody will be seriously affected as the articulatory or phonatory gesture is interrupted by the spontaneous movements.

are constant the vocal folds vibrate at the same frequency. Alteration of mass and elasticity changes the frequency of vibration.

Several important terms describe aspects of perceived pitch. Unfortunately, most of these terms refer to perceived pitch when they really describe physical frequency! Let us take a look at optimal and habitual pitch, average fundamental frequency, and range of fundamental frequency.

prosody: *Combination of changes in fundamental frequency and vocal intensity that provides linguistically relevant information.*

hypertonus: *Abnormal increase in muscle tone.*

Optimal Pitch

The term **optimal pitch** is used to refer to the pitch (actually, the frequency) of vocal fold vibration that is optimal or most appropriate for an individual. This frequency of vibration is the most efficient for a given pair of vocal folds and is a function of the mass and elasticity of the vocal folds. Some voice scientists and clinicians estimate optimal pitch directly from the individual's range of phonation because it is considered to be approximately 20–25% above an individual's lowest frequency of vibration. Others estimate it from a cough or throat-clearing because frequency of the vibrating vocal folds during throat-clearing approximates conditions associated

optimal pitch: *The frequency of vibration of the vocal folds that is most efficient for the vocal folds.*

with conversational frequency but without social conditions associated with use of phonation for communication.

Optimal pitch varies as a function of sex and age. You can expect an adult female to have a fundamental frequency of approximately 212 Hz during a reading task, whereas the optimal fundamental frequency for adult males can be much lower, around 132 Hz for the same task.

The reason for the difference in fundamental frequency between males and females has to do with tissue mass and length of vocal folds. Children of both sexes have fundamental frequency in the range of 300 Hz, but that frequency changes during puberty. During puberty, males undergo a significant growth of muscle and cartilage, resulting in greater muscle mass even in the vocal mechanism. This results in the prominent "Adam's apple" and a drop in fundamental frequency arising from the increased mass of the folds (see Figure 3–28).

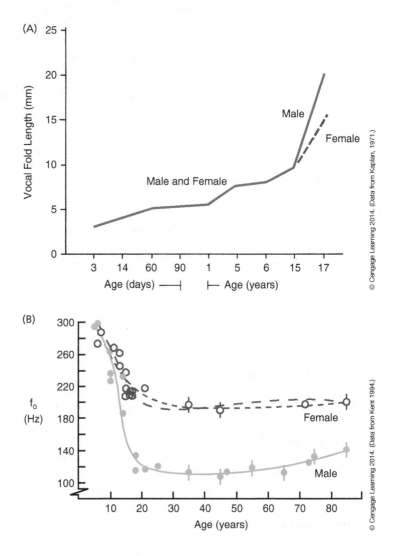

© Cengage Learning 2014. (Data from Kaplan, 1971.)

© Cengage Learning 2014. (Data from Kent 1994.)

Figure 3–28. (A) Changes in vocal fold length for males and females as a function of age. Note that males and females have essentially the same length of vocal folds until puberty, at which time both sexes undergo marked physical development. (B) Fundamental frequency change over the lifespan for males and females.

Laryngeal Stridor

Laryngeal stridor refers to a harsh sound produced during respiration. The sound is associated with some obstruction in the respiratory passageway and is always a sign of dysfunction. Stridor may arise from a growth in the larynx or trachea, causing turbulence during respiration, or it may arise from the dysfunction of vocal folds. If the vocal folds are paralyzed in the adducted position (abductor paralysis), they not only obstruct the airway but also vibrate as the air of inspiration passes by them. In this case, the harsh sound is referred to as inspiratory tridor. You may want to imitate this yourself so that you can learn to recognize this sign of obstruction. Phonate while breathing out, and then, without abducting your vocal folds, force your inspiration through the closed vocal folds. You will notice not only a harsh sound but also the extreme difficulty of inhaling through an obstruction.

Habitual Pitch

We use the term **habitual pitch** to refer to the frequency of vibration of vocal folds that is habitually used during speech. In the ideal condition, this would be the same as optimal pitch. Some individuals alter their everyday pitch in speech beyond the range expected for their age, size, or gender. Although the choice to use an abnormally higher or lower fundamental frequency is often not a conscious decision, it has an effect on phonatory efficiency and effort. When the vocal folds are forced into the extremes of their range of ability, greater effort is required to sustain phonation, and this results in vocal and physical fatigue.

laryngeal stridor: *Harsh sound produced upon inhalation or exhalation.*

habitual pitch: *The frequency of vibration of the vocal folds habitually used by an individual during speech.*

Average Fundamental Frequency

The **average fundamental frequency** of vibration of the vocal folds during phonation can be measured during a variety of tasks (e.g., reading aloud, conversational speech, counting aloud). Different tasks result in variations of average fundamental frequency, but they all provide measures of habitual pitch.

average fundamental frequency: *The average frequency of vibration taken over a given time period of phonation.*

Pitch Range

Pitch range refers to the range of fundamental frequency for an individual and is calculated as the difference between the highest and lowest frequencies. The vocal mechanism is capable of approximately two to three octaves of change

pitch range: *The range of phonation possible, calculated as the highest frequency of vibration minus the lowest frequency of vibration.*

in fundamental frequency from the lowest possible to the highest frequency. An individual with a lowest-possible fundamental frequency of 90 Hz can reach a high of about 360 Hz (octave 1 = 90 Hz to 180 Hz; octave 2 = 180 Hz to 360 Hz).

Pitch Changing Mechanism

Fundamental frequency increase comes from stretching and tensing the vocal folds using the cricothyroid and thyrovocalis muscles. Here is the mechanism of this change.

Tension, Length, and Mass

The changeable elements of the vocal folds are tension, length, and mass. We can change the *mass per unit length* by spreading the muscle, mucosa, and ligament out over more distance. We can change the *tension* of the vocal folds by stretching them tighter or relaxing them. Both of these changes arise from elongation.

When the cricothyroid muscle is contracted, the thyroid tilts down, lengthening the vocal folds and increasing the fundamental frequency, although lengthening has no real effect on increasing fundamental frequency. The real benefit of the cricothyroid contraction is to apply tension to the vocal folds. When the tension on the vocal folds is increased, the natural frequency of vibration increases. When vocal folds are lengthened they are stretched thinner and made more tense, and it is this increase in tension and decrease in cross-sectional mass that results in increased fundamental frequency.

The thyrovocalis is also a tenser of the vocal folds. Contraction of this muscle pulls both cricoid and thyroid closer together, an action opposed by the simultaneously contracted cricothyroid.

Lowering fundamental frequency requires the opposite manipulation. Contraction of the thyromuscularis shortens the vocal folds so they become more massive and less tense.

Subglottal Pressure and Frequency Change

Increasing pitch requires increasing the tension of the system, thereby increasing the glottal resistance to airflow. If airflow is to remain constant through the glottis, air pressure must increase. It appears, however, that increases in subglottal pressure are a response to, rather than a cause of, the increased tension required for frequency change. Subglottal pressure does increase, but by itself has little effect on frequency change.

Summary

- Pitch is the perceptual correlate of frequency of vibration, although the term has come to refer in common usage to phenomena associated with the physical vibration of the vocal folds.

- Optimal pitch is the frequency of vibration that is most efficient for a given pair of vocal folds, and habitual pitch is the frequency of vibration habitually used by an individual.

- Fundamental frequency is the lowest component of a harmonic series. In phonation, it is the lowest frequency of the voiced source.

- The pitch range of an individual spans approximately two octaves.

- Changes in vocal fundamental frequency are governed by the tension of the vocal folds and their mass per unit length.

- Increasing the length of the vocal folds increases vocal fold tension and decreases the mass per unit area, which increases the fundamental frequency.

- The respiratory system responds to increased vocal fold tension with increased subglottal pressure, so that pitch and subglottal pressure tend to vary in relation to each other.

- Increased subglottal pressure is a response to increased vocal fold tension.

INTENSITY AND INTENSITY CHANGE

Just as pitch is the perceptual correlate of frequency, loudness is the perceptual correlate of intensity. Intensity (or its correlate, sound pressure level) is the physical measure of power (or pressure) ratios, but loudness is how we perceive power or pressure differences. As with pitch and frequency, there is a close relationship between loudness and intensity.

loudness: *The perceptual correlate of intensity.*

To increase the vocal intensity of vibrating vocal folds, one must somehow increase the vigor with which the vocal folds are forced open by air pressure. In sustained phonation, the vocal folds move only as a result of the air pressure beneath them and the flow between them. Subglottal pressure and flow provide the energy for this vocal engine, so to increase the intensity or strength of the phonatory product we will have to increase the energy that drives it. We increase subglottal pressure to increase vocal intensity. To prove this to yourself, do the following. You need to feel what you do to produce loud speech. You may be in a quiet setting right now and you really may not want to yell, but that is fine. Pay attention to your lungs and larynx as you prepare to yell as loudly as you can to someone across the room. Without even yelling, you should have been able to feel your lungs take in a large charge of air, and you also should have felt your vocal folds tighten. These are the two gestures of significance for increasing vocal intensity: increased subglottal pressure and medial compression.

To explain the effect that medial compression has on vocal intensity requires a return to discussion of a cycle of vocal fold vibration. We can break a cycle of vibration into stages. There is an opening stage, in which the vocal folds are opening; a closing stage, in which the vocal folds are returning to the point of approximation; and a closed stage, in which there is no air escaping between the vocal folds (see Figures 3–29 and 3–30). In modal phonation at

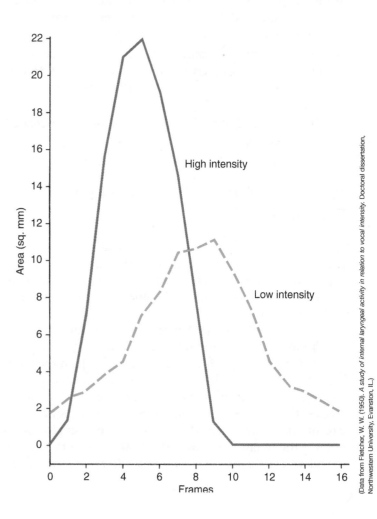

Figure 3–29. Effect of vocal intensity on vocal fold vibration. During low-intensity speech the opening and closing phases occupy most of the vibratory cycle, as revealed in the area of the glottis. During high-intensity speech the opening phase is greatly compressed, as is the closing phase, while the time spent in the closed phase is greatly increased.

(Data from Fletcher, W. W. (1950). A study of internal laryngeal activity in relation to vocal intensity. Doctoral dissertation, Northwestern University, Evanston, IL.)

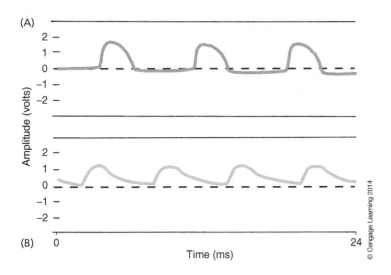

Figure 3–30. Effect of vocal intensity shown on electroglottographic trace. The electroglottograph measures impedance across the vocal folds; the peak represents the closed phase of the glottal cycle. (A) Conversational-level sustained vowel. (B) High-level sustained vowel.

conversational intensities, it has been found that the vocal folds spend about 50% of their time in the opening phase, 37% of the time in the closing phase, and 13% of the cycle completely closed. When the vocal folds are tightly adducted for increased vocal intensity, they tend to return to the closed position more quickly and to stay closed for a longer time. The opening phase reduces to approximately 33%, while the closed phase increases to more than 30%, depending on the intensity increase (Fletcher, 1950).

The concept you should retain is this: To increase vocal intensity, the vocal folds are tightly compressed, it takes more force to blow them open, they close more rapidly, and they tend to stay closed because they are tightly compressed. This is the cause side of the equation. The effect portion is that because so much energy is required to hold the folds in compression, the release of the folds from this condition is going to be markedly stronger. Each time the folds open, they do so with vigor, producing an explosive compression of the air medium. The harder that eruption of the vocal folds is, the greater is the amplitude of the cycle of vibration. If you remember that as the amplitude of the signal increases so does the intensity, you will recognize the difference of intensity in Figure 3–30A and 3–30B.

The two waveforms in Figure 3–31 are different in intensity, but not in frequency. The time between the cycles is exactly the same, so the frequency must be the same. From this situation comes a very important point: Intensity and frequency are controlled independently, and you can increase intensity without increasing frequency. Here is the paradox. Increases in intensity and fundamental frequency depend on the same basic mechanism (tension/compression and subglottal pressure), so it is difficult to increase intensity without increasing pitch, but trained or well-controlled speakers can do this. The tendency is for frequency and

Figure 3–31. Oscillogram of sustained vowel at two vocal intensities. (A) Sustained vowel at conversational level. (B) Sustained vowel at increased vocal intensity. Although the vocal intensity increases, the period of each cycle of vibration remains constant at 9.2 milliseconds.

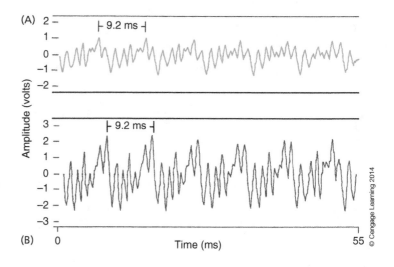

intensity to increase together, which is a natural phenomenon that you can demonstrate for yourself. Find a place where you can shout, and then say a word before shouting it. Your pitch will most certainly go up when you shout, unless you try very hard to avoid it.

The relationship between subglottal pressure and the actual sound pressure output of the vocal folds depends on the speaker. However, it appears that for every doubling of subglottal pressure there is an increase of between 8 and 12 decibels in vocal intensity.

Summary

- Vocal intensity is to the increase in sound pressure of the speech signal.
- To increase vocal intensity of phonation, the speaker must increase medial compression through the muscles of adduction.
- This increased adductory force requires greater subglottal pressure to produce phonation and forces the vocal folds to remain closed for a longer time.
- The increased laryngeal tension required for increasing intensity also increases the vocal fundamental frequency, although the trained voice is capable of controlling fundamental frequency and vocal intensity independently.

LINGUISTIC ASPECTS OF PITCH AND INTENSITY

suprasegmental: *Information within the speech signal that spans two or more phonemes, generally called prosodic elements.*

Pitch and intensity are elements of suprasegmental aspects of communication. **Suprasegmental** elements are the parameters of speech above the segment (phonetic) level. The phonetic level of speech refers to the *phonemes*, or unique sounds, of speech (although some speech scientists consider segments to be the components of phonemes, such as aspiration, frequency transitions, etc.). The term *segment* arises from the need to parse out the independent and unique sounds that represent meaning in speech (phonemes), but we would be remiss if we did not note that the subsegmental elements, such as the specific frequency transition of a stop phoneme, are critical to the accurate identification of the segment. The term *suprasegmental* generally refers to elements of prosody, the system of phoneme, syllable, and word stress (emphasis) used to vary meaning in speech. The prosodic elements include pitch, intonation, loudness, stress, duration, and rhythm. These elements convey much of the emotion, intent, and meaning of speech. Even though it is beyond the scope of this text to deeply examine these suprasegmental elements, pitch and intensity play such a large role in speech that we will discuss them here.

Suprasegmental elements are largely a product of phonation. Intonation refers to the changes in pitch in speech, and stress refers to syllable or word emphasis relative to an entire utterance. For example, say the following sentence out loud: "My cat's name is Mary." You end it with a falling intonation and put more stress on "cat's" than on "name" or "Mary." To a large extent, these elements both arise out of variation in vocal intensity and fundamental frequency. Intonation can be considered the melodic envelope that contains the sentence and serves to mark sentence type. Generally, statements have falling intonation at the end and questions have rising intonation. For example, Figure 3–32 shows traces of the fundamental frequency for the productions of "Bev bombed Bob." and "Bev bombed Bob?" If you say these two sentences, you can hear the changes that are so strong in the second sentence. Hirano, Ohala, and Vennard (1969) used this sentence contrast to show that the lateral cricoarytenoid, thyrovocalis, and cricothyroid are all quite active in these rapid laryngeal adjustments.

Stress helps punctuate speech, providing emphasis to syllables or words through both intensity and frequency changes. To increase stress, we increase fundamental frequency and intensity through increasing subglottal pressure, medial compression, and glottal tension. Remember from our earlier discussion that both frequency and intensity involve adjustments of these variables. We capitalize on the fact that both intensity and fundamental frequency vary together, so that stressed syllables or words show changes in both.

You should realize that these suprasegmental aspects, like all linguistic forms, are very language-specific. Different languages capitalize on different suprasegmental characteristics,

intonation: *The changes in pitch in continuous speech.*

stress: *The emphasis on a word produced in continuous speech, relative to the emphasis of the entire utterance.*

Figure 3–32. Fundamental
frequency fluctuation for
declarative statement and
question form. Note the
difference in falling and rising
intonation between these two
sentence forms.

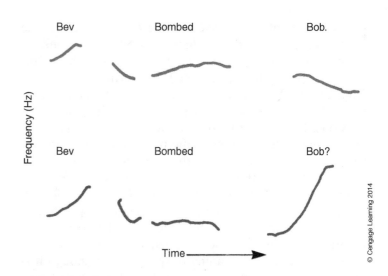

Figure 3–32. Fundamental frequency fluctuation for declarative statement and question form. Note the difference in falling and rising intonation between these two sentence forms.

so that a meaning derived from an intonational contour in one language will not necessarily translate into meaningful information in another. Similarly, voice onset time, which relies on microstructure control of phonatory adduction and abduction, is very language-specific. Timings vary from language to language, but that's a story for another time!

The musculature involved in stress is similar to that of intonation, with an increase in subglottal pressure. The changes in fundamental frequency are on the order of 50 Hz (Netsell, 1973), governed by the lateral cricoarytenoid, thyrovocalis, and cricothyroid. The changes in subglottal pressure will be small but rapid, or pulsatile (Hixon, 1973). Because they require bursts of increased expiratory force, they are driven by expiratory muscles.

Although stress and intonation are not essential for communication, they are essential for natural sounding speech. Clearly you can speak in a **monopitch** (unvarying vocal pitch) or **monoloud** voice (unvarying vocal loudness), but the effect is so distracting that it interferes with communication. You may find individuals with neurological impairments who show both of these characteristics. Treatment directed toward increased muscular effort at points requiring stress will greatly enhance the naturalness of speech because increasing vocal effort at the points inevitably increases both fundamental frequency and vocal intensity.

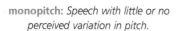

monopitch: *Speech with little or no perceived variation in pitch.*

monoloud: *Of unvarying vocal loudness.*

THEORIES OF PHONATION

One of the earliest theories of phonation, the neurochronaxic theory, hypothesized that the vibration of the vocal folds occurred as a result of pulsed muscular contractions. The theory had appeal because it gave total control of phonation to the nervous system (to be discussed in Chapter 5), but it soon became clear that the nervous system was not capable of contracting muscles at the rate required for speech. In contrast, the myoelastic-aerodynamic theory of phonation states that vibration of the vocal folds depends on the elements embodied in the name of the theory. The *myoelastic element* is the elastic component of muscle (*myo* = muscle) and associated soft tissues of the larynx, and the aerodynamic component is that of the airflow and pressure through this constricted tube. Van den Berg (1958) recognized that the combination of tissue elasticity, which causes the vocal folds to return to their original position after being distended, and the Bernoulli effect, which helped promote this return by dropping the pressure at the constriction, could account for the sustained vibration shown in even a cadaverous specimen provided with an artificial source of expiratory charge.

Titze's cover-body theory (1994) has sought to explain how complex acoustic output can come from a seemingly simple oscillator such as the vocal folds. We have long recognized that the vocal folds undulate in the modes discussed earlier. Titze recognized that this complex vibration arises from the loosely bound masses associated with the membranous cover of the vocal folds (the epithelium and superficial layer of the lamina propria) and the body of the vocal folds (the intermediate and deep layers of lamina propria and thyrovocalis muscle). The loosely bound elastic tissue supports oscillation, and viewing the soft tissue as an infinite (or at least uncountable) number of masses reveals that a very large number of modes of vibration is possible. This discussion in no way gives justice to the elegance of this theory, and we recommend that you take time for the exceptionally readable work of Titze.

The phonatory mechanism is an important component of the speaking mechanism, providing the voiced source for speech. In the next chapter, we explore what happens to the voice source after it leaves the larynx.

CHAPTER SUMMARY

Phonation is the product of vibrating vocal folds in the larynx. The vocal folds vibrate as air flows past them, capitalizing on the Bernoulli principle and tissue elasticity to maintain phonation. The interaction of subglottal pressure, tissue elasticity, and constriction of the airflow caused by the vocal folds produces sustained phonation as long as pressure, flow, and vocal fold approximation are maintained.

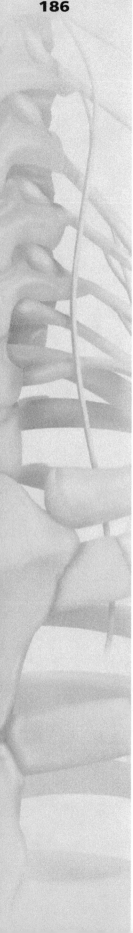

The larynx comprises the cricoid, thyroid, and epiglottis cartilages, as well as the paired arytenoid, corniculate, and cuneiform cartilages. The thyroid and cricoid cartilages articulate by means of the cricothyroid joint, which lets the two cartilages come closer together in front. The arytenoid and cricoid cartilages also articulate with a joint, which permits a wide range of arytenoid motion. The epiglottis is attached to the thyroid cartilage and base of the tongue. The corniculate cartilages rest on the upper surface of the arytenoids, and the cuneiform cartilages reside in the aryepiglottic folds.

The cavity of the larynx is a constricted tube with a smooth surface. Sheets and cords of ligaments connect the cartilages, and smooth mucous membrane covers the medial-most surface of the larynx. The valleculae are found between the tongue and the epiglottis, in folds formed by the lateral and median glossoepiglottic ligaments. The fibroelastic membrane is composed of the upper quadrangular membranes and aryepiglottic folds, the lower conus elasticus, and the vocal ligament, which is actually the upward free extension of the conus elasticus.

The vocal folds are five layers of tissue, the deepest being muscle. The aditus is the entryway of the larynx.

Intrinsic muscles of the larynx include the thyrovocalis, thyromuscularis, cricothyroid, lateral and posterior cricoarytenoid, transverse arytenoid and oblique interarytenoid, and superior thyroarytenoid muscles. Extrinsic muscles of the larynx include infrahyoid and suprahyoid muscles. The digastricus anterior and posterior elevate the hyoid, and the stylohyoid retracts it. The mylohyoid and hyoglossus elevate the hyoid, and the geniohyoid elevates the hyoid and draws it forward. The thyropharyngeus and cricopharyngeus muscles elevate the larynx, and the sternohyoid, sternothyroid, and omohyoid muscles depress the larynx.

Movement of the vocal folds into and out of approximation requires coordinated effort of the intrinsic muscles of the larynx. The lateral cricoarytenoid muscle rocks the arytenoid cartilage on its axis, tipping the vocal folds in and slightly down. The posterior cricoarytenoid muscle rocks the arytenoid out. The transverse arytenoid muscle draws the posterior surfaces of the arytenoids closer together. The oblique arytenoid assists the vocal folds to dip downward when they are adducted. Vocal fundamental frequency is increased by increasing tension, a function of the thyrovocalis and cricothyroid muscles.

We must adduct the vocal folds to initiate phonation, and this may take several forms, including breathy, simultaneous, and glottal attacks. Termination of phonation requires abduction of the vocal folds, a process that must occur with the transition of voiced to voiceless speech sounds. Sustained phonation can take several forms, depending on the laryngeal configuration. Falsetto occupies the upper range of laryngeal function, and glottal fry is found in the lower range. Vocal fold vibration among phonatory modes and the differences are governed by laryngeal tension, medial compression, and subglottal pressure.

Pitch is the perceptual correlate of frequency of vibration, although the term has come into common usage when referring to phenomena associated with the physical vibration of the vocal folds. Optimal pitch refers to the frequency of vibration that is most efficient for a given pair of vocal folds, and habitual pitch is the frequency of vibration habitually used by an individual. Fundamental frequency is the lowest component of a harmonic series. In phonation, it is the lowest frequency of the voiced source. The pitch range of an individual spans approximately two octaves. Changes in vocal fundamental frequency are governed by the tension of the vocal folds and their mass per unit length. Increasing the length of the vocal folds increases vocal fold tension and decreases the mass per unit area, which increases the fundamental frequency. The respiratory system responds to increased vocal fold tension with increased subglottal pressure, so that pitch and subglottal pressure tend to vary in relation to each other.

Increased subglottal pressure is a response to increased vocal fold tension. Vocal intensity refers to the increase in sound pressure of the speech signal. To increase vocal intensity of phonation, the speaker must increase medial compression through the muscles of adduction. This increased adductory force requires greater subglottal pressure to produce phonation and forces the vocal folds to remain in the closed portion of the phonatory cycle for a longer time. The increased laryngeal tension required for increasing intensity also increases the vocal fundamental frequency, although the trained voice is capable of controlling fundamental frequency and vocal intensity independently.

Suprasegmental elements are the parameters of speech above the segment (phonetic) level, generally referring to elements of prosody (pitch, intonation, loudness, stress, duration, and rhythm). Intonation refers to the changes in pitch in speech, and stress refers to syllable or word emphasis relative to an entire utterance. Intonation can be considered the melodic envelope that contains the sentence and can mark sentence type. Stress provides emphasis to syllables or words through both intensity and frequency changes.

The myoelastic-aerodynamic theory of phonation states that vibration of the vocal folds depends on the elements embodied in the name of the theory. Titze (1994) enlarged this theory to encompass the complex vibratory modes responsible for the rich acoustics of speech.

STUDY QUESTIONS

1. Identify the structures indicated on the figure.

   A. _____ cartilage

   B. _____ cartilage

   C. _____ cartilage

   D. _____ cartilage

   E. _____ cartilage

   F. _____ bone

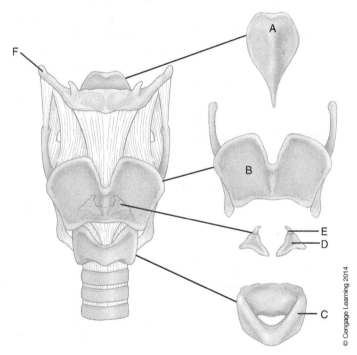

© Cengage Learning 2014

2. Identify the landmarks indicated on the figure.

A. _____

B. _____

C. _____

D. _____

E. _____

F. _____

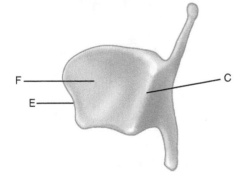

3. Identify the landmarks indicated on the figure.

    A. _____ process

    B. _____ process

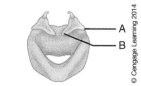

4. Identify the muscles indicated in the accompanying figure.

    A. _____

    B. _____

    C. _____

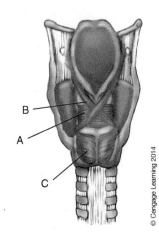

5. Identify the muscles indicated in the accompanying figure.

A. _____

B. _____

C. _____

D. _____

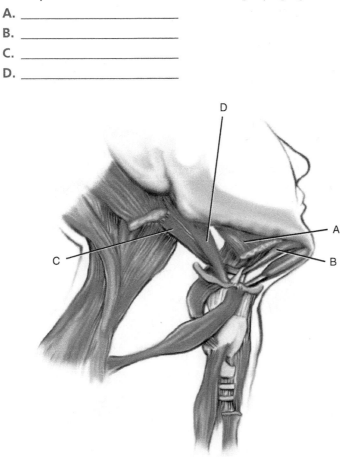

© Cengage Learning 2014

6. Identify the muscles indicated in the accompanying figure.

A. _____

B. _____

C. _____

D. _____

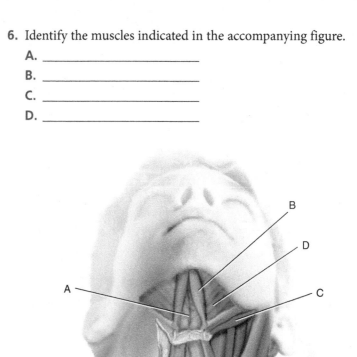

7. This is a view of the laryngeal opening from above. Identify the indicated structures.

   A. _____

   B. _____

   C. _____

   D. _____

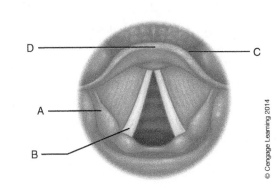

8. Identify the two muscles in the accompanying figure.

   A. _____

   B. _____

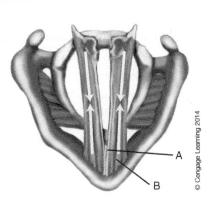

9. The _____ muscle is the primary muscle responsible for change of vocal fundamental frequency.

10. The space between the vocal folds is the _____.

11. The _____ effect states that given a constant volume flow of air or fluid, at a point of constriction there will be a decrease in air (or fluid) pressure perpendicular to the flow and an increase in velocity of the flow.

12. Laryngeal cancer sometimes necessitates complete removal of the larynx. Because the respiratory and digestive systems share the pharynx, removal of this protective mechanism poses a problem for the needs of breathing and swallowing. What surgical changes would permit both processes?

13. _____ is the process of capturing air in the thorax to provide the muscles with a structure upon which to push or pull.

14. In _____ attack, the vocal folds are adducted before initiation of expiratory flow.

15. In _____ attack, the vocal folds are adducted after the initiation of expiratory flow.

16. In _____ attack, the vocal folds are adducted simultaneous with initiation of expiratory flow.

17. During modal phonation, the vocal folds open from (inferior/superior) to _____ (inferior/superior). The folds close from _____ (inferior/superior) to (inferior/superior).

18. The minimum subglottal driving pressure for speech is _____ cm H_2O.

19. In the mode of vibration known as _____, the vocal folds vibrate at a much lower rate than in modal phonation, and the folds exhibit a syncopated vibratory pattern.

20. In the mode of vibration known as _____, the vocal folds lengthen and become extremely thin and reedlike.

21. Presence of vocal nodules or other space-occupying laryngeal pathology may result in _____ phonation.

22. To increase vocal intensity, one must _____ (increase/decrease) subglottal pressure and _____ (increase/decrease) medial compression.

23. To increase vocal fundamental frequency, one must vocal fold tension by _____ (lengthening/shortening) the vocal folds.

24. _____ is the pitch of phonation that is optimal or most appropriate for an individual.

25. _____ is the vocal pitch habitually used during speech.

26. As vocal intensity increases, the closed phase of the vibratory cycle
_____ (increases/decreases).

27. We had occasion to record the speech of an individual with a
maxillary fistula secondary to squamous cell carcinoma. The
cancerous condition had required removal of part of her maxilla,
which meant that the oral cavity was continuous with the nasal cavity.
While working with the physician who was fitting her for an oral
prosthesis, we recorded her speech, only to find that when speech was
produced with the open fistula, the fundamental frequency was highly
irregular but became regular again when the oral prosthesis was in
place. What could be the link between the vocal folds and the oral-
nasal communication?

REFERENCES

Abrahams, P. H., McMinn, R. M. H., Hutchings, et al. (2003). *McMinn's color atlas of human anatomy* (5th ed.). Philadelphia: Mosby.

Adair, R. K. (1990). *The physics of baseball* (3rd ed.). New York: HarperCollins.

Adair, R. K. (1995). The physics of baseball. *Physics Today, 48*(5), 26–31.

Aronson, E. A. (1985). *Clinical voice disorders.* New York: Thieme.

Baer, T., Sasaki, C., & Harris, K. (1985). *Laryngeal function in phonation and respiration.* Boston: College-Hill Press.

Baken, R. J., & Orlikoff, R. F. (1999). *Clinical measurement of speech and voice,* (2nd ed.). San Diego: Singular Publishing Group.

Bateman, H. E. (1977). *A clinical approach to speech anatomy and physiology.* Springfield, IL: Charles C. Thomas.

Beck, E. W., Monson, H., & Groer, M. (1982). *Mosby's atlas of functional human anatomy.* St. Louis: Mosby.

Berkovitz, B. K. B., & Moxham, B. J. (2002). *Head and neck anatomy: A clinical reference.* London: Martin Dunitz.

Bless, D. M., & Abbs, J. H. (1983). *Vocal fold physiology.* San Diego: College-Hill Press.

Bly, L. (1994). *Motor skills acquisition in the first year.* Tucson, AZ: Therapy Skill Builders.

Boone, D. R. (1999). *The voice and voice therapy.* Englewood Cliffs, NJ: Prentice-Hall.

Broad, D. J. (1973). Phonation. In F. D. Minifie, T. J. Hixon, & F. Williams, (Eds.), *Normal aspects of speech, hearing, and language.* Englewood Cliffs, NJ: Prentice-Hall.

Carrau, R. L., & Murry, T. (1999). *Comprehensive management of swallowing disorders.* San Diego: Singular Publishing Group.

Childers, D. G., Hicks, D. M., Moore, G. P., et al. (1990). Electroglottography and vocal fold physiology. *Journal of Speech and Hearing Research, 33,* 245–254.

Chusid, J. G. (1985). *Correlative neuroanatomy and functional neurology* (17th ed.). Los Altos, CA: Lange Medical Publications.

Daniloff, R. G. (1989). *Speech science.* San Diego: College-Hill Press.

Dejaeger, E., Pelemans, W., Ponette, E., & Joosten, E. (1997). Mechanisms involved in postdeglutition retention in the elderly. *Dysphagia, 12*(2), 63–67.

Doyle, P. C., Grantmyre, A., & Myers, C. (1989). Clinical modification of the tracheostoma breathing valve for voice restoration. *Journal of Speech and Hearing Disorders, 54,* 189–192.

Durrant, J. D., & Lovrinic, J. H. (1995). *Bases of hearing science.* Baltimore: Williams & Wilkins.

Eckel, F., & Boone, D. (1981). The s/z ratio as an indicator of laryngeal pathology. *Journal of Speech and Hearing Disorders, 46,* 147–149.

Fink, B. R. (1975). *The human larynx.* New York: Raven Press.

Fink, B. R., & Demarest, R. J. (1978). *Laryngeal biomechanics.* Cambridge, MA: Harvard University Press.

Fletcher, W. W. (1950). *A study of internal laryngeal activity in relation to vocal intensity.* Doctoral dissertation, Northwestern University, Evanston, IL.

Fucci, D. J., & Lass, N. J. (1999). *Fundamentals of speech science.* Boston: Allyn & Bacon.

Frable, M. A. (1961). Computation of motion of the cricoarytenoid joint. *Archives of Otolaryngology, 73,* 551–556.

Fujimura, O. (1988). *Vocal fold physiology. Vol. 2. Vocal physiology.* New York: Raven Press.

Fukida, H., Kawaida, M., Tatehara, T., et al. (1988). A new concept of lubricating mechanisms of the larynx. In Fujimura, O. (Ed.), *Vocal physiology: Voice production, mechanisms and functions* (pp. 83–92). New York: Raven Press.

Ganong, W. F. (2003). *Review of medical physiology* (2nd ed.). New York: McGraw-Hill/Appleton & Lange.

Gosling, J. A., Harris, P. F., Humpherson, J. R., et al. (1985). *Atlas of human anatomy.* Philadelphia: J. B. Lippincott.

Gray, H., Bannister, L. H., Berry, M. M., & Williams, P. L. (Eds.). (1995). *Gray's anatomy.* London: Churchill Livingstone.

Grobler, N. J. (1977). *Textbook of clinical anatomy* (Vol. 1). Amsterdam: Elsevier Scientific.

Hirano, M. (1974). Morphological structure of the vocal cord as a vibrator and its variations. *Folia Phoniatrica, 26,* 89–94.

Hirano, M., Kirchner, J. A., & Bless, D. M. (1987). *Neurolaryngology.* Boston: College-Hill Press.

Hirano, M., Kiyokawa, K., & Kurita, S. (1988). Laryngeal muscles and glottic shaping. In O. Fujimura (Ed.), *Vocal physiology: Voice production, mechanisms and functions* (pp. 49–65). New York: Raven Press.

Hirano, M., Ohala, J., & Vennard, W. (1969). The function of laryngeal muscles in regulation of fundamental frequency and intensity of phonation. *Journal of Speech and Hearing Research, 12,* 616–628.

Hixon, T. J. (1973). Respiratory function in speech. In F. D. Minifie, T. J. Hixon, & F. Williams (Eds.), *Normal aspects of speech, hearing, and language* (pp. 73–126). Englewood Cliffs, NJ: Prentice-Hall.

Hixon, T. J. (1982). Speech breathing kinematics and mechanism inferences therefrom. In S. Grillner, A. Persson, B. Lindblom, & J. Lubker (Eds.), *Speech motor control* (pp. 75–94). New York: Pergamon.

Hixon, T. J., Hawley, J. L., & Wilson, K. J. (1982). An around-the-house device for the clinical determination of respiratory driving pressure: A note on making simple even simpler. *Journal of Speech and Hearing Disorders, 47,* 413–415.

Hollien, H., & Moore, G. P. (1968). Stroboscopic laminography of the larynx during phonation. *Acta Otolaryngologica, 65,* 209–215.

Hufnagle, J., & Hufnagle, K. K. (1988). S/Z ratio in dysphonic children with and without vocal cord nodules. *Language, Speech, and Hearing Services in Schools, 19,* 418–422.

Husson, R. (1953). Sur la physiologie vocale. *Annals of Otolaryngology, 69,* 124–137.

Isshiki, N. (1964). Regulatory mechanisms of voice intensity variation. *Journal of Speech and Hearing Research, 7,* 17–29.

Jones-Owens, J. L. (1991). Prespeech assessment and treatment strategies. In M. B. Langley, & L. J. Lombardino (Eds.), *Neurodevelopmental strategies for managing communication disorders in children with severe motor dysfunction.* Austin: Pro-Ed.

Kaplan, H. M. (1971). *Anatomy and physiology of speech.* New York: McGraw-Hill.

Kazarian, A. G., Sarkissian, L. S., & Isaakian, D. G. (1978). Length of the human vocal folds by age. *Zhurnal Eksperimentalnoi Klinicheskoi Meditsiny, 18,* 105–109.

Kent, R. (1994). *Reference manual for communicative sciences and disorders. Vocal fundamental frequency in males and females from childhood to old age.* Austin, TX: Pro-Ed, p. 160.

Kent, R. D. (1997). *The speech sciences.* San Diego: Singular Publishing Group.

Kent, R. D., Kent, J. F., & Rosenbek, J. C. (1987). Maximum performance tests of speech production. *Journal of Speech and Hearing Disorders, 52,* 367–387.

Kirchner, J. A., & Suzuki, M. (1968). Laryngeal reflexes and voice production. In M. Krauss (Ed.), *Sound production in man. Annals of the New York Academy of Sciences, 155,* 98–109.

Kuehn, D. P., Lemme, M. L., & Baumgartner, J. M. (1989). *Neural bases of speech, hearing, and language.* Boston: Little, Brown.

Langley, M. B., & Lombardino, L. J. (1991). *Neurodevelopmental strategies for managing communication disorders in children with severe motor dysfunction.* Austin: Pro-Ed.

Lieberman, P. (1968a). *Intonation, perception, and language.* Research monograph No. 38. Cambridge, MA: M.I.T. Press.

Lieberman, P. (1968b). Vocal cord motion in man. *Annals of the New York Academy of Sciences, 155,* 28–38.

Lieberman, P. (1977). *Speech science and acoustic phonetics: An introduction.* New York: Macmillan.

Liebgott, B. (2001). The anatomical basis of dentistry. St. Louis, MO: Mosby.

Logemann, J. (1998). *Evaluation and treatment of swallowing disorders* (2nd ed.). Austin: Pro-Ed.

McMinn, R. M. H., Hutchings, R. T., & Logan, B. M. (1994). *Color atlas of head and neck anatomy.* London: Mosby-Wolfe.

Mu, L., & Sanders, I. (2008). Newly revealed cricothyropharyngeus muscle in the human laryngopharynx. *Anatomical Record,* June 2.

Netsell, R. (1973). Speech physiology. In F. D. Minifie, T. J. Hixon, & F. Williams (Eds.), *Normal aspects of speech, hearing, and language* (pp. 134–211). Englewood Cliffs, NJ: Prentice-Hall.

Netsell, R., & Hixon, T. J. (1978). A noninvasive method for clinically estimating subglottal air pressure. *Journal of Speech and Hearing Disorders, 43,* 326–330.

Netter, F. H. (1983a). *The CIBA collection of medical illustrations. Vol. 1. Nervous System. Part I. Anatomy and physiology.* West Caldwell, NJ: CIBA Pharmaceutical Company.

Netter, F. H. (1983b). *The CIBA collection of medical illustrations. Vol. 1. Nervous system. Part II. Neurologic and neuromuscular disorders.* West Caldwell, NJ: CIBA Pharmaceutical Company.

Netter, F. H. (1989). *Atlas of human anatomy.* West Caldwell, NJ: CIBA Pharmaceutical Company.

Netter, F. H. (1997). *Atlas of human anatomy.* Los Angeles: Icon Learning Systems.

Nishizawa, N., Sawashima, M., & Yonemoto, K. (1988). Vocal fold length in vocal pitch change. In O. Fujimua (Ed.), *Vocal physiology: Voice production, mechanisms and functions* (pp. 49–65). New York: Raven Press.

Proctor, D. F. (1968). The physiologic basis of voice training. In M. Krauss (Ed.), *Sound production in man. Annals of the New York Academy of Sciences, 155*, 208–228.

Ptacek, P. H., & Sander, E. K. (1963). Maximum duration of phonation. *Journal of Speech and Hearing Disorders, 28*(2), 171–182.

Ramig, L. A., & Ringel, R. L. (1983). Effects of physiological aging on selected acoustic characteristics of voice. *Journal of Speech and Hearing Research, 26*, 22–30.

Rastatter, M. P., & Hyman, M. (1982). Maximum phoneme duration of /s/ and /z/ by children with vocal nodules. *Language, Speech, and Hearing Services in Schools, 13*, 197–199.

Rohen, J. W., Yokochi, C., Lutjen-Drecoll, E. L., & Romrell, L. J. (2002). *Color atlas of anatomy: A photographic study of the human body* (5th ed.). Philadelphia: Lippincott, Williams & Wilkins.

Rosse, C., Gaddum-Rosse, P., & Rosse, G. (1997). *Hollinshead's textbook of anatomy.* Philadelphia: Lippincott-Raven.

Sapienza, C. M., & Stathopoulos, E. T. (1994). Respiratory and laryngeal measures of children and women with bilateral vocal fold nodules. *Journal of Speech and Hearing Research, 37*, 1229–1243.

Shepard, T. H. (1998). *Catalog of teratogenic agents* (9th ed.). Baltimore: Johns Hopkins University Press.

Sonninen, A. (1968). The external frame function in the control of pitch in the human voice. In M. Krauss (Ed.), *Sound production in man. Annals of the New York Academy of Sciences, 155*, 68–89.

Sorensen, D. N., & Parker, P. A. (1992). The voiced/voiceless phonation time in children with and without laryngeal pathology. *Language, Speech, and Hearing Services in Schools, 23*, 163–168.

Tait, N. A., Michel, J. F., & Carpenter, M. A. (1980). Maximum duration of sustained /s/ and /z/ in children. *Journal of Speech and Hearing Disorders, 15*, 239–246.

Timcke, R., Von Leden, H., & Moore, G. P. (1958). Laryngeal vibrations: Measurements of the glottic wave I: The normal vibratory cycle. *Archives of Otolaryngology, 68*, 1–19.

Titze, I. R. (1973). The human vocal cords: A mathematical model, Part I. *Phonetica, 28*, 129–170.

Titze, I. R. (1988). The physics of small amplitude oscillation of the vocal folds. *Journal of the Acoustical Society of America, 83*(4), 1536–1552.

Titze, I. R. (1994). *Principles of voice production.* Englewood Cliffs, NJ: Prentice-Hall.

Van den Berg, J. W. (1958). Myoelastic-aerodynamic theory of voice production. *Journal of Speech and Hearing Research, 1*, 227–244.

Van den Berg, J. W. (1968). Sound production in isolated human larynges. In M. Krauss (Ed.), *Sound production in man. Annals of the New York Academy of Sciences, 155*, 18–27.

Van den Berg, J. W., & Tan, T. S. (1959). Results of experiments with human larynxes. *Practica Oto-rhino-laryngologica, 21*, 425–450.

Verdolini, K., Titze, I. R., & Fennell, A. (1994). Dependence of phonatory effort on hydration level. *Journal of Speech and Hearing Research, 37*, 1001–1007.

Whillis, J. (1946). Movements of the tongue in swallowing. *Journal of Anatomy, 80*, 115–116.

Zemlin, W. R. (1998). *Speech and hearing science. Anatomy and physiology* (4th ed.). Needham Heights, MA: Allyn & Bacon.

4

Anatomy and Physiology of Articulation, Resonation, and Deglutition

OUTLINE

e. Nasal conchae
f. Vomer
g. Zygomatic
h. Hyoid
2. Bones of the cranial skeleton
a. Ethmoid
b. Sphenoid
c. Frontal
d. Parietal
e. Occipital
f. Temporal
E. Dentition
1. Dental alveoli
2. Teeth categorized as incisors, cuspids, bicuspids, and molars
3. Each tooth has a root and crown, the crown's surface composed of enamel overlying dentin
4. Each tooth has medial (or mesial), distal, lingual, buccal (or labial), and occlusal surfaces
5. Clinical eruption
6. The permanent arch
7. Types of occlusion
a. Class I occlusion
b. Class II malocclusion
c. Class III malocclusion
8. Aberrant orientation
a. Torsiversion
b. Labioversion
c. Linguaversion
d. Distoversion
e. Mesioversion
f. Infraversion
g. Supraversion
F. Cavities of the vocal tract
1. Pharynx
a. Oropharynx
b. Nasopharynx
c. Laryngopharynx
2. Oral cavity
3. Buccal cavity
4. Nasal cavities
G. Muscles of the face and mouth
1. Muscles of the face
a. Orbicularis oris
b. Risorius
c. Buccinator
d. Levator labii superioris
e. Zygomatic minor

   f. Levator labii superioris alaeque nasi
   g. Levator anguli oris
   h. Zygomatic major, zygomatic minor
   i. Depressor labii inferioris
   j. Depressor anguli oris
   k. Mentalis
   l. Platysma
  2. Tongue
   a. Intrinsic tongue muscles
   b. Extrinsic tongue muscles
  3. Muscles of mastication
   a. Mandibular elevators
   b. Mandibular depressors
  4. Muscles of the soft palate
   a. Palatal elevators
   b. Palatal depressors
  5. Muscles of the pharynx
   a. Superior pharyngeal constrictor
   b. Middle pharyngeal constrictor
   c. Inferior pharyngeal constrictor
   d. Cricopharyngeal muscle
   e. Stylopharyngeus

II. Physiology of Articulation, Resonation, and Deglutition

 A. Biological functions: Mastication and deglutition
  1. Oral preparatory stage
  2. Oral stage
  3. Pharyngeal stage
  4. Esophageal stage
 B. Speech function
  1. Extralabial force of mentalis muscle
  2. Mandible adjustments
  3. Tongue function
 C. Pressures of deglutition

If you asked most people what is involved in the process of speaking, they would probably mention the elements of articulation. You now know, of course, that there is much more to speech than moving the lips, tongue, and mandible. Still, the articulatory system is an extremely important element in our communication system.

Articulation is the process of bringing the mobile and immobile articulators into contact for the purpose of shaping the sounds of speech produced by laryngeal vibration. Laryngeal vibration produces the sound required for voicing in speech.

articulation: *The process of bringing the mobile and immobile articulators into contact for the purpose of shaping the sounds of speech.*

BIOLOGICAL FUNCTION OF ARTICULATORS

Articulators are the oral and pharyngeal structures we use to form the sounds of speech, but they have a more basic function that we will discuss. While speech is clearly a very important role, the primary role of the articulators is for mastication (chewing) and deglutition (swallowing). After we talk about the structures of articulation, we'll delve into some aspects of this important biological function before discussing the role of articulators in speech.

SOURCE-FILTER THEORY OF VOWEL PRODUCTION

A widely accepted description of how the oral cavity creates some speech sounds is the *source-filter theory* of vowel production. The theory states that a voicing source is generated by the vocal folds and routed through the vocal tract where it is shaped into the sounds of speech. Changes in the shape and configuration of the tongue, mandible, soft palate, and other articulators govern the resonance characteristics of the vocal tract, and the resonances of the tract determine the sound of a vowel.

vocal tract: *The oral cavity, the pharynx, and the nasal cavity.*

The **vocal tract**, consisting of the mouth (oral cavity), the region behind the mouth (pharynx), and the nasal cavity, can be thought of as a series of linked tubes (see Figure 4–1). You probably know that if you blow carefully across the top of a glass or plastic bottle, you will hear a tone. If you decrease the volume of the air in the bottle by adding fluid to it, the frequency of vibration of the tone increases. Likewise, if you blow across the top of a bottle with larger air volume, the tone decreases in frequency. As the volume of the air in the bottle increases, the frequency of the tone decreases. As the volume decreases, the frequency increases. You are experimenting with the resonant frequency of a cavity, which is the frequency of sound to which the cavity most effectively responds. You might think of the bottle as a filter that lets only one frequency of sound through and rejects the other frequencies, much as a coffee filter lets the liquid through but traps the grounds. The airstream blowing across the top of the bottle is actually producing a very broad-spectrum signal, but the bottle selects the frequency components that are at its resonant frequency. The resonant frequency of a cavity is largely governed by its volume and length.

When you move your tongue around in your mouth, you are changing the shape of your oral cavity. This, then, is the source-filter theory of speech production. The vocal folds

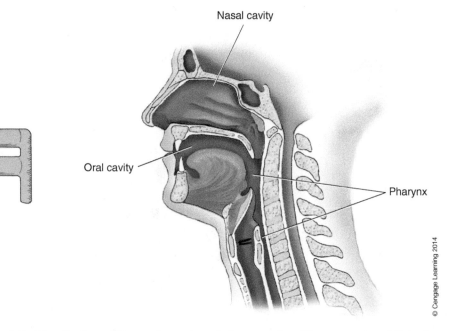

Figure 4–1. Visualization of the oral, nasal, and pharyngeal cavities as a series of linked tubes. This linkage provides the variable resonating cavity that produces speech.

produce a tone that is passed through the filter of your vocal tract. Because the vocal tract filter is changeable, you are able to reconfigure its shape and therefore change the sound.

Summary

- The source-filter theory states that speech is the product of sending an acoustic source, such as the sound produced by the vibrating vocal folds, through the filter of the vocal tract, which shapes the output.
- The ever-changing speech signal is the product of moving articulators.

Let us now examine the structures of the articulatory system. As with the phonatory system, we must examine the support structure (the skull and bones of the face) and the muscles that move the articulators. Before we begin, we will define the articulators used in speech production.

THE ARTICULATORS

Articulators can be mobile or immobile. In speech we often move one articulator to make contact with another, thus positioning a mobile articulator in relation to an immobile articulator. The largest mobile articulator is the tongue, with the lower jaw (mandible) a close second (see Figure 4–2).

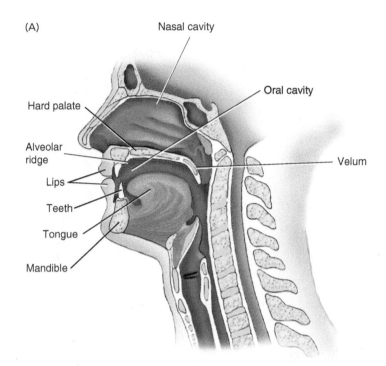

(A)

Nasal cavity

Oral cavity

Hard palate

Alveolar
ridge

Lips

Teeth

Tongue

Mandible

Velum

SAGITTAL VIEW

(B)

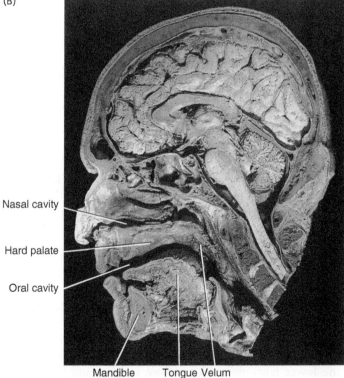

Nasal cavity

Hard palate

Oral cavity

Mandible   Tongue Velum

© Cengage Learning 2014

Figure 4–2. (A) Relationship
among articulators.
(B) Photograph of articulators
seen through sagittal section.

The velum, or soft palate, is another mobile articulator, used to differentiate nasal sounds such as /m/ and /n/ from non-nasal sounds. The lips are moved to produce different speech sounds, and the cheeks play a role in changes of resonance of the cavity. The region behind the oral cavity (the *fauces*, shown in a later figure, and the pharynx) can be moved through muscular action, and the larynx and hyoid bone both change to accommodate different articulatory postures.

There are three immobile articulators. The alveolar ridge of the upper jaw (maxilla, pl. maxillae) and the hard palate are both significant articulatory surfaces. The teeth are used to produce a variety of speech sounds.

Of these mobile and immobile articulators, the tongue, mandible, teeth, hard palate, and velum are the major players, although all surfaces and cavities in the articulatory-resonatory system contribute to the production of speech. You may wish to refer to Figures 4–3 through 4–7 as we

(A)   ANTERIOR VIEW

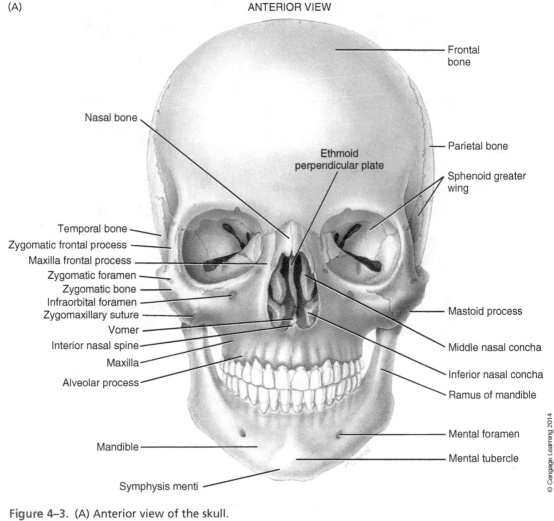

Labels: Frontal bone, Nasal bone, Ethmoid perpendicular plate, Parietal bone, Sphenoid greater wing, Temporal bone, Zygomatic frontal process, Maxilla frontal process, Zygomatic foramen, Zygomatic bone, Infraorbital foramen, Zygomaxillary suture, Vomer, Interior nasal spine, Maxilla, Alveolar process, Mastoid process, Middle nasal concha, Inferior nasal concha, Ramus of mandible, Mental foramen, Mental tubercle, Mandible, Symphysis menti

© Cengage Learning 2014

Figure 4–3. (A) Anterior view of the skull.
(continues)

(B)

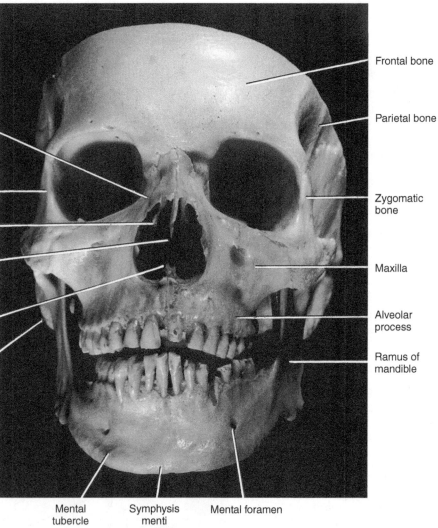

Frontal bone

Maxilla
frontal process

Parietal bone

Zygomatic
frontal process

Zygomatic
bone

Middle
nasal concha

Perpendicular
plate

Maxilla

Anterior
nasal spine

Alveolar
process

Mastoid
process

Ramus of
mandible

Mental
tubercle

Symphysis
menti

Mental foramen

© Cengage Learning 2014

Figure 4–3. continued (B) Photograph of anterior skull.

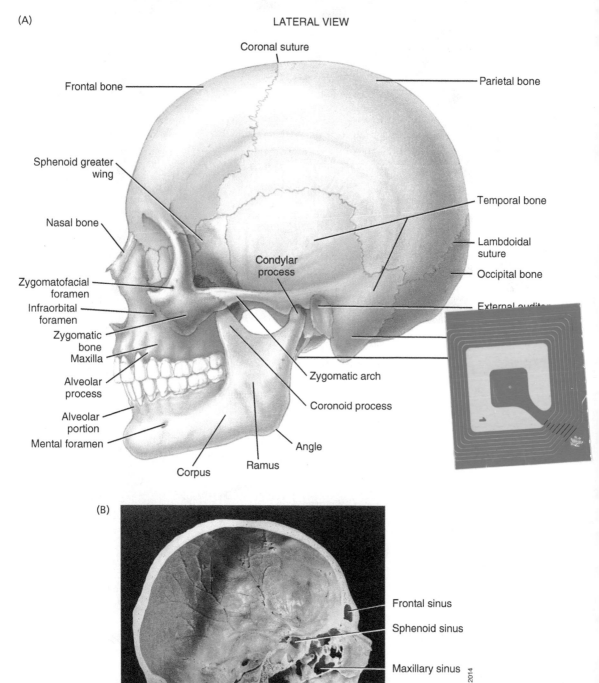

(A) LATERAL VIEW

Coronal suture

Frontal bone

Parietal bone

Sphenoid greater wing

Temporal bone

Nasal bone

Condylar process

Lambdoidal suture

Occipital bone

Zygomatofacial foramen

Infraorbital foramen

External auditory

Zygomatic bone
Maxilla

Zygomatic arch

Alveolar process

Coronoid process

Alveolar portion
Mental foramen

Angle

Corpus

Ramus

(B)

Frontal sinus

Sphenoid sinus

Maxillary sinus

© Cengage Learning 2014

Figure 4–4. (A) Lateral view of the skull. (B) Medial surface of the skull.

(continues)

(C)

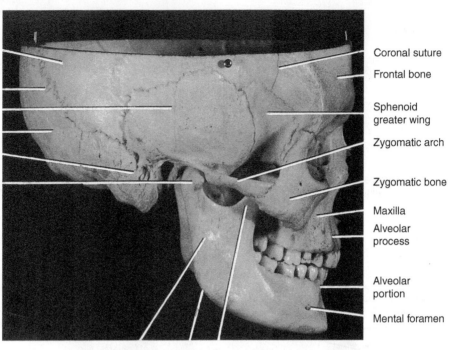

Parietal bone

Lambdoidal suture

Temporal bone

Occipital bone

Mastoid process

Condylar process

Coronal suture

Frontal bone

Sphenoid greater wing

Zygomatic arch

Zygomatic bone

Maxilla

Alveolar process

Alveolar portion

Mental foramen

Ramus   Angle   Coronoid process

© Cengage Learning 2014

Figure 4–4. continued (C) Photograph of lateral skull.

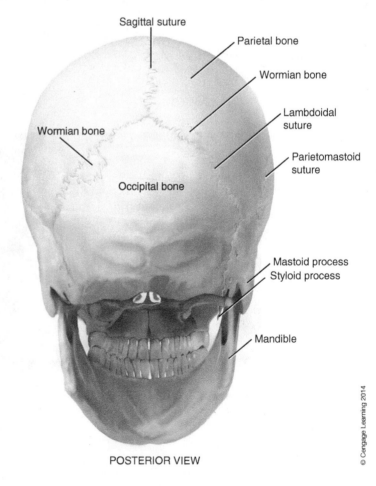

Sagittal suture

Parietal bone

Wormian bone

Lambdoidal suture

Parietomastoid suture

Wormian bone

Occipital bone

Mastoid process
Styloid process

Mandible

Figure 4–5. Posterior view of the skull.

POSTERIOR VIEW

© Cengage Learning 2014

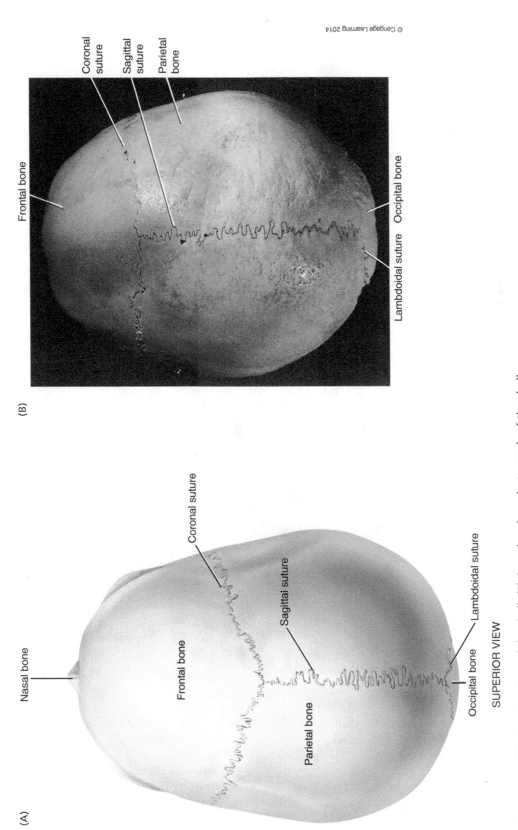

(B)

Coronal suture

Sagittal suture

Parietal bone

Frontal bone

Occipital bone

Lambdoidal suture

(A)

Nasal bone

Coronal suture

Frontal bone

Sagittal suture

Parietal bone

Occipital bone

Lambdoidal suture

SUPERIOR VIEW

Figure 4–6. (A) Superior view of the skull. (B) Superior view photograph of the skull.

(A)

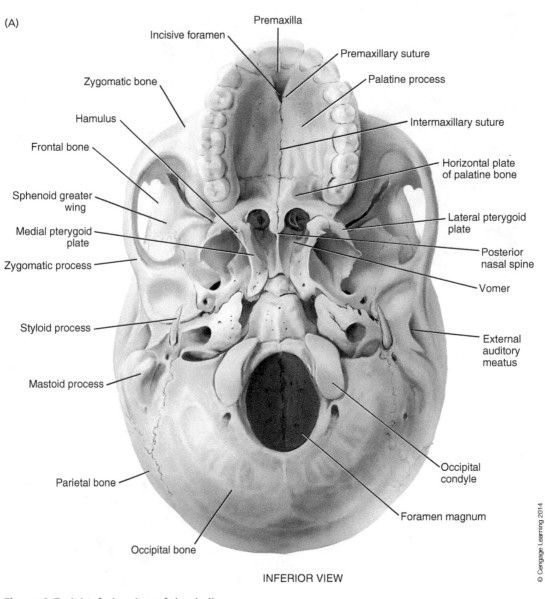

Premaxilla

Incisive foramen

Premaxillary suture

Zygomatic bone

Palatine process

Hamulus

Intermaxillary suture

Frontal bone

Horizontal plate
of palatine bone

Sphenoid greater
wing

Medial pterygoid
plate

Lateral pterygoid
plate

Zygomatic process

Posterior
nasal spine

Vomer

Styloid process

External
auditory
meatus

Mastoid process

Parietal bone

Occipital
condyle

Occipital bone

Foramen magnum

INFERIOR VIEW

Figure 4–7. (A) Inferior view of the skull.
(continues)

© Cengage Learning 2014

210

(B)

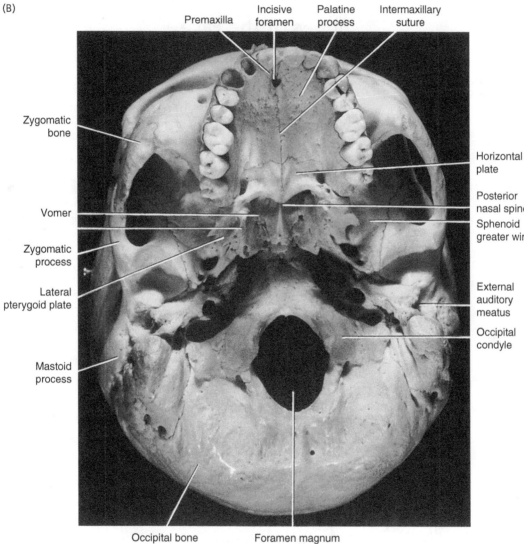

Premaxilla

Incisive foramen

Palatine process

Intermaxillary suture

Zygomatic bone

Horizontal plate

Posterior nasal spine

Vomer

Sphenoid greater wing

Zygomatic process

Lateral pterygoid plate

External auditory meatus

Occipital condyle

Mastoid process

Occipital bone

Foramen magnum

© Cengage Learning 2014

Figure 4–7. continued (B) Photograph of skull, inferior view.

begin our discussion of the bones of the facial and cranial skeleton. In addition, Table 4–1 may help you to organize this body of material.

BONES OF THE FACE AND CRANIAL SKELETON

Bones of the Face

The face has numerous bones, with which you should become familiar (see Table 4–1).

The *mandible* is the massive bone making up the lower jaw of the face. It begins as a paired bone but fuses at the midline by the child's first birthday. As you can see in Figure 4–8, there are several landmarks of interest on both

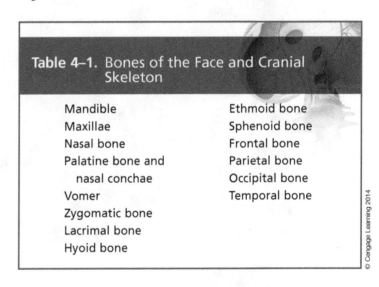

Table 4–1. Bones of the Face and Cranial Skeleton	
Mandible	Ethmoid bone
Maxillae	Sphenoid bone
Nasal bone	Frontal bone
Palatine bone and	Parietal bone
nasal conchae	Occipital bone
Vomer	Temporal bone
Zygomatic bone	
Lacrimal bone	
Hyoid bone	

© Cengage Learning 2014

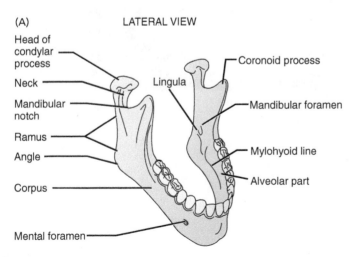
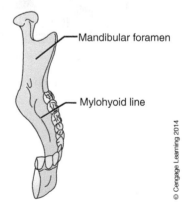

(A)   LATERAL VIEW

Head of condylar process
Neck
Mandibular notch
Ramus
Angle
Corpus
Mental foramen
Lingula
Coronoid process
Mandibular foramen
Mylohyoid line
Alveolar part

(B)   MEDIAL VIEW

Mandibular foramen
Mylohyoid line

© Cengage Learning 2014

Figure 4–8. (A and B) Lateral and medial views of the mandible.

(C)

LATERAL VIEW | Coronoid process / Condylar process | ANTERIOR VIEW

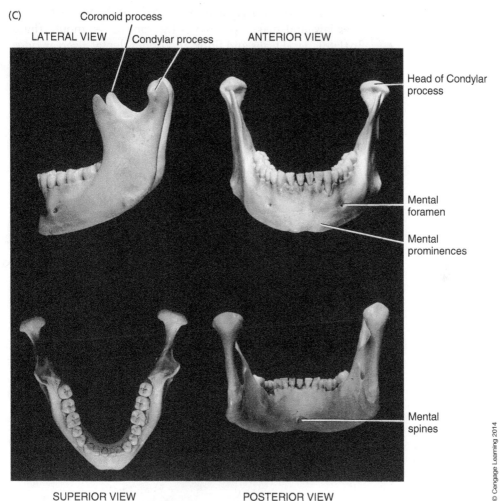

Head of Condylar process

Mental foramen

Mental prominences

Mental spines

SUPERIOR VIEW   POSTERIOR VIEW

© Cengage Learning 2014

Figure 4–8. continued (C) photographs of mandible.

outer and inner surfaces. The point of fusion of the two halves of the mandible is the *symphysis menti,* or mental symphysis. Lateral to this on either side is the *mental foramen,* the hole through which the mental nerve, a branch of the trigeminal nerve (cranial nerve V), passes in life. On the side is the corpus, or body, and the point at which the mandible bends upward is the *angle.* The plate rising up from the mandible is the *ramus,* and the *condylar process* is an important landmark because the head of the condylar process articulates with the skull, permitting rotation of the mandible. Teeth are found in small *dental alveoli* (sacs, not shown) on the upper surface of the *alveolar part* of the mandible.

On the inner surface of the mandible is the *mandibular foramen,* which houses the inferior alveolar nerve that provides sensory innervation for the teeth and gums.

The left and right maxillae are the bones of the upper jaw, and make up most of the roof of the mouth (hard palate), nasal walls and floor, and upper dental alveolar ridge (see Figure 4–9). Supporting the eye is the *orbital process*, the lower portion of the orbital surface. The *zygomatic process* of

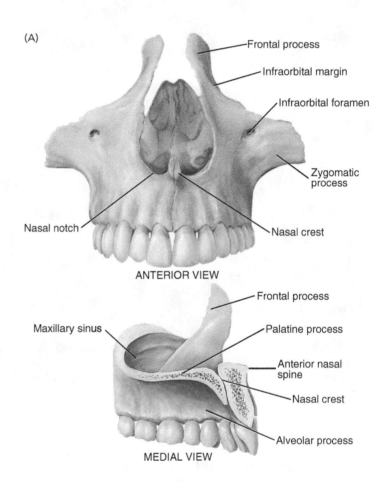

(A)

Frontal process

Infraorbital margin

Infraorbital foramen

Zygomatic process

Nasal notch

Nasal crest

ANTERIOR VIEW

Maxillary sinus

Frontal process

Palatine process

Anterior nasal spine

Nasal crest

Alveolar process

MEDIAL VIEW

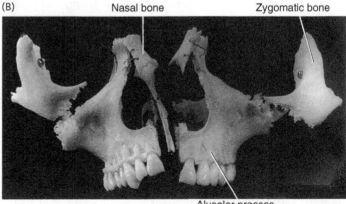

(B)

Nasal bone

Zygomatic bone

Alveolar process

ANTERIOR VIEW

Figure 4–9. (A) Anterior and medial views of maxilla. (B) Anterior photograph of maxillae showing relationship with nasal and zygomatic bones.

© Cengage Learning 2014

the maxilla bone articulates with the zygomatic bone. At the midline, you can see the *anterior nasal spine* and *nasal crest*, and lateral to this is the *nasal notch*. The alveolar process contains alveoli that hold teeth in the intact adult maxilla. A medial view reveals the *maxillary sinus,* the *palatine process,* and the inner margin of the *alveolar process.*

Figure 4–9 shows an anterior view of the maxillae. As you can see, the two *palatine processes* of the maxillae articulate at the *intermaxillary suture.* This suture marks the point of a cleft of the hard palate. The palatine process makes up three fourths of the hard palate; the other one fourth is the *horizontal plate of the palatine bone.*

The *incisive foramen* in the anterior aspect of the hard palate is a conduit for the nasopalatine nerve serving the nasal mucosa. Trace the *premaxillary suture* forward from the incisive foramen to the alveolar process and you have identified the borders of the *premaxilla.* The premaxilla is difficult to see on the adult skull, but it is an important landmark. Note that the premaxillary suture neatly separates the lateral incisors from the cuspids.

The *nasal bones* are small, making up the superior nasal surface. Recall that the posterior one fourth of the hard palate is made up of the horizontal plate of the palatine bone (see Figure 4–11). When viewed from the front, you can see that the articulated palatine bones echo the nasal cavity defined by the maxillae.

The *inferior nasal conchae* (inferior *turbinates*) are small, scroll-like bones on the lateral surface of the nasal cavity. These small bones articulate with the maxilla, palatine, and ethmoid bones. The middle and superior nasal conchae, processes of the ethmoid bone (to be discussed), are above the inferior conchae. The mucosal lining covering the nasal conchae is the thickest of the nose and is richly endowed with vascular supply. Air passing over the nasal conchae is warmed and humidified before reaching the delicate tissues of the lower respiratory system. The shape of the conchae greatly increases the surface area, which promotes rapid heat exchange.

There is only one *vomer* because it is a midline bone. It makes up the inferior and posterior nasal septum, which is the dividing plate between the two nasal cavities (see Figure 4–12). The bony nasal septum is made of two elements: the vomer and the perpendicular plate of the ethmoid bone. With the addition of the midline septal cartilage, the nasal septum is complete.

The *zygomatic bone* makes up the prominent structure we identify as the cheekbone. As you can see from Figure 4–13, the zygomatic bone articulates with the maxillae, frontal bone, and temporal bone (you cannot see the

(A)

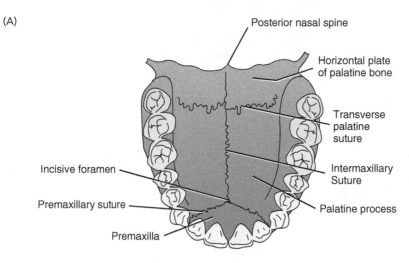

Posterior nasal spine

Horizontal plate
of palatine bone

Transverse
palatine
suture

Intermaxillary
Suture

Incisive foramen

Premaxillary suture

Premaxilla

Palatine process

(B)   INFERIOR VIEW

Posterior nasal spine

Horizontal plate

Palatine process

Transverse
palatine suture

Intermaxillary suture

Incisive foramen

Premaxillary suture

Zygomatic
process

Premaxilla

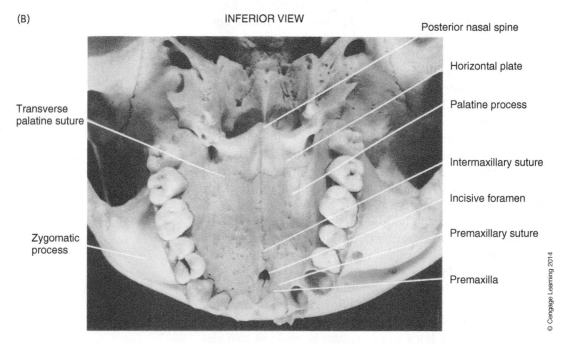

Figure 4–10. Schematic drawing (A) and photograph (B) of inferior view of the hard palate.

(A)   RIGHT PALATINE BONE

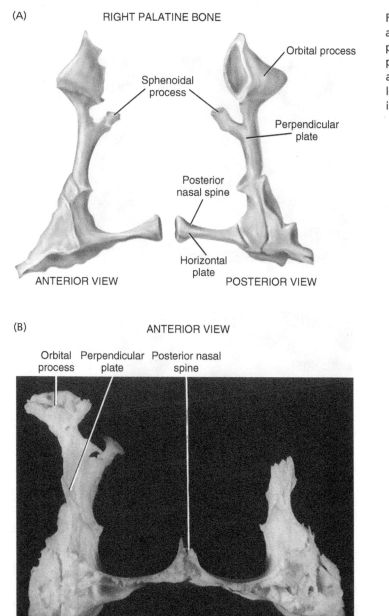

Orbital process

Sphenoidal process

Perpendicular plate

Posterior nasal spine

Horizontal plate

ANTERIOR VIEW   POSTERIOR VIEW

Figure 4–11. (A) Anterior and posterior views of palatine bones. (B) Articulated palatine bones from front and beneath. Note that the left perpendicular plate is incomplete. *(continues)*

(B)   ANTERIOR VIEW

Orbital process   Perpendicular plate   Posterior nasal spine

Horizontal plate

INFERIOR VIEW

© Cengage Learning 2014

(C)

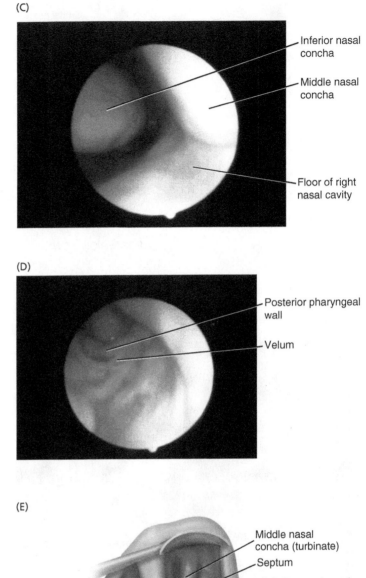

Inferior nasal concha

Middle nasal concha

Floor of right nasal cavity

(D)

Posterior pharyngeal wall

Velum

(E)

Middle nasal concha (turbinate)

Septum

Columella nasi

Inferior nasal concha

Floor of nasal cavity

SPECULUM VIEW

© Cengage Learning 2014

Figure 4–11. continued (C) Nasoendoscopic view of entry to right naris. Note the prominent inferior nasal concha arising from the left side (medial wall of the nasal cavity). (D) Nasoendoscopic view of nasopharynx as seen from the right nares, showing superior surface of velum and posterior pharyngeal wall. (E) View of left naris opened using speculum for visualization, showing inferior and middle conchae.

(A)

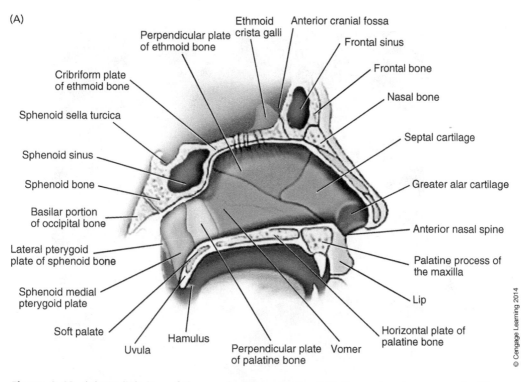

Ethmoid crista galli

Anterior cranial fossa

Perpendicular plate of ethmoid bone

Frontal sinus

Frontal bone

Cribriform plate of ethmoid bone

Nasal bone

Sphenoid sella turcica

Septal cartilage

Sphenoid sinus

Sphenoid bone

Greater alar cartilage

Basilar portion of occipital bone

Anterior nasal spine

Lateral pterygoid plate of sphenoid bone

Palatine process of the maxilla

Sphenoid medial pterygoid plate

Lip

Soft palate

Hamulus

Horizontal plate of palatine bone

Uvula

Perpendicular plate of palatine bone

Vomer

© Cengage Learning 2014

Figure 4–12. (A) Medial view of the nasal septum. Notice that the septum is composed of the perpendicular plate of ethmoid, the vomer, and the septal cartilage. *(continues)*

articulation with the sphenoid bone) and makes up the lateral orbit. The *zygomatic arch* consists of the temporal process of the zygomatic bone and the zygomatic process of the temporal bone.

These small bones are almost hidden in the intact skull. They articulate with the maxillae, frontal bone, nasal bone, and inferior conchae. They constitute a small portion of the lateral nasal wall and form a small portion of the medial orbit as well.

The *hyoid bone* is discussed in Chapter 3, but it rightfully belongs in this chapter as well. Its presence in this listing should remind you of the interconnectedness of the phonatory and articulatory systems.

Bones of the Cranial Skeleton

The bones of the cranium include those that define the cranial cavity. The *ethmoid bone* is a complex, delicate structure with a presence in the cranial, nasal, and orbital spaces

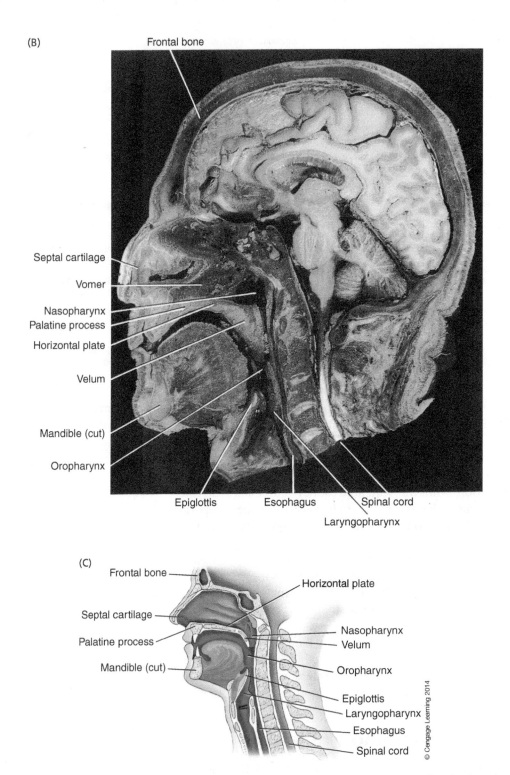

(B)

Frontal bone

Septal cartilage

Vomer

Nasopharynx
Palatine process

Horizontal plate

Velum

Mandible (cut)

Oropharynx

Epiglottis   Esophagus   Spinal cord

Laryngopharynx

(C)

Frontal bone

Horizontal plate

Septal cartilage

Palatine process

Mandible (cut)

Nasopharynx
Velum

Oropharynx

Epiglottis
Laryngopharynx

Esophagus

Spinal cord

© Cengage Learning 2014

Figure 4–12. continued (B) Sagittal section through the nasal septum. (C) Drawing of sagittal section through the nasal septum.

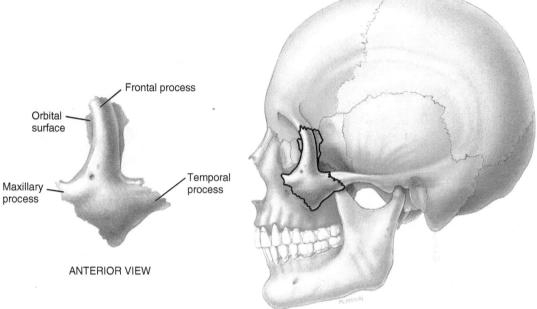

Frontal process

Orbital surface

Maxillary process

Temporal process

ANTERIOR VIEW

© Cengage Learning 2014

Figure 4–13. Anterior view of the zygomatic bone.

(Figure 4–14). If the cranium and facial skeleton were an apple, the ethmoid would be the core. When the ethmoid is viewed from the front, it is easy to identify the *crista galli*, which protrudes into the cranial space. The *perpendicular plate* makes up the *superior nasal septum*. The *cribriform plates* separate the nasal and cranial cavities and provide the conduit for the *olfactory nerves* as they enter the cranial space.

Figure 4–15 shows that the *sphenoid* consists of a corpus and three pairs of processes, the *greater wings of sphenoid, lesser wings of sphenoid,* and *pterygoid processes*. When the sphenoid is viewed from above, you can see the *hypophyseal fossa*, the indentation that holds the pituitary gland (hypophysis).

Projecting downward from the greater wing and corpus are the *lateral* and *medial pterygoid plates*. These plates and the fossa between them are important points of attachment for one of the muscles of mastication and a muscle of the soft palate. A *hamulus* (hook) projects from each medial lamina, and the tendon of the tensor veli palatini of the soft palate passes around this on its course to the velum, as will be discussed.

The frontal bone shown in Figure 4–16 makes up the bony forehead, anterior cranial case, and supraorbital region. The *coronal suture* (see Figure 4-4B) is where the frontal and parietal bones articulate.

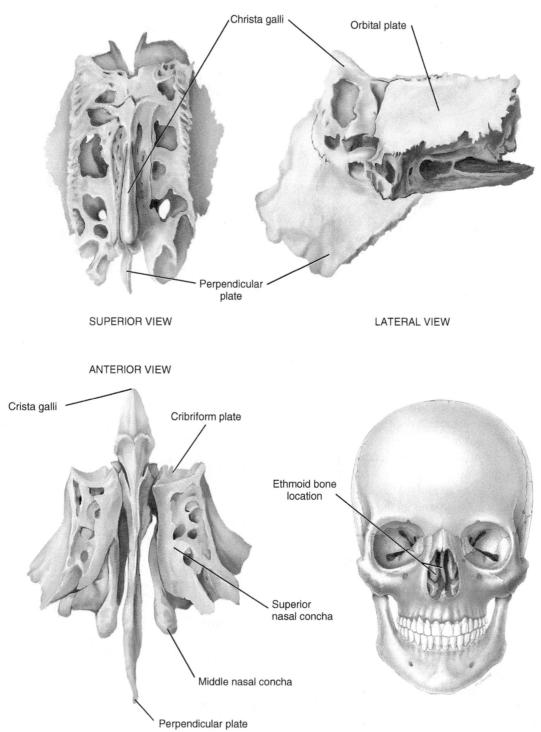

Christa galli

Orbital plate

Perpendicular plate

SUPERIOR VIEW

LATERAL VIEW

ANTERIOR VIEW

Crista galli

Cribriform plate

Ethmoid bone location

Superior nasal concha

Middle nasal concha

Perpendicular plate

Figure 4–14. Views of the ethmoid bone.

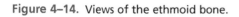

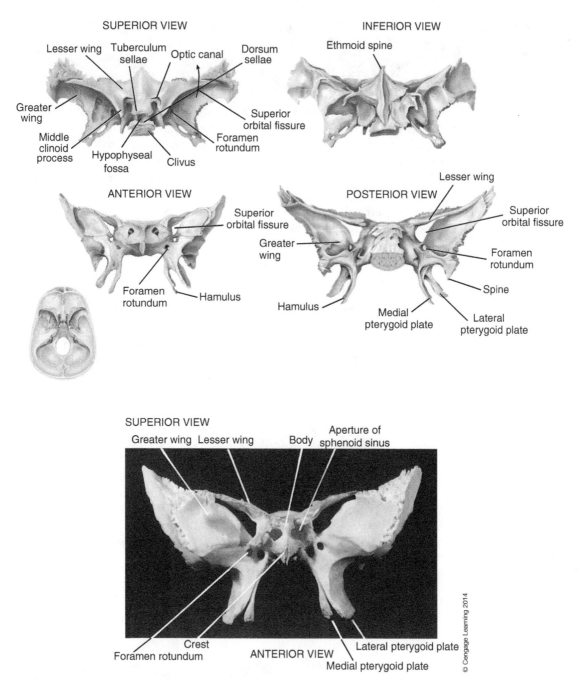

SUPERIOR VIEW

Lesser wing • Tuberculum sellae • Optic canal • Dorsum sellae

Greater wing

Middle clinoid process • Hypophyseal fossa • Clivus

Superior orbital fissure

Foramen rotundum

INFERIOR VIEW

Ethmoid spine

ANTERIOR VIEW

Superior orbital fissure

Foramen rotundum • Hamulus

POSTERIOR VIEW

Lesser wing

Superior orbital fissure

Greater wing

Foramen rotundum

Spine

Hamulus

Medial pterygoid plate • Lateral pterygoid plate

SUPERIOR VIEW

Greater wing • Lesser wing • Body • Aperture of sphenoid sinus

Crest

Foramen rotundum

Lateral pterygoid plate

Medial pterygoid plate

ANTERIOR VIEW

© Cengage Learning 2014

Figure 4–15. Photograph of anterior view of sphenoid bone, and schematic drawings of sphenoid from four views.

Mandibular Hypoplasia and Micrognathia

Congenital mandibular hypoplasia is a condition of inadequate development of the mandible. Although some specific genetic syndromes have this as a trait (e.g., Pierre Robin syndrome), micrognathia (small jaw) may occur without a known mediating condition. The misalignment of the mandibular and maxillary arches can be corrected through surgery to extend the mandible. It is hypothesized that during development, micrognathia leads to cleft palate: The mandible may not develop adequately to accommodate the tongue, which in turn blocks the extension of the palatine processes of the maxillae.

The *parietal bones* form the upper middle portion of the braincase (see Figure 4–17). These bones are joined at the *sagittal suture*, and join the occipital bones by means of the *lambdoidal suture*. The temporal bone articulates with the parietal bone by means of the *squamosal suture*.

The *occipital bone* (see Figure 4–18) makes up the posterior braincase. It articulates with the temporal, parietal, and sphenoid bones. From beneath you can see that the occipital bone forms the base of the skull, wrapping beneath the brain. The *foramen magnum* provides the conduit for the spinal cord and beginning of the medulla oblongata, and the *condyles* mark the resting point for the first cervical vertebra.

The *temporal bone* is an important structure for students of speech pathology and audiology. The temporal

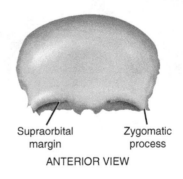

Supraorbital
margin

Zygomatic
process

ANTERIOR VIEW

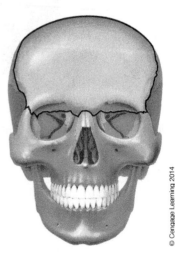

© Cengage Learning 2014

Figure 4–16. Anterior view of frontal bone.

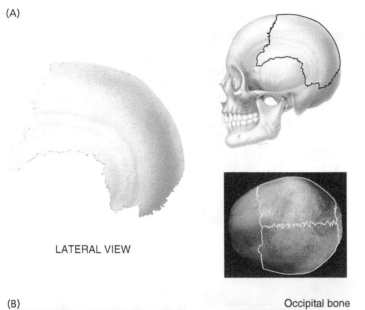

(A)

LATERAL VIEW

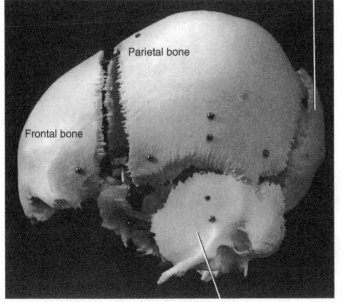

(B)

Occipital bone

Parietal bone

Frontal bone

Temporal bone

© Cengage Learning 2014

Figure 4–17. (A) Lateral view of parietal bone. (B) Photograph of disarticulated parietal, frontal, temporal, and occipital bones.

226

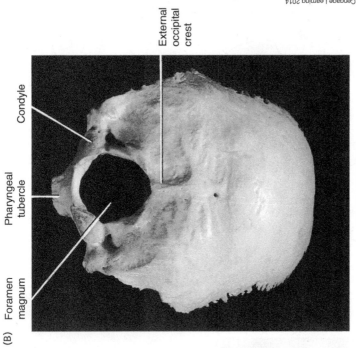

(B)

Condyle

Pharyngeal tubercle

Foramen magnum

External occipital crest

INFERIOR VIEW

© Cengage Learning 2014

Figure 4–18. (A) Occipital bone seen from inferior and superior aspects. (B) Photograph of occipital bone, inferior view.

(A)

LATERAL VIEW

Cerebellar fossa

Clivus

SUPERIOR VIEW

POSTERIOR VIEW

Condyle

Foramen magnum

INFERIOR VIEW

Cleft Lip and Cleft Palate

Cleft lip and cleft palate occur during early fetal development. Cleft lip is either unilateral or bilateral, occurring along the premaxillary suture. Cleft lip is rarely midline, but it can involve soft tissue alone or include a cleft of the maxilla up to the incisive foramen. Cleft palate can involve both hard and soft palates.

Cleft lip results from a failure of embryonic facial and labial tissue to fuse during development. It is assumed that tissues migrate and develop normally, but for some reason either fail to fuse or the fusion of the migrating medial nasal, maxillary, and lateral nasal processes breaks down. Cleft palate apparently results from some mechanical intervention in development. Prior to the seventh embryonic week, the palatine processes of the maxillae have been resting alongside the tongue so the tongue separates the processes. As the oral cavity and mandible grow, the tongue drops away from the processes, and the processes can extend, make midline contact, and fuse. If something blocks the movement of the tongue (such as micrognathia), the palatine processes will not move in time to make contact. The head grows rapidly, and the plates will have missed their chance to become an intact palate.

bone is extremely dense and is remarkably rich in important landmarks (see Figure 4–19). This complex bone is divided into four segments: the squamous, tympanic, mastoid, and petrous portions. The *squamous portion* is fan-shaped and thin. The lower margin includes the roof of the *external auditory meatus*, the conduit for sound energy to the middle ear. The *zygomatic process* also arises from the squamous portion, forming part of the *zygomatic arch* (not shown). Beneath the base of the zygomatic process is the *mandibular fossa* of the temporal bone with which the condyloid process of the mandible articulates.

The *mastoid portion* is the posterior part of the temporal bone. Air cells deep within the mastoid portion communicate with the *tympanic antrum*. Above the antrum is the *tegmen tympani*, a thin plate of bone, and medial to it is the *lateral semicircular canal*. On the anterior surface of the temporal bone is the *mastoid process*, which arises from the *mastoid portion*. The *tympanic portion* of the temporal bone includes the anterior and inferior walls of the external auditory meatus (or ear canal). The *styloid process* protrudes beneath the external auditory meatus and medial to the mastoid process. The *petrous portion* includes the *cochlea* and *semicircular canals*.

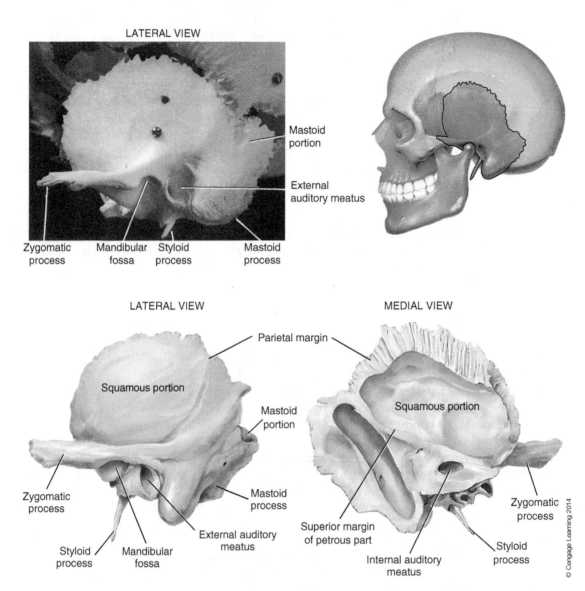

LATERAL VIEW

Mastoid
portion

External
auditory meatus

Zygomatic
process

Mandibular
fossa

Styloid
process

Mastoid
process

LATERAL VIEW

MEDIAL VIEW

Squamous portion

Parietal margin

Mastoid
portion

Squamous portion

Zygomatic
process

Mastoid
process

Zygomatic
process

Styloid
process

Mandibular
fossa

External auditory
meatus

Superior margin
of petrous part

Internal auditory
meatus

Styloid
process

© Cengage Learning 2014

Figure 4–19. Schematic drawing and photograph of lateral view of the temporal bone.

The *temporal fossa* is a region that includes a portion of the temporal, parietal, and occipital bones, and is the point of origin of the fan-shaped temporalis muscle used for mastication (chewing). The medial surface of the temporal bone reveals the *internal auditory meatus* through which the eighth cranial nerve passes on its way to the brainstem.

Summary

- The mandible provides the lower dental arch, alveolar region, and the resting location for the tongue.
- The maxillae provide the hard palate, point of attachment for the soft palate, alveolar ridge, upper dental arch, and dominant structures of the nasal cavities.
- The midline vomer articulates with the perpendicular plate of ethmoid and the cartilaginous septum to form the nasal septum.
- The zygomatic bone articulates with the frontal bone and maxillae to form the cheekbone. The small nasal bones provide the upper margin of the nasal cavity.
- The ethmoid bone serves as the core of the skull and face, with the prominent crista galli protruding into the cranium and the perpendicular plate dividing the nasal cavities.
- The frontal, parietal, temporal, and occipital bones of the skull overlie the lobes of the brain of the same names.
- The sphenoid bone has a marked presence in the braincase, with the prominent greater and lesser wings of sphenoid lateral to the corpus.
- The hypophyseal fossa houses the pituitary gland.

DENTITION

The teeth are vital components of the speech mechanism. Housed in the alveoli of the maxillae and mandible, teeth provide the mechanism for mastication, as well as articulatory surfaces for several speech sounds. Before we discuss the specific teeth, let us begin with an orientation to the dental arch. The upper and lower dental arches contain equal numbers of teeth of four types: incisors, cuspids, bicuspids, and molars (Figure 4–20 and Table 4–2).

Generally, teeth in the upper arch are larger than those in the lower arch, and the upper arch typically overlaps the lower arch in front. Each tooth has a *root* and *crown* (see Figure 4–20).

(A)

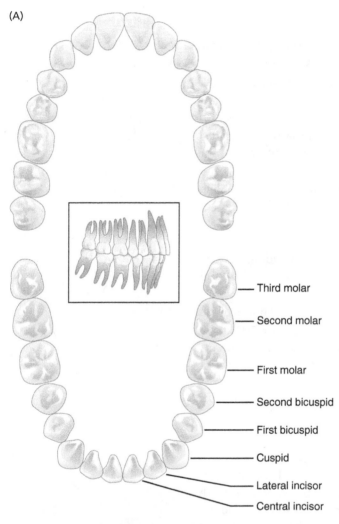

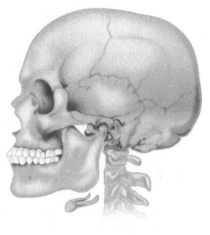

Third molar

Second molar

First molar

Second bicuspid

First bicuspid

Cuspid

Lateral incisor

Central incisor

© Cengage Learning 2014

Figure 4–20. (A) Permanent dental arches.
(continues)

Figure 4–20. continued
(B) Anterior and lateral views of normal adult dental arch. (C) Anterior and lateral views of deciduous dental arch. (D) Dental arch of child with significant oromyofunctional disorder. Note significant the marked labioversion of the incisors. (E) Deciduous dental arch of child with significant oromyofunctional disorder. Note significant cross-bite, open bite, and malocclusion.

(B)
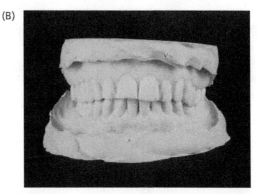

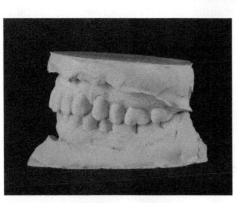
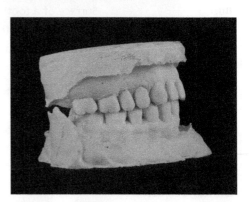

(C)
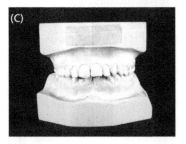
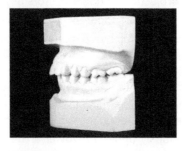
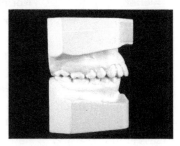

(D)
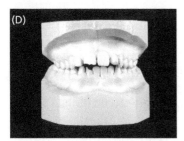
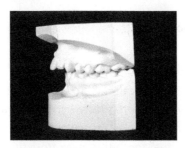
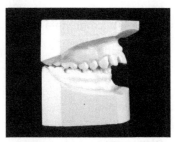

(E)
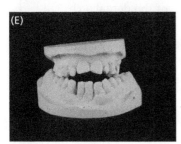
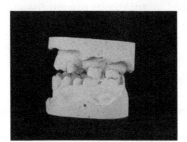
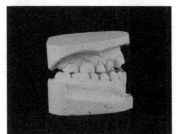

Table 4–2. Terms Related to Dentition

Term	Meaning
Surfaces	
Medial/mesial	Surface of individual tooth closest to midline point on arch between central incisors
Distal	Surface of individual tooth most distant from midline point on arch between central incisors
Buccal	Surface of a tooth that could come in contact with the buccal wall
Lingual	Surface of a tooth that could come in contact with the tongue
Occlusal	The contact surface between teeth of the upper and lower arches
Development	
Intraosseous eruption	Eruption of teeth through the alveolar process
Clinical eruption	Eruption of teeth into the oral cavity
Successional teeth	Teeth that replace deciduous teeth
Superadded teeth	Teeth in the adult arch not present within the deciduous arch
Supernumerary teeth	Teeth in excess of the normal number for an arch
Dental Occlusion	
Overjet	Normal projection of upper incisors beyond lower incisors
Overbite	Normal overlap of upper incisors relative to lower incisors
Class I occlusal relationship	Relationship between upper and lower teeth in which the first molar of the mandibular arch is one-half tooth advanced of the maxillary molar
Class I malocclusion	Occlusal relationship in which there is normal orientation of the molars but an abnormal orientation of the incisors
Class II malocclusion	Relationship of upper and lower arches in which the first mandibular molars are retracted at least one tooth from the first maxillary molars
Class III malocclusion	Relationship of upper and lower arches in which the first mandibular molar is advanced greater than one tooth beyond the first maxillary molar
Relative micrognathia	Condition in which mandible is small in relation to the maxillae
Axial Orientation	
Torsiversion	An individual tooth is rotated or twisted on its long axis
Labioversion	An individual tooth tilts toward the lips
Linguaversion	An individual tooth tilts toward the tongue
Buccoversion	An individual tooth tilts toward cheek
Distoversion	An individual tooth tilts away from midline of dental arch
Mesioversion	An individual tooth tilts toward the midline of the dental arch
Infraversion	A tooth is inadequately erupted
Supraversion	A tooth protrudes excessively into the oral cavity, causing inadequate occlusion of other dentition
Persistent open bite	Front teeth do not occlude because of excessive eruption of posterior teeth
Persistent closed bite	Posterior teeth do not occlude because of excessive eruption of anterior dentition

Craniosynostosis

As an infant develops, the sutures of the skull become ossified, a process called synostosis. Complete synostosis normally occurs well into childhood, but in some instances synostosis occurs prenatally. Continued normal growth of the brain, especially during the first postnatal year, places pressure on the skull. The effects of premature synostosis on skull development, or craniosynostosis, are profound. With premature sagittal synostosis, the child's head becomes peaked along the suture and elongated in back. In Apert syndrome, a genetic condition, the affected child's stereotypic "peaked head" is the result of premature closure of the coronal suture, resulting in pronounced bulging along that articulation.

Five surfaces are important to remember when discussing teeth. To understand the terminology you need to alter your thinking about the dental arch a bit. Examine Figure 4–21 and you will see that the center of the dental arch is the point between the two central incisors, in front. Follow the arch around toward the molars in back and you have traced a path distal to those incisors. That is, *medial* refers to movement along the arch toward the midline between the central incisors, and *distal* refers to movement along the arch away from that midpoint. From this you can see that the *medial*, or *mesial, surface* of any tooth is the surface "looking" along the arch toward the midpoint between the central incisors. The *distal surface* is the surface of any tooth that is farthest from that midline point. Every tooth has a medial and a distal surface. The *buccal surface* of a tooth is that which could come in contact with the buccal wall (cheek), and the *lingual surface* is the surface facing the tongue. The *occlusal*

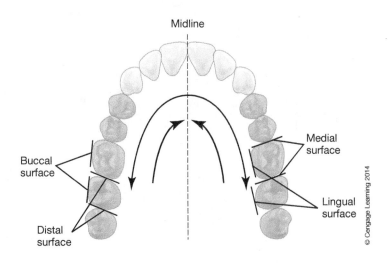

Figure 4–21. Surface referents of teeth and the dental arch.

surface is the contact surface between teeth of the upper and lower arches. Not surprisingly, the thickest enamel overlays the occlusal surface because it receives the most abrasion.

Incisors clearly are designed for cutting, as their name implies. The *central incisors* of the upper dental arch present a large, spadelike tooth with a thin cutting surface. The *lateral incisors* present a smaller but similar surface.

The *cuspid* (see Figure 4–22) (also canine; eyetooth) is well named. It has a single *cusp*, or point, that is used for tearing. In carnivores this tooth is particularly well suited for separating the fibers of muscle to permit meat eating. Lateral to the cuspids are the *first* and *second bicuspids*, or *premolars*. These teeth have two cusps on the occlusal surface, and they are absent from the deciduous dental arch.

Molars are large teeth with great occlusal surfaces designed to grind material, and their placement in the posterior arch capitalizes on the significant force available in the muscles of mastication. This mix of cutting teeth (incisors, cuspids, bicuspids) and grinding teeth (molars) is just right for *omnivorous* humans: We will eat virtually anything! There are three molars in each half of the adult dental arch.

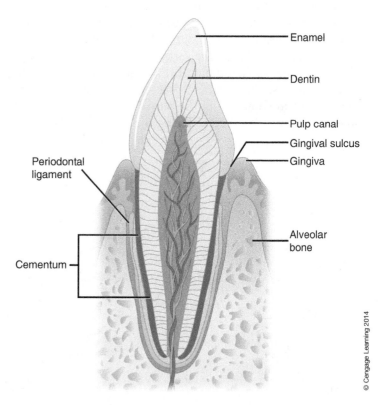

Enamel

Dentin

Pulp canal

Gingival sulcus

Gingiva

Periodontal ligament

Alveolar bone

Cementum

© Cengage Learning 2014

Figure 4–22. Components of a tooth.

Dental Development

Dental development clearly parallels that of the individual. Infants develop **deciduous**, or **shedding, teeth** (also known as milk teeth) that give way to the *permanent teeth* that must last a lifetime. Not only are deciduous teeth much smaller than adult teeth but there are fewer of them. You will notice that in deciduous teeth there is no third molar or first or second bicuspid. These teeth are reserved for the adult arch. Each deciduous arch has 10 teeth, whereas the adult arch has 16 (see Figure 4–23).

Your first-grade school photograph will remind you of the period during which *shedding* begins. That gap-toothed grin of the 6-year-old child comes from shedding of the deciduous arch, beginning with the incisors (6 through 9 years), followed by first molars and cuspids (9 to 12 years), and finally second molars (beginning around 10 years of age).

deciduous (shedding) teeth: *The primary set of teeth.*

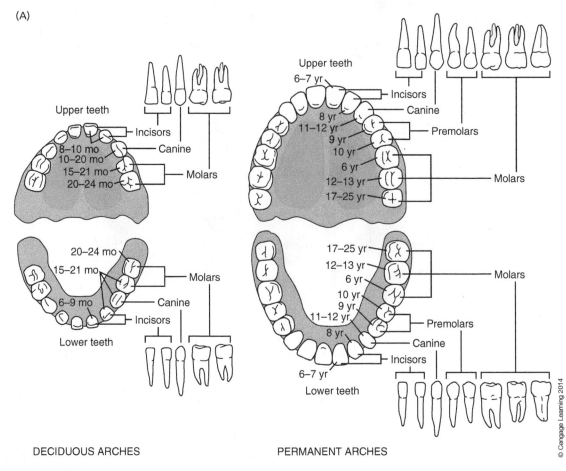

(A)

DECIDUOUS ARCHES   PERMANENT ARCHES

© Cengage Learning 2014

Figure 4–23. (A) Age of eruption of teeth in the permanent and deciduous arches. *(continues)*

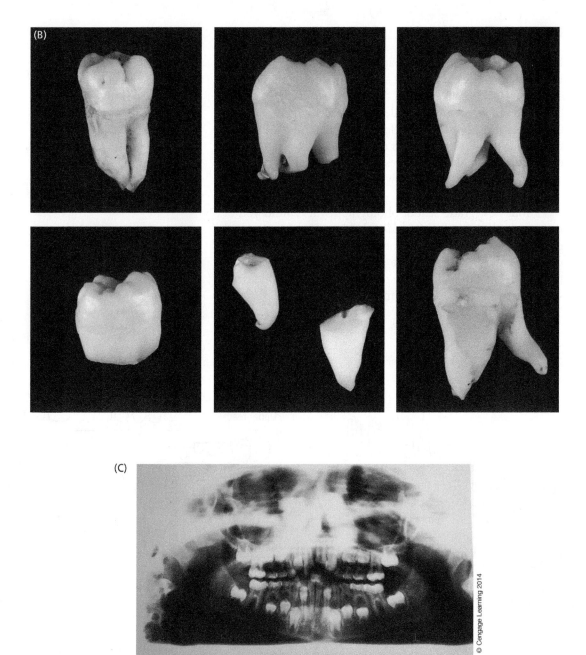

Figure 4–23. continued (B) Individual deciduous and permanent teeth. Top row: adult third molars; bottom row, left to right: deciduous molar, deciduous cuspids, deciduous molar. (C) Pantograph of mixed dentition. Note the presence of unerupted permanent teeth within the maxilla and mandible.

© Cengage Learning 2014

Dental Anomalies

There are numerous developmental dental anomalies. Children may be born with supernumerary teeth (teeth in addition to the normal number), or teeth may be smaller than appropriate for the dental arch (microdontia). Teeth may fuse together at the root or crown. In addition, enamel may be extremely thin or even missing from the surface of the tooth (amelogenesis imperfecta), or the enamel may be stained from excessive use of the antibiotic tetracycline or fluoride.

Supernumerary teeth arise from a developmental anomaly in which the embryonic dental lamina produces excessive numbers of tooth buds. When this occurs, the individual is born with more teeth than predicted, often resulting in "twinning" of incisors. Below is a report from J. M. Harris, D.D.S., of a child he saw in his dental practice in Idaho Falls, Idaho.

> An 8-year-old girl was brought to Dr. Harris's clinic with the complaint that one of her deciduous teeth needed to be extracted due to the patient's age. Dr. Harris performed panelipse radiography to verify that the permanent teeth were present prior to the extraction, but the X ray revealed supernumerary teeth in the left mandibular arch in the bicuspid region.
>
> Extraction of the decayed deciduous tooth revealed a pocket of 15 supernumerary teeth: Some were simply tooth buds, but some had developed small roots and looked like fully formed molars. In an arch built ultimately for 16 teeth, that would be a significant addition!
>
> The cluster was removed, Gelfoam was placed in the cavity, and sutures closed the space. There were no complications.

The permanent teeth that replace deciduous teeth are called **successional teeth**. The third molar and bicuspids erupt in addition to the original constellation, and thus are referred to as *superadded*.

successional teeth: *Teeth in the mature dental arch that replace corresponding teeth of the deciduous arch.*

Dental Occlusion

Occlusion is the process of bringing the upper and lower teeth into contact, and proper occlusion is essential for successful mastication. A **Class I occlusal relationship** between your upper and lower teeth is that in which the first molar of the mandibular arch is one-half tooth advanced of the first maxillary molar. The upper incisors project beyond the lower incisors vertically by a few millimeters (**overjet**), and the upper incisors naturally hide the lower incisors (overbite) so that only a little of the lower teeth will show. This Class I occlusion (also known as **neutroclusion**) (see Figure 4–24) is the normal relationship between the molars of the dental arches. Extreme overbite, however, can be clinically significant.

occlusion: *Closing.*

Class I occlusal relationship (neutroclusion): *The normal occlusal relationship characterized by the maxillary and mandibular molar relationship in which the maxillary first molar is retracted one-half tooth relative to the mandibular first molar.*

overjet: *Condition of normal dentition in which the upper incisors project beyond the lower incisors.*

neutroclusion: *The normal occlusal relationship characterized by the maxillary and mandibular molar relationship in which the maxillary first molar is retracted one-half tooth relative to the mandibular first molar.*

Class II malocclusion: *The occlusal relationship characterized by the maxillary and mandibular molar relationship in which the maxillary first molar is retracted at least one tooth relative to the mandibular first molar.*

Class III malocclusion: *The occlusal relationship characterized by the maxillary and mandibular molar relationship in which the maxillary first molar is advanced at least one tooth relative to the mandibular first molar.*

torsiversion: *Twisted on the long axis.*

labioversion: *Tilted toward the lip.*

linguaversion: *Tilted toward the tongue.*

buccoversion: *Tilted toward the cheek.*

distoversion: *Tilted away from the midline of the dental arch.*

mesioversion: *Tilted toward the midline of the dental arch.*

infraversion: *Inadequate eruption relative to the other teeth in the arch.*

supraversion: *Excessive eruption relative to the majority of teeth in the arch.*

persistent open bite: *Anterior dentition fails to occlude properly as a result of supraversion of the posterior teeth.*

persistent closed bite: *Posterior dentition fails to occlude properly as a result of supraversion of the anterior teeth.*

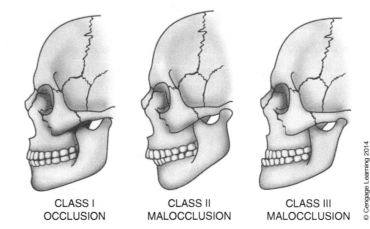

CLASS I OCCLUSION   CLASS II MALOCCLUSION   CLASS III MALOCCLUSION

© Cengage Learning 2014

Figure 4–24. Types of malocclusion.

In **Class II malocclusion**, the first mandibular molars are retracted at least one tooth behind the first maxillary molars. A **Class III malocclusion** is identified if the first mandibular molar is advanced farther than one tooth ahead of the first maxillary molar. If a tooth is rotated or twisted on its long axis, it has undergone **torsiversion**. If it tilts toward the lips, it is as **labioverted**, whereas tilting toward the tongue is **linguaverted** (see Figure 4–25). When molars tilt toward the cheeks, it is called **buccoversion**. A tooth that tilts away from the midline along the arch is **distoverted**, whereas one tilting toward that midline between the two central incisors is **mesioverted**. When a tooth does not erupt sufficiently to make occlusal contact with its pair in the opposite arch it is **infraverted**, whereas the tooth that erupts too far is **supraverted**. In some cases the front teeth do not demonstrate the proper occlusion because teeth in the posterior arch prohibit anterior contact, which is termed **persistent open bite**. If supraversion prohibits the posterior teeth from occlusion, it is called **persistent closed bite**.

Summary

- The teeth are housed in the alveoli of the maxillae and mandible and they consist of incisors, cuspids, bicuspids, and molars.

- Each tooth has a root and crown, with the surface of the crown composed of enamel overlying dentin.

- Each tooth has a medial (or mesial), distal, lingual, buccal (or labial), and occlusal surface, and the occlusal surface reflects the function of the teeth in the omnivorous human dental arch.

- Class I occlusion refers to normal orientation of mandible and maxillae; Class II malocclusion refers to a

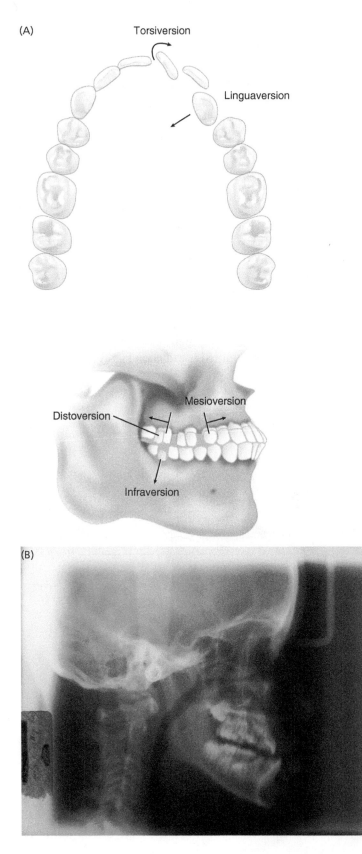

(A)

Torsiversion

Linguaversion

Distoversion

Mesioversion

Infraversion

(B)

Figure 4–25. (A) Graphic representation of torsiversion, linguaversion, infraversion, distoversion, and mesioversion. (B) Radiograph of prognathic mandible that was later surgically corrected.

239

relatively retracted mandible; and Class III malocclusion refers to a relatively protruded mandible.

- Individual teeth may have aberrant orientation in the alveolus, including torsiversion, labioversion, linguaversion, distoversion, and mesioversion.
- Inadequately erupted or hypererupted teeth are referred to as infraverted and supraverted.

CAVITIES OF THE VOCAL TRACT

We mentioned that the source-filter theory depends on cavities to shape the acoustic output. Before we show you the muscles associated with articulation, let us discuss the cavities that are shaped by moving those muscles. These are the oral, buccal, nasal, and pharyngeal cavities (see Figure 4–26).

The *oral cavity* extends from the oral opening, or mouth, in front to the *faucial pillars* (also *fauces, faucial arches*) in back. The oral opening is strongly involved in articulation, being the point of exit of sound for all orally emitted phonemes (i.e., all sounds except those emitted nasally: see Figure 4–27).

(A)

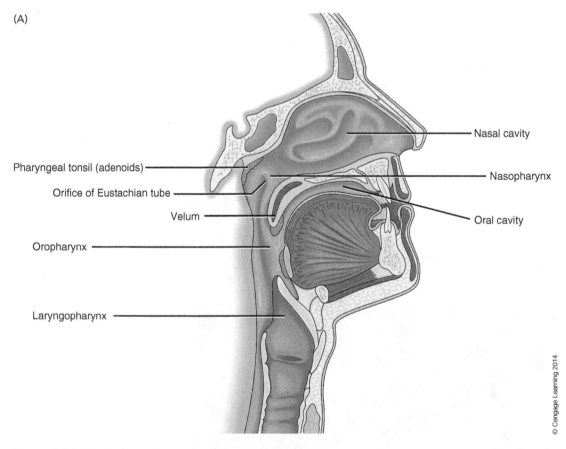

Figure 4–26. (A) Oral, nasal, and pharyngeal cavities.   *(continues)*

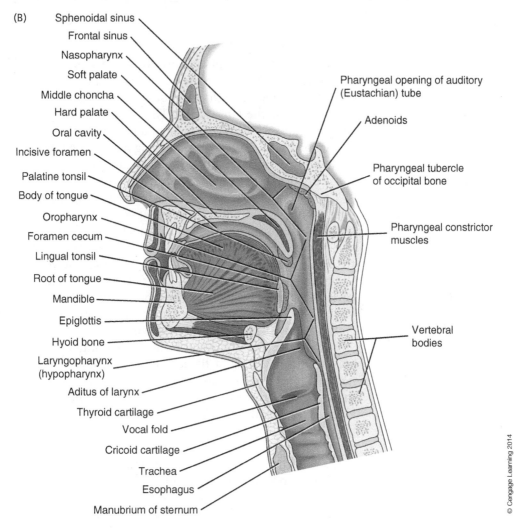

(B)

Sphenoidal sinus
Frontal sinus
Nasopharynx
Soft palate
Middle choncha
Hard palate
Oral cavity
Incisive foramen
Palatine tonsil
Body of tongue
Oropharynx
Foramen cecum
Lingual tonsil
Root of tongue
Mandible
Epiglottis
Hyoid bone
Laryngopharynx
(hypopharynx)
Aditus of larynx
Thyroid cartilage
Vocal fold
Cricoid cartilage
Trachea
Esophagus
Manubrium of sternum

Pharyngeal opening of auditory
(Eustachian) tube
Adenoids
Pharyngeal tubercle
of occipital bone
Pharyngeal constrictor
muscles
Vertebral
bodies

© Cengage Learning 2014

Figure 4–26. continued (B) Detail of structures and cavities.

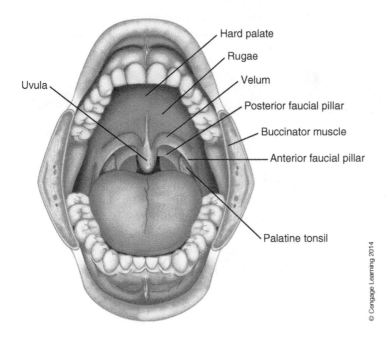

Uvula

Hard palate
Rugae
Velum
Posterior faucial pillar
Buccinator muscle
Anterior faucial pillar

Palatine tonsil

© Cengage Learning 2014

Figure 4–27. Anterior view of
oral cavity.

241

This is a good opportunity to take a guided tour of your own mouth. Palpate the roof of your mouth (you can use your tongue to feel this if you wish). The hard roof of your mouth is the *hard palate*. The prominent ridges running laterally are the *rugae*, potentially useful structures in formation of the **bolus** of food during deglutition (swallowing) and serving as a landmark in articulation. The *median raphe* divides the hard palate into halves.

bolus: *A mass of masticated food ready to be swallowed.*

As you run your tongue or finger back along the roof of your mouth, you can feel the point at which the hard palate suddenly becomes soft. This is the juncture of the hard and soft palate. The soft portion is the *soft palate*, or *velum*, with the *uvula* marking the terminus of the velum. The velum is the movable muscle mass that separates the oral and nasal cavities (or more technically, the oropharynx and nasopharynx). The velum is attached in front to the palatine bone and is thus a muscular extension of the hard palate.

On each side of the soft palate and continuous with it are prominent bands of tissue. These are the *anterior* and *posterior faucial pillars* (also *posterior faucial arches*), and they mark the posterior margin of the oral cavity. The teeth and alveolar ridge of the maxillae make up the lateral margins of the oral cavity. The tongue occupies most of the lower mouth.

Between the anterior and posterior faucial pillars you may see the *palatine tonsils*. These masses of lymphoid tissue are situated between the pillars on each side and even invade the lateral undersurface of the soft palate. Medial to these tonsils, on the surface of the tongue, are the *lingual tonsils*.

The *buccal cavity* lies lateral to the oral cavity, composed of the space between the posterior teeth and the cheeks of the face. It is bounded by the cheeks laterally, the lips in front, and the teeth medially. The posterior margin is at the third molar.

Eustachian Tube Development

The eustachian tube is the communicative port between the nasopharynx and the middle ear cavity. It is opened during deglutition and yawning and provides a means of aeration of the middle ear cavity. In the adult, the eustachian tube courses down at an angle of about 45°. In the infant, the tube is more horizontal, with the shift in angle of descent brought about by head growth. It is thought that this horizontal course in the infant contributes to middle ear disease, the assumption being that liquids and bacteria have a low-resistance path to the middle ear from the nasopharynx of an infant being bottle-fed in the supine position.

Although the oral cavity is fairly easy to view and palpate, only a small portion of the pharyngeal cavity is. The *pharyngeal cavity*, or pharynx, is broken into the oropharynx, laryngopharyx, and nasopharynx. The *oropharynx* is the portion of the pharynx immediately posterior to the fauces and bounded above by the velum. The lower boundary of the oropharynx is the hyoid bone. The *laryngopharynx* is bounded anteriorly by the epiglottis and inferiorly by the esophagus. The third pharyngeal space is the *nasopharynx*, the space above the soft palate. It is bounded in back by the pharyngeal protuberance of the occipital bone and in front by the nasal *choanae*. The lateral nasopharyngeal wall contains the orifice of the *eustachian*, or *auditory, tube*.

Although minute, the eustachian tube serves an extremely important function in that it provides a means of aerating the middle ear cavity. Recognize that the nasopharynx is on a level with the ears, so that the tube connecting the nasopharynx with the middle ear space must course slightly up, back, and out to reach that cavity. The eustachian tube is actively opened through contraction of the tensor veli palatini muscle, as will be discussed.

Also in the nasopharynx is the pharyngeal tonsil (also known as adenoids). This mass of lymphoid tissue typically is found to arise from the base of the posterior nasopharynx. Removal of the adenoids from children with short or hypotrophied soft palates may result in persistent hypernasality.

The final cavities of concern to articulation are the nasal cavities (see Figure 4–28). The nasal cavities are produced by the paired maxillae, palatine, and nasal bones, and are divided by the nasal septum (made up of the singular vomer bone, the perpendicular plate of ethmoid, and the cartilaginous septum). The nasal cavities and turbinates are covered with mucous membrane endowed with beating and secreting epithelia, as well as a rich vascular supply. Air entering the nasal cavities is quickly warmed and humidified to protect the lungs, and fine nasal hairs help prevent particulate matter from entering the lower respiratory passageway. Beating epithelia propel encapsulated pollutants toward the nasopharynx, from which point they slowly work their way toward the esophagus, to be swallowed (a much better fate than to be deposited in the lungs).

The **nares**, or nostrils, mark the anterior boundaries of the nasal cavities, and the nasal choanae are the posterior portals connecting the nasopharynx and nasal cavities. The floor of the nasal cavity is the hard palate of the oral cavity, specifically the palatine processes of maxillae and horizontal plates of the palatine bones.

nares: *Nostrils.*

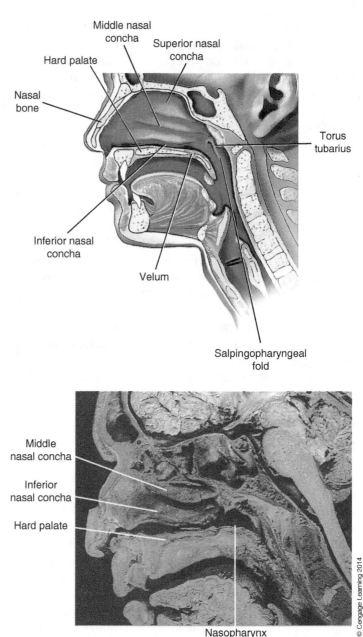

Figure 4–28. Nasal cavity and nasopharynx.

Summary

- The most posterior oral cavity is the vertically directed pharynx, made up of the laryngopharynx, oropharynx, and nasopharynx.
- The horizontally coursing tube representing the nasal cavities arises from the nasopharynx, with the nasal and nasopharyngeal regions entirely separated from the oral cavity by elevation of the soft palate.

- The large tube representing the oral cavity is flanked by the small buccal cavities.
- The shape and size of the oral cavity is altered through movement of the tongue and mandible, and the nasal cavity may be coupled with the oral/pharyngeal cavities by means of the velum.
- The shape of the pharyngeal cavity is altered primarily by use of the pharyngeal constrictor muscles and by elevation or depression of the larynx.

Let us now examine the muscles involved in the articulatory system.

MUSCLES OF THE ARTICULATORY SYSTEM

The articulatory system is dominated by three significant structures: the lips, the tongue, and the velum. Movement of the lips for speech is a product of the muscles of the face. The tongue capitalizes on its own musculature and that of the mandible and hyoid for its movement. The muscles of the velum elevate that structure to separate the oral and nasal regions. Table 4–3 may assist you in organizing the muscles of the face and mouth, while Figure 4–29 will help you recognize their functions.

Muscles of the Face

The lips form the focus of the facial muscles; their movement largely determines their function in both facial expression and speech (see Figure 4–30). The lips comprise muscle and mucous membrane that is richly invested with vascular supply, a trait made apparent by the translucent superficial epithelia.

The *orbicularis oris* is really two muscles, the upper orbicularis oris and the lower orbicularis oris. The upper and lower orbicularis oris muscles act much like a drawstring to pull the lips together and effect a labial seal. Both upper and lower orbicularis oris muscles are innervated by the seventh cranial, or facial, nerve.

The upper and lower orbicularis oris serves as the point of insertion for many other muscles and interacts with the muscles of the face to produce the wide variety of facial gestures of which we are capable. The muscles inserting into the orbicularis oris have different effects, based on their course and point of insertion into the lips. The *risorius* and *buccinator* muscles insert into the corners of the mouth and retract the lips. The *depressor labii inferioris* depresses the lower lip, and the *levator labii superioris, zygomatic minor,*

Table 4–3. Muscles of Articulation

Muscles of the Face

Orbicularis oris
Risorius
Buccinator
Levator labii superioris muscle
Zygomatic minor muscle
Levator labii superioris alaeque nasi muscle

Levator anguli oris muscle
Zygomatic major muscle
Depressor labii inferioris muscle
Depressor anguli oris muscle
Mentalis
Platysma

Muscles of the Mouth

The Tongue

Intrinsic Tongue Muscles
Superior longitudinal muscle of tongue
Inferior longitudinal muscle of tongue
Transverse muscle of tongue
Vertical muscle of tongue

Extrinsic Tongue Muscles
Genioglossus muscle
Hyoglossus muscle
Styloglossus muscle
Chondroglossus muscle
Palatoglossus muscle

Muscles of Mastication

Mandibular Elevators
Masseter
Temporalis muscle
Medial pterygoid muscle

Mandibular Depressors
Digastricus muscle
Mylohyoid muscle

Geniohyoid muscle
Platysma

Mandibular Protrusion
Lateral pterygoid muscle

Muscles of the the Soft Palate

Levator veli palatini muscle
Musculus uvulae
Tensor veli palatini muscle

Palatoglossus muscle
Palatopharyngeus muscle

Pharyngeal Musculature
Superior pharyngeal constrictor
Middle pharyngeal constrictor
Inferior pharyngeal constrictor
Cricopharyngeal muscle

Thyropharyngeus muscle
Salpingopharyngeus muscle
Stylopharyngeus muscle

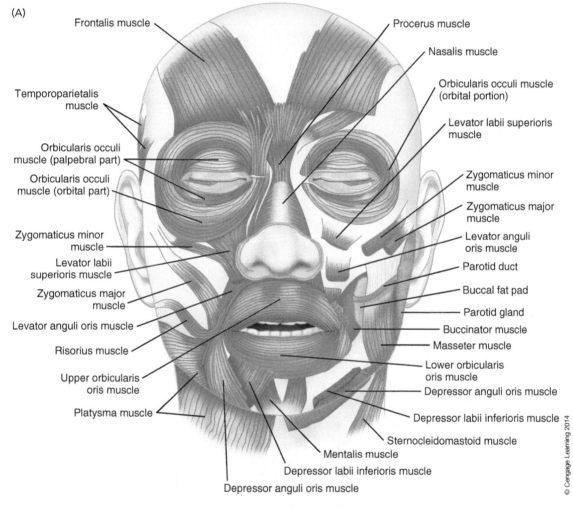

(A)

Frontalis muscle

Procerus muscle

Nasalis muscle

Orbicularis occuli muscle
(orbital portion)

Temporoparietalis
muscle

Levator labii superioris
muscle

Orbicularis occuli
muscle (palpebral part)

Zygomaticus minor
muscle

Orbicularis occuli
muscle (orbital part)

Zygomaticus major
muscle

Levator anguli
oris muscle

Zygomaticus minor
muscle

Parotid duct

Levator labii
superioris muscle

Buccal fat pad

Zygomaticus major
muscle

Parotid gland

Levator anguli oris muscle

Buccinator muscle

Risorius muscle

Masseter muscle

Upper orbicularis
oris muscle

Lower orbicularis
oris muscle

Depressor anguli oris muscle

Platysma muscle

Depressor labii inferioris muscle

Sternocleidomastoid muscle

Mentalis muscle

Depressor labii inferioris muscle

Depressor anguli oris muscle

Figure 4–29. (A) Muscles of the face.

(continues)

© Cengage Learning 2014

247

(B)

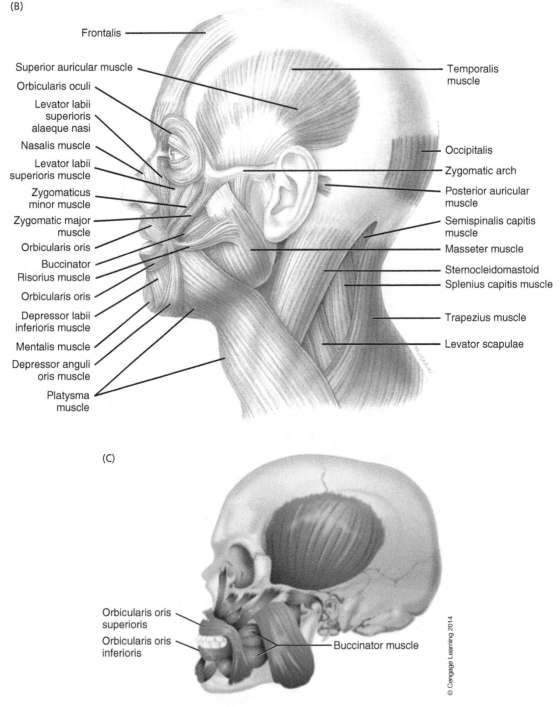

Frontalis

Superior auricular muscle

Orbicularis oculi

Levator labii superioris alaeque nasi

Nasalis muscle

Levator labii superioris muscle

Zygomaticus minor muscle

Zygomatic major muscle

Orbicularis oris

Buccinator

Risorius muscle

Orbicularis oris

Depressor labii inferioris muscle

Mentalis muscle

Depressor anguli oris muscle

Platysma muscle

Temporalis muscle

Occipitalis

Zygomatic arch

Posterior auricular muscle

Semispinalis capitis muscle

Masseter muscle

Sternocleidomastoid

Splenius capitis muscle

Trapezius muscle

Levator scapulae

(C)

Orbicularis oris superioris

Orbicularis oris inferioris

Buccinator muscle

© Cengage Learning 2014

Figure 4–29. continued (B) Lateral view of facial muscles. (C) Relationship among facial muscles and pharyngeal constrictor muscles. Note that the orbicularis oris muscles are continuous with the buccinator muscle and ultimately with the superior pharyngeal constrictor.

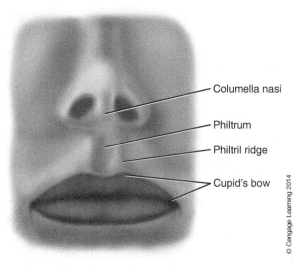

Columella nasi

Philtrum

Philtril ridge

Cupid's bow

© Cengage Learning 2014

Figure 4–30. Landmarks of the lips.

and *levator labii superioris alaeque nasi* muscles elevate the upper lip. The *zygomatic major* muscle elevates and retracts the lips, whereas the *depressor anguli oris* depresses the corner of the mouth. The *levator anguli oris* pulls the corner of the mouth up and medially.

The *buccinator muscle* ("bugler's muscle") lies deep to the risorius, following a parallel course. It originates on the *pterygomandibular ligament*, a tendinous slip running from the hamulus of the internal pterygoid plate of the sphenoid to the posterior mylohyoid line of the inner mandible. The posterior fibers are continuous with those of the superior pharyngeal constrictor. The buccinator courses forward to insert into the upper and lower orbicularis oris.

The buccinator, like the risorius, is involved primarily in mastication. The buccinator is used to move food onto the grinding surfaces of the molars, and contraction of this muscle tends to constrict the oropharynx. The risorius and buccinator are innervated by the facial nerve. The risorius muscle is superficial to the buccinator, originating from the posterior region of the face along the fascia of the masseter muscle. Besides assisting in mastication, the risorius muscles retract the lips at the corners, facilitating smiling.

The *levator labii superioris, zygomatic minor*, and *levator labii superioris alaeque nasi* share a point of insertion into the mid-lateral region of the upper lip. The three hold the major responsibility for elevation of the upper lip. The levator labii superioris alaeque nasi arises from the frontal process of maxilla, the levator labii superioris arises from the infraorbital margin of the maxilla, and the zygomatic minor arises from the zygomatic bone. Working together, these muscles dilate the oral opening, and fibers from the levator labii superioris alaeque nasi that insert into the wing of the nostril can flare the nasal opening. The levator labii superioris, zygomatic minor, and levator labii superioris alaeque nasi are innervated by the facial nerve.

The *levator anguli oris* arises from the canine fossa of the maxilla, coursing to insert into the upper and lower lips. This muscle is hidden by the levator labii superioris. The levator anguli oris draws the corner of the mouth up and medial. The levator anguli oris is innervated by the facial nerve.

The *zygomatic major* muscle arises lateral to the *zygomatic minor* on the zygomatic bone and inserts into the corner of the orbicularis oris. The zygomatic major elevates and retracts the angle of the mouth, as in smiling. The zygomatic major muscle is innervated by the buccal branches of the facial nerve.

The *depressor labii inferioris* originates from the mandible at the oblique line, coursing up and into the lower lip. Contraction of the depressor labii inferioris dilates the orifice of the mouth by pulling the lips down and out. The depressor labii inferioris is innervated by the facial nerve.

The *depressor anguli oris* originates along the lateral margins of the mandible on the oblique line. Its fanlike fibers converge on the orbicularis oris and upper lip at the corner. Contraction of the depressor anguli oris depresses the corners of the mouth and helps compress the upper lip against the lower lip. The depressor anguli oris is innervated by the facial nerve.

The *mentalis muscle* arises from the region of the incisive fossa of the mandible, inserting into the skin of the chin below. Contraction of the mentalis elevates and wrinkles the chin and pulls the lower lip out. The mentalis receives its innervation by means of facial nerve.

The *platysma* is more typically considered a muscle of the neck, but it is discussed here because of its function as a mandibular depressor. The platysma arises from the fascia overlying the pectoralis major and deltoid, coursing up and into the corner of the mouth, the region below the symphysis menti, and the lower margin of the mandible, fanning as well to insert into the skin near the masseter. The platysma is highly variable but appears to assist in depression of the mandible. The platysma is innervated by the facial nerve.

Summary

- Numerous muscles insert into the orbicularis oris inferior and superior muscles, providing a flexible system for lip protrusion, closure, retraction, elevation, and depression.

- The risorius and buccinator muscles assist in retraction of the lips.
- Contraction of the levator labii superioris, zygomatic minor, and levator labii superioris alaeque nasi elevate the upper lip, and contraction of the depressor labii inferioris depresses the lower lip.
- Contraction of the zygomatic major muscle elevates and retracts the corner of the mouth, and the depressor labii inferioris pulls the lips down and out.
- The depressor anguli oris muscle depresses the corner of the mouth, the mentalis muscle pulls the lower lip out, and the platysma depresses the mandible.

Muscles of the Mouth

Musculature of the mouth is dominated by intrinsic and extrinsic muscles of the tongue, as well as those responsible for elevation of the soft palate.

The Tongue

The *tongue* is a massive structure that occupies the floor of the mouth (see Figure 4–31). We divide the muscles of the tongue into intrinsic and extrinsic musculature. The extrinsic muscles move the tongue into the general region desired and the intrinsic muscles tend to provide the fine, graded control of the articulatory gesture. Aside from its role in speech, the tongue is involved primarily in mastication and deglutition, being responsible for movement of food within the oral cavity to position it for chewing and to propel it backward for swallowing.

The tongue is divided longitudinally by the *median fibrous septum*, a wall between right and left halves that serves as the point of origin for the transverse muscle of the

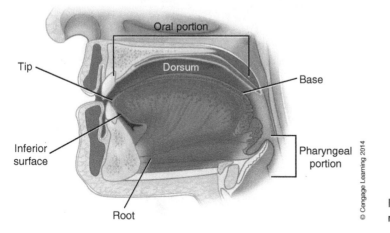

© Cengage Learning 2014

Figure 4–31. Demarcation of regions of the tongue.

tongue. The septum originates on the body of the hyoid bone via the *hyoglossal membrane*, forming the tongue attachment with the hyoid. The septum courses the length of the tongue.

It is useful to divide the tongue into regions as we discuss its characteristics (see Figure 4–32). The superior surface is the *dorsum*, and the anterior-most portion is the *tip*, or *apex*. The base of the tongue is the portion of the tongue that resides in the oropharynx. The portion of the tongue surface in the oral cavity is the *oral*, or *palatine, surface*, which makes up about two thirds of the surface of the tongue. The other third of the tongue surface, the *pharyngeal surface*, lies in the oropharynx.

Beneath the membranous lining of the pharyngeal surface of the tongue are *lingual tonsils*, groups of lymphoid tissue. Taken in conjunction with the pharyngeal and palatine tonsils, the lingual tonsils form the final portion of the ring of lymph tissue in the oral and pharyngeal cavities. Tonsils tend to *atrophy* (lose mass) over time. Although the pharyngeal and palatine tonsils may be quite prominent during childhood, they are markedly diminished by puberty.

The tongue is invested with sensors, or "taste buds." The tip of the tongue is sensitive to both sweet and sour tastes, and the sides of the tongue are sensitive only to sour tastes. Bitter tastes are sensed in the posterior tongue.

If you examine the inferior surface of your tongue in a mirror, you will see three important landmarks (see Figure 4–33). Notice the rich vascular supply on the undersurface. Medications administered under the tongue (sublingually) are absorbed very quickly into the bloodstream. The band of tissue running from the inner mandibular mucosa to the underside of the tongue is the *lingual frenulum*, or

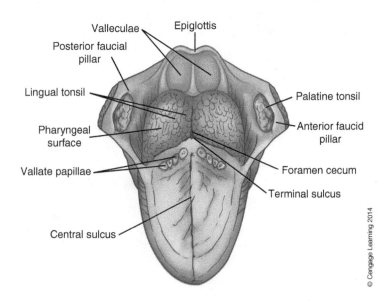

Figure 4–32. Landmarks of the tongue.

Valleculae
Epiglottis
Posterior faucial pillar
Lingual tonsil
Palatine tonsil
Pharyngeal surface
Anterior faucid pillar
Vallate papillae
Foramen cecum
Terminal sulcus
Central sulcus

© Cengage Learning 2014

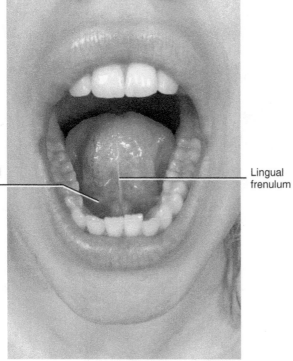

Sublingual folds

Lingual frenulum

© Cengage Learning 2014

Figure 4–33. Inferior surface of tongue.

lingual frenum. Notice also the transverse band of tissue on the sides of the tongue (the *sublingual fold*). At this point reside the ducts for the sublingual salivary glands. Lateral to the lingual frenulum are the ducts for the *submandibular salivary glands* that are hidden under the mucosa on the inner surface of the mandible.

Intrinsic Tongue Muscles. The intrinsic muscles of the tongue include two pairs of muscles running longitudinally, as well as muscles coursing transversely and vertically. The intrinsic muscles interact in a complex fashion to produce the rapid, delicate articulations for speech and nonspeech activities. As we discuss each muscle, we will tell you its basic function. Examination of Figure 4–34 will assist you in our discussion of these very important lingual muscles.

The paired *superior longitudinal muscles* course the length of the tongue, composing the upper layer of the tongue. These muscles originate from the fibrous submucous layer near the epiglottis, the hyoid, and from the median fibrous septum. The fibers fan forward and outward to insert into the lateral margins of the tongue and region of the apex. The superior longitudinal muscles elevate the tip of the tongue. If one superior longitudinal muscle is contracted without the other, it pulls the tongue toward the side of contraction.

LATERAL VIEW

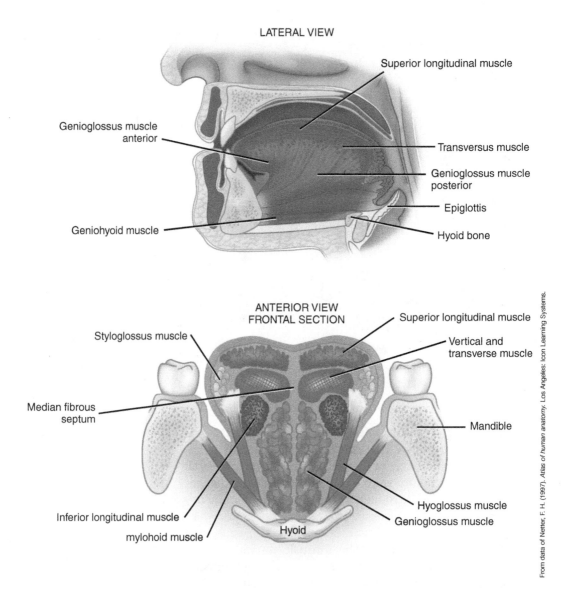

Figure 4–34. Intrinsic muscles of the tongue

The *inferior longitudinal muscle* originates at the root of the tongue and corpus hyoid, with fibers coursing to the apex of the tongue. This muscle occupies the lower sides of the tongue but is absent in the medial tongue base. The inferior longitudinal muscle pulls the tip of the tongue downward and assists in retraction of the tongue if co-contracted with the superior longitudinal. As with the superior longitudinal, unilateral contraction of the inferior longitudinal causes the tongue to turn toward the contracted side and downward.

The *transverse muscles of the tongue* provide a mechanism for narrowing the tongue. Fibers of these muscles

"Tongue Tie"

The lingual frenulum is a band of tissue that connects the tongue to the floor of the mouth. It appears to assist in stabilizing the tongue during movement, but occasionally it is too short for proper lingual function. This condition, colloquially referred to as "tongue tie," is termed *ankyloglossia*. Ankyloglossia results in difficulty elevating the tongue for phonemes that require palatal or alveolar contact. The tongue may appear heart-shaped when protruded, resulting from the excessive tension on the midline by the short frenulum. A surgical procedure to correct the condition might be useful, although the surgery is not minor.

Tongue Thrust

As with other motor functions, swallowing changes and matures as the organism develops. The immature swallow capitalizes on the needs of the moment. An infant needs to compress his or her mother's nipple to stimulate release of milk, so the tongue moves forward naturally during this process. As the infant develops teeth, anterior movement of the tongue is blocked even as the need for it diminishes. The child begins eating semi-solid and solid food, and chewing becomes more important than sucking. The mature swallow propels a bolus back toward the oropharynx, a maneuver that requires posterior direction of the tongue.

If the child fails to develop the mature swallow, he or she has a condition known as tongue thrust. The anterior direction of the tongue causes labioversion of the incisors. This child may have flaccid oral musculature, weak masseter action during swallow, and a disorganized approach to generation of the bolus. Considering that we swallow between 400 and 600 times per day, the immature swallow is difficult (but far from impossible) to reorganize into a mature swallow. Many speech-language pathologists specialize in oral myofunctional therapy directed toward remediation of such problems, a rewarding practice that results in (literally) smiling clients (see Zickefoose, 1989).

originate at the median fibrous septum and course laterally to insert into the side of the tongue in the submucous tissue. The transverse muscle of the tongue pulls the edges of the tongue toward the midline, effectively narrowing the tongue.

The *vertical muscles of the tongue* run at right angles to the transverse muscles and flatten the tongue. Fibers of the vertical muscle course from the base of the tongue and insert into the membranous cover. The fibers of the transverse and vertical muscles interweave. Contraction of the vertical muscles of the tongue pulls the tongue down into the floor of the mouth. Innervation of all intrinsic muscles of the tongue is by means of the hypoglossal nerve (cranial nerve XII).

Extrinsic Tongue Muscles. The extrinsic muscles of the tongue tend to move the tongue as a unit. It appears that they set the general posture for articulation, with the intrinsic muscles performing the refined perfection of that gesture.

The *genioglossus* is the prime mover of the tongue, making up most of its bulk. The genioglossus (see Figure 4–35)

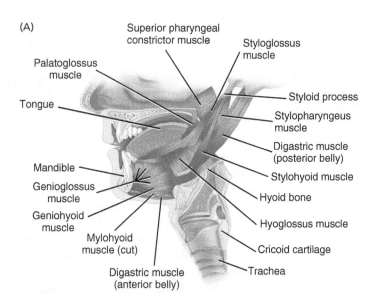

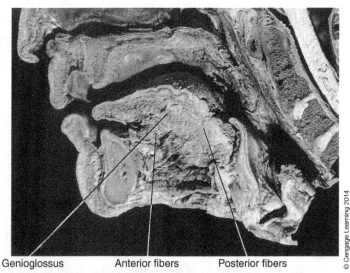

Figure 4–35. (A) Drawing and photograph of sagittal section, revealing anterior and posterior fibers of the genioglossus muscle of tongue.   *(continues)*

(B)

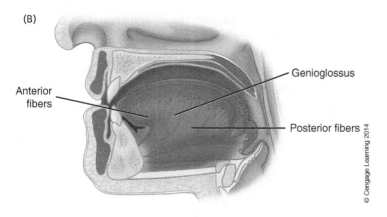

Figure 4–35. continued (B) Diagram representing anterior and posterior fibers of the genioglossus muscle.

arises from the inner mandibular surface at the symphysis and fans to insert into the tip and dorsum of the tongue, as well as to the corpus of the hyoid bone.

The genioglossus muscle occupies a medial position in the tongue, with the inferior longitudinal muscle, hyoglossus, and the styloglossus lateral to it. Fibers of the genioglossus insert into the entire surface of the tongue but are sparse to absent in the tip. Contraction of the anterior fibers of the genioglossus muscle retracts the tongue, whereas contraction of the posterior fibers draws the tongue forward to aid protrusion of the apex. If both anterior and posterior portions are contracted, the middle portion of the tongue will be drawn down into the floor of the mouth, functionally cupping the tongue along its length. The genioglossus is innervated by the hypoglossal nerve.

As the name implies, the *hyoglossus* arises from the length of the greater cornu and lateral body of the hyoid bone, coursing upward to insert into the sides of the tongue between the styloglossus and the inferior longitudinal muscles. The hyoglossus pulls the sides of the tongue down, in direct antagonism to the palatoglossus. The hyoglossus is innervated by the hypoglossal nerve.

If you examine Figure 4–35 again, you will see that the *styloglossus* originates from the anterolateral margin of styloid process of the temporal bone, coursing forward and down to insert into the inferior sides of the tongue. It divides into two portions, with one interdigitating with the inferior longitudinal muscle and the other with the fibers of the hyoglossus. Contraction of the styloglossus draws the tongue back and up. The styloglossus is innervated by the hypoglossal nerve.

The *chondroglossus muscle* is often considered part of the hyoglossus muscle. As with the hyoglossus, the chondroglossus arises from the hyoid (lesser cornu), coursing up to interdigitate with the intrinsic muscles of the tongue medial to the point of insertion of the hyoglossus. The chondroglossus is a depressor of the tongue. The chondroglossus is innervated by the hypoglossal nerve.

The *palatoglossus* can be functionally defined as a muscle of the tongue or of the velum, although it is more closely allied with palatal architecture and origin. It is described in a later section, but you should realize that it serves the dual purpose of depressing the soft palate or elevating the back of the tongue.

Summary

- The tongue is a massive structure that occupies the floor of the mouth. It is divided by a median fibrous septum that provides the origination for the transverse intrinsic muscle of the tongue.
- The tongue is divided into dorsum, apex (tip), and base.
- Fine movements are produced by contraction of the intrinsic musculature (transverse, vertical, inferior longitudinal, and superior longitudinal muscles of the tongue).
- Larger adjustments of lingual movement are completed through use of extrinsic muscles. The genioglossus retracts, protrudes, or depresses the tongue. The hyoglossus and chondroglossus depress the tongue, and the styloglossus and palatoglossus elevate the posterior tongue.

Muscles of Mastication: Mandibular Elevators and Depressors

mastication: The process of chewing food.

The process of chewing food, or mastication, requires movement of the mandible so the molars can make a solid, grinding contact. The muscles of mastication are among the body's strongest, and the coordinated contraction of these muscles is required for proper preparation of food for swallowing. The muscles of mastication include the mandibular elevators (masseter, temporalis, medial pterygoid), muscles of protrusion (lateral pterygoid), and depressors (digastricus, mylohyoid, geniohyoid, platysma).

The *masseter* (see Figure 4–36) is the most superficial of the muscles of mastication. This massive muscle originates on the lateral, inferior, and medial surfaces of the zygomatic arch, coursing down to insert primarily into the ramus of the mandible, but some of the deeper fibers terminate on the coronoid process. The course and attachments of the masseter make it ideally suited for placing maximum force on the molars. Contraction of this muscle elevates the mandible. The masseter

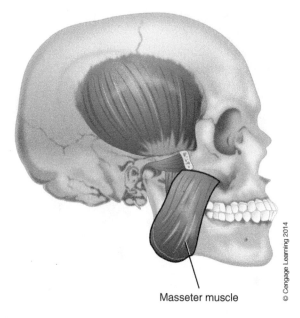

Masseter muscle

© Cengage Learning 2014

Figure 4–36. Graphic representation of the masseter muscle.

is innervated by the anterior trunk of the mandibular nerve arising from the trigeminal nerve (cranial nerve V).

The *temporalis muscle* is deep to the masseter, arising from a region of the temporal and parietal bones known as the temporal fossa (see Figure 4–37). The terminal tendon of the temporalis passes through the zygomatic arch and inserts in the coronoid process and ramus of the mandible. The temporalis elevates the mandible and draws it back if protruded. The temporalis is innervated by the temporal branches arising from the mandibular branch of the trigeminal nerve.

The *medial*, or *internal*, *pterygoid muscle* originates from the medial pterygoid plate and lateral fossa of the sphenoid. Fibers from the muscle course down and back to insert into the mandibular ramus. The medial pterygoid muscle elevates the mandible.

The *lateral*, or *external*, *pterygoid muscle* arises from the lateral pterygoid plate and the greater wing of sphenoid (see Figure 4-38). Fibers course back to insert into the pterygoid fovea of the mandible. Contraction of the lateral pterygoid muscle protrudes the mandible. The lateral and medial pterygoid muscles are innervated by the mandibular branch of the trigeminal nerve.

The dual-bellied *digastricus* was shown in Figure 3–20, so it is discussed only briefly here. Digastricus anterior originates on the inner surface of the mandible at the digastricus fossa, near the symphysis, and the digastricus posterior originates on the mastoid process of the temporal bone. The anterior fibers and posterior fibers join by means of an intermediate tendon that inserts into the hyoid at the juncture of the hyoid corpus and greater cornu. If the hyoid bone is held

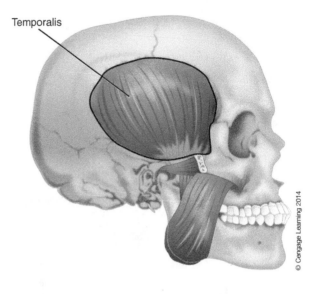

Temporalis

Figure 4–37. Graphic
representation of the
temporalis muscle.

© Cengage Learning 2014

Palpation of the Oral Cavity

This palpation exercise would be well performed with one of your friends, and requires aseptic procedures, which include ensuring that your hands are clean and that you have on gloves that have not come in contact with any material once having been removed from their protective packaging. You will want to perform it under the guidance of your instructor, because this is a procedure that will carry into the oral peripheral examination in your clinical practice. A flashlight will help you identify structures.

Have your friend open her mouth as you look inside. Ensure that your nondominant hand (e.g., left hand if you are right-handed) is the only hand that holds or touches the flashlight; the other hand is gloved and must not touch anything but your friend. Ask your friend to say "ah" and watch the velum in back elevate. Look for presence or absence of the palatine tonsils between the faucial pillars. Shine the light on the hard palate and note the median raphe and rugae. Now palpate both of these structures, running your finger back along both sides of the median raphe of the hard palate. Palpate the margin of the hard and soft palates, being sensitive to the fact that this may elicit a gag reflex in some people. As you palpate the hard palate, be sensitive to the possible presence of occult (hidden; submucous) clefts of the hard palate.

Have your friend bite lightly on her molars and hold her teeth closed but lips open for an /i/ vowel. With the gloved finger, palpate the lateral margins of the teeth and gums. With a tongue depressor, move the cheeks away from the teeth and examine the relationship between the upper and lower teeth for occlusion.

Pull the lower lip down gently and examine the labial frenulum. Ask your friend to open her mouth and elevate her tongue, and examine the lingual frenulum.

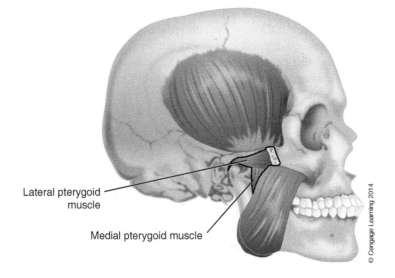

Lateral pterygoid
muscle

Medial pterygoid muscle

© Cengage Learning 2014

Figure 4–38. Lateral and
medial pterygoid muscles.

in position by other muscles, contraction of the digastricus
depresses the mandible. The anterior belly is innervated by
the mandibular branch of the trigeminal nerve. The posterior belly is innervated by the facial nerve.

The *mylohyoid* (see Figure 3–20) originates on the mylohyoid line of the mandible and inserts into the median fibrous raphe and hyoid bone, forming the floor of the mouth.
With the hyoid fixed in position, the mylohyoid depresses the
mandible. The mylohyoid is innervated by the alveolar nerve,
arising from the trigeminal nerve, mandibular branch.

Also shown in Figure 3–20, the *geniohyoid muscle* originates at the mental spines of the mandible and inserts into the
corpus hyoid. Contraction of the geniohyoid depresses the
mandible if the hyoid is fixed. The geniohyoid is innervated
by means of the hypoglossal nerve. The *platysma* is discussed
earlier in this chapter under Muscles of the Face.

Summary

- Mandibular elevators include the masseter, temporalis,
  and medial pterygoid muscles, and the lateral pterygoid
  protrudes the mandible.
- Depression of the mandible is performed by the mylohyoid, geniohyoid, and platysma muscles. The grinding
  action of the molars requires coordinated and synchro-
  nized contraction of the muscles of mastication.

Muscles of the Soft Palate

Only three speech sounds in English require that the soft
palate be depressed (/m/, /ŋm/, and /n/). During most speaking

time, the soft palate is actively elevated. We will discuss the general configuration of the soft palate and then discuss how we elevate and depress this important structure.

The *soft palate*, or *velum*, is actually a combination of muscle, aponeurosis, nerves, and blood supply covered by mucous membrane lining. The *palatal aponeurosis* makes up the mid-front of the soft palate, being an extension of an aponeurosis arising from the tensor veli palatini (described later). The palatal aponeurosis divides around the musculus uvulae, but serves as the point of insertion for other muscles of the soft palate. The *mucous membrane lining* is invested with lymph and mucous glands, and the oral side of the lining also has taste buds.

Muscles of the soft palate include elevators (levator veli palatini, musculus uvulae), a tensor (tensor veli palatini), and depressors (palatoglossus and palatopharyngeus). Although the superior constrictor muscle is a pharyngeal muscle, it is an important muscle for function of the soft palate. We will discuss the muscles of the pharynx following discussion of the muscles of the soft palate (see Figures 4–39).

The *levator veli palatini*, or *levator palati*, is the palatal elevator, making up the bulk of the soft palate (see Figure 4–39). This muscle arises from the petrous portion of the temporal bone and from the medial wall of the eustachian tube cartilage. The levator veli palatini courses down and forward to insert into the palatal aponeurosis of the soft palate. Contraction elevates and retracts the posterior velum. The levator veli palatini is innervated by the pharyngeal plexus, arising from the accessory nerve (cranial nerve XI) and vagus nerve (cranial nerve X).

The uvula makes up the medial and posterior portions of the soft palate, and the *musculus uvulae* is the muscle it embodies. This muscle arises from the posterior nasal spines of the palatine bones and from the palatal aponeurosis, and it inserts into the mucous membrane cover of the velum. Contraction of the uvula shortens the soft palate, effectively bunching it up. The musculus uvulae is innervated by the pharyngeal plexus, arising from the accessory and vagus nerves.

The *tensor veli palatini* (tensor veli palati) may add some stability to the velum, but it is a major dilator of the eustachian tube. This muscle arises from the scaphoid fossa of the sphenoid bone and from the lateral eustachian tube wall. The fibers converge to course down to terminate in a tendon. The tendon passes around the pterygoid hamulus and then is directed medially. This tendon expands to become the palatal aponeurosis. Contraction of the tensor veli palatini stabilizes the soft palate and flattens it. It assists in dilating or opening the eustachian tube, thereby permitting aeration (exchange of air) of the middle ear cavity. This muscle is innervated by the trigeminal nerve (cranial nerve V).

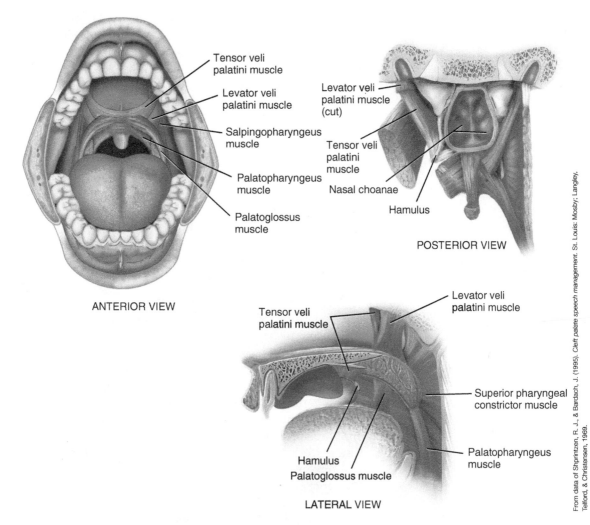

Figure 4–39. Muscles of the soft palate from superior-posterior (left), posterior (top right), and the side (lower right) views.

The *palatoglossus muscle* was discussed briefly as a muscle of the tongue. This muscle originates at the anterolateral palatal aponeurosis, coursing down to insert into the sides of the posterior tongue. This muscle helps to either elevate the tongue or depress the soft palate. The palatoglossus is innervated by the pharyngeal plexus, arising from the accessory and vagus nerves.

Although classically considered a pharyngeal muscle, the *palatopharyngeus* is included in this discussion because of its role in velar function. Anterior fibers of the palatopharyngeus originate from the anterior hard palate, and posterior fibers arise from the midline of the soft palate posterior to the fibers of the levator veli palatini, attached to the palatal aponeurosis. Fibers of each muscle course laterally and down, forming the posterior faucial pillar and inserting into the posterior thyroid cartilage. It assists in narrowing

From data of Shprintzen, R. J., & Bardach, J. (1995). *Cleft palate speech management.* St. Louis: Mosby; Langley, Telford, & Christensen, 1969.

the pharyngeal cavity and lowering the soft palate. The palatopharyngeus is innervated by the pharyngeal plexus, arising from the accessory nerve and pharyngeal branch of the vagus nerve.

Pharyngeal Musculature

Muscles of the pharynx are closely allied with those of the tongue, face, and larynx. It will help if you imagine the pharynx as a vertical tube. This tube is made of muscles wrapping more or less horizontally from the front to a midline point in the back, as well as by muscles and connective tissue running from skull structures. Thus, the pharynx is composed of a complex of muscles that, when contracted, constrict the pharynx to assist in deglutition.

Pharyngeal Constrictor Muscles

The superior, middle, and inferior constrictor muscles are the means by which the pharyngeal space is reduced in diameter. Of these, the superior constrictor is an important muscle of velopharyngeal function (see Figure 4–40).

The *superior pharyngeal constrictor* forms a tube originating at the *pterygomandibular raphe* (the point of attachment of the buccinator), the mylohyoid line of the mandible, and the sides of the tongue. It projects back from this structure on both sides to the median *pharyngeal raphe*, the midline tendinous component of the pharyngeal aponeurosis. This aponeurosis arises from the pharyngeal tubercle of the occipital bone and forms the upper sleeve of the pharyngeal wall by attaching to the temporal bone (petrous portion), medial pterygoid plate, and eustachian tube.

The median pterygoid plate gives rise to the uppermost fibers of the muscle, and these fibers are the "landing pad" for the soft palate, known as *Passavant's pad*. This pad of muscle at the posterior pharyngeal wall appears as a ridge at the point of articulation of the soft palate with the wall.

Contraction of the superior pharyngeal constrictor muscle pulls the pharyngeal wall forward and constricts the pharyngeal diameter, an especially prominent movement during swallowing. It assists in effecting the velopharyngeal seal. The superior pharyngeal constrictor is innervated by the accessory nerve in conjunction with the vagus nerve, via the pharyngeal plexus.

The *middle pharyngeal constrictor* arises from the horns of the hyoid bone and inserts into the median pharyngeal raphe. It narrows the diameter of the pharynx. The middle pharyngeal constrictor is innervated by the accessory nerve in conjunction with the vagus nerve, via the pharyngeal plexus.

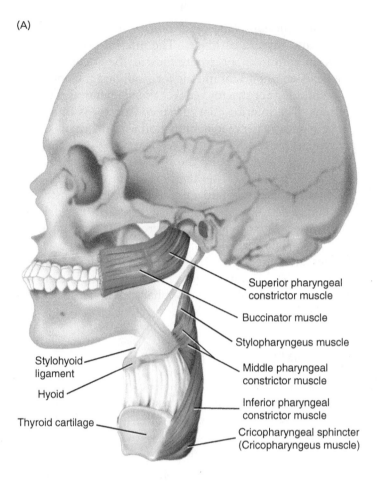

Superior pharyngeal
constrictor muscle

Buccinator muscle

Stylopharyngeus muscle

Middle pharyngeal
constrictor muscle

Inferior pharyngeal
constrictor muscle

Cricopharyngeal sphincter
(Cricopharyngeus muscle)

Stylohyoid
ligament

Hyoid

Thyroid cartilage

(B)

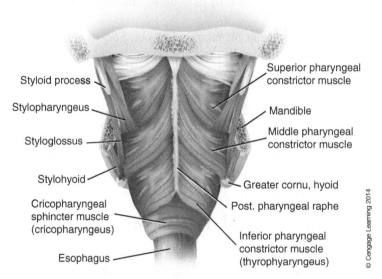

Styloid process

Stylopharyngeus

Styloglossus

Stylohyoid

Cricopharyngeal
sphincter muscle
(cricopharyngeus)

Esophagus

Superior pharyngeal
constrictor muscle

Mandible

Middle pharyngeal
constrictor muscle

Greater cornu, hyoid

Post. pharyngeal raphe

Inferior pharyngeal
constrictor muscle
(thyrophyaryngeus)

© Cengage Learning 2014

Figure 4–40. (A) Lateral view
of pharyngeal constrictor
muscles. (B) Posterior view
of pharyngeal constrictor
musculature.

The *inferior pharyngeal constrictor* arises from the cricoid and thyroid cartilages. The inferior portion, sometimes referred to as a separate muscle, the cricopharyngeal muscle, is an important muscle for swallowing. Contraction of the inferior constrictor reduces the diameter of the lower pharynx. The inferior pharyngeal constrictor is innervated by the accessory nerve in conjunction with the vagus, via the pharyngeal plexus.

As the name implies, the *stylopharyngeus* arises from the styloid process of the temporal bone, coursing down between the superior and middle pharyngeal constrictors (see Figure 4–40). Some fibers insert into the constrictors, others insert into the posterior thyroid cartilage in concert with the palatopharyngeus muscle. The stylopharyngeus elevates and opens the pharynx, particularly during deglutition. The stylopharyngeus muscle is innervated by the muscular branch of the glossopharyngeal nerve (cranial nerve IX).

Summary

- The levator veli palatini muscle elevates the soft palate, the musculus uvulae bunches the soft palate, and the tensor veli palatini tenses and shortens the palate.
- The soft palate is depressed by the palatoglossus and palatopharyngeus muscles.
- The superior pharyngeal constrictor assists in gaining velopharyngeal closure, and peristaltic movement of food is facilitated by the middle and inferior pharyngeal constrictors.
- The cricopharyngeal muscle, a component of the inferior constrictor, forms the muscular orifice of the esophagus.
- The stylopharyngeus assists in elevation of the pharynx.

Clearly, the structures of the articulatory system are extremely complex and mobile. We are capable of myriad movements that are incorporated into nonspeech and speech functions. Let us move on to articulatory physiology.

PHYSIOLOGY OF ARTICULATION, RESONATION, AND DEGLUTITION

In preparation for our discussion of the physiology of speech production, we will first discuss the biological functions from which the speech functions arise: mastication and deglutition. *Mastication* refers to the processes involved in food preparation, including moving unchewed food onto the grinding surface of the teeth, chewing it, and mixing it with saliva in preparation for swallowing. *Deglutition* refers to swallowing. We'll cross these biological functions one more time in Chapter 6, when we talk about reflexes that support mastication and deglutition.

Biological Function: Mastication and Deglutition

Mastication and deglutition consist of a sequence of four events or stages: oral preparatory stage, oral stage of swallow, pharyngeal stage, and esophageal stage (see Figure 4–41).

Oral Preparatory Stage

In the *oral preparatory stage*, food is prepared for swallowing. First, we introduce food into the mouth and keep it there by tightly occluding the lips as we breathe through the nose. The tongue bunches up in back and the soft palate is pulled down to keep the food in the oral cavity with the aid of the palatoglossus muscle.

The food must be ground up so that it can pass through the esophagus for digestion. This is performed by the coordinated activity of the muscles of mastication and the lingual

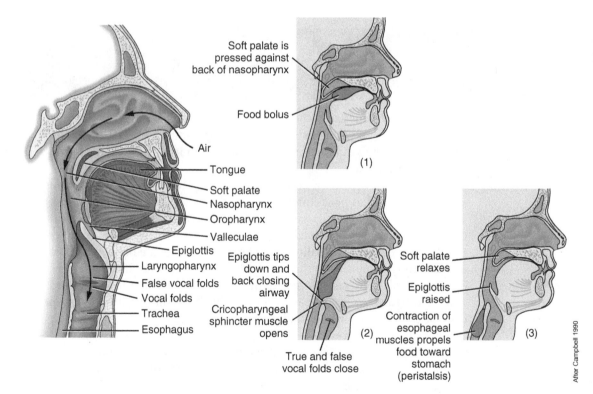

Figure 4–41. Stages of deglutition.

muscles. The tongue keeps food in the oral cavity by making a seal along the alveolar ridge. As it holds the food in place, it compresses it against the hard palate, partially crushing it in preparation for the teeth. The tongue then begins moving the food onto the grinding surfaces of the teeth, pulling the food back into the oral cavity to be mixed with saliva, and then moving it back to the teeth for more mastication. The salivary glands secrete saliva into the oral cavity to help form the mass of food into a bolus for swallowing. The risorius and buccinator muscles contract to keep the food from entering the lateral buccal cavity.

Oral Stage

When the bolus of food is finally ready to swallow, the *oral stage of swallowing* begins. Several processes must occur sequentially. Mastication stops and the anterior tongue elevates to the hard palate and squeezes the bolus back toward the faucial pillars.

Pharyngeal Stage

Propelling the bolus posteriorly during the oral stage causes the bolus to contact the fauces and the depressed velum. In younger individuals, the contact with the fauces and velum appears to trigger the reflexes of the pharyngeal stage; for

dysphagia: *Disorder of swallowing.*

Deficits of the Oral Preparatory Stage

Numerous problems arise when neuromuscular control and muscle strength associated with mastication are compromised. In addition, physical changes in the structure of the oral cavity can lead to problems of the oral preparation stage.

Loss of oral sensation and awareness, coupled with weak buccal musculature, can lead to pocketing of food in the buccal cavity (lateral sulcus) or between the teeth and the lip (anterior sulcus). Weak muscles of mastication can cause inadequately chewed food, and weak lingual muscles will result in poor mixture of saliva with the food, inadequate bolus generation, and difficulty compressing the bolus onto the hard palate. If the muscles of the soft palate are compromised, the velum may not be fully depressed and the tongue may not be elevated in the back, permitting food to escape into the pharynx prior to initiation of the pharyngeal reflexes. This is life-threatening because food entering the pharynx in absence of reflexive response may reach the open airway. Aspiration pneumonia (pneumonia secondary to aspirated matter) is a constant concern for individuals with dysphagia (a disorder of swallowing).

Deficits of the Oral Stage

Deficits of the oral stage can arise from sensory and motor dysfunction, as well as from structural problems. Weakened movements cause increased posterior transit time of the bolus toward the pharynx. Indeed, some people are so weak that they have difficulty propelling a thick bolus (for instance, mashed potatoes) to the pharynx. Structural problems, such as partial glossectomy (removal of a portion of the tongue) or palatal fistula (opening in the hard palate that is either developmentally present or secondary to a surgical procedure) can result in oral stage deficit as well.

the elderly these reflexes appear to be triggered as the bolus passes the region of the mandibular angle (viewed through fluoroscopy, in Logemann, 1998). The soft palate, which was depressed, elevates to close off the oropharynx from the nasopharynx. Respiration stops reflexively at this point. Both oral and nasal outlets are closed so air cannot escape or enter for respiration and food is ready to enter the pharynx. The airway must be protected. The vocal folds tightly adduct, and elevation of the larynx relative to the tongue base causes the epiglottis to drop over the laryngeal aditus. Simultaneously, the cricopharyngeus muscle relaxes, allowing the upper esophagus to open. When you are not swallowing it remains closed to keep food and gastric juices from escaping into the laryngopharynx (esophageal reflux). Elevation of the larynx during the pharyngeal stage facilitates opening of the upper esophageal sphincter.

Food is propelled down the pharynx toward the esophagus by means of contraction of the pharyngeal constrictors. As food is forced into the oropharynx, the posterior faucial pillars move medially, effectively channeling the bolus downward.

After about 1 second of pharyngeal transit, the bolus reaches the laryngopharynx where it passes over the epiglottis. The bolus is divided into two roughly equal masses, passing on the sides of the larynx, through the piriform sinuses, to recombine at the esophageal entrance.

Esophageal Stage

The *esophageal stage* is out of voluntary control. It begins when the bolus reaches the orifice of the esophagus. The bolus is transported through the esophagus to the inferior esophageal sphincter by peristaltic contraction and gravity, arriving at the stomach for the process of digestion after 10 to 20 seconds of transit time. When the bolus enters the esophagus, the cricopharyngeus again contracts, the larynx

Deficits of the Pharyngeal Stage

Sensory, motor, and structural deficits contribute to pharyngeal stage dysphagia. Slowed velar elevation during the pharyngeal swallow may result in **nasal regurgitation** (loss of food or liquid through the nose); reduced sensation at the fauces, posterior tongue, pharyngeal wall, and soft palate may result in an elevated threshold for triggering the swallowing reflex. Reduced function of the pharyngeal constrictors may result in slowed pharyngeal transit time of the bolus, in which case the individual may prematurely re-initiate respiration. Laryngeal elevation relative to the tongue normally causes the epiglottis to invert, covering the laryngeal aditus. Reduced laryngeal elevation during swallow may prevent the epiglottis from covering the larynx, resulting in residue left in the valleculae. Further, laryngeal elevation helps to open the relaxed esophageal sphincter, so that failure of elevation may result in food remaining in the airway at the level of the upper esophageal sphincter after respiration has resumed. This food can easily find its way into the airway, resulting in aspiration and life-threatening pneumonia.

nasal regurgitation: *Loss of masticated food or liquid through the nasal cavity.*

and soft palate drop down, and respiration begins again. In the normal swallow, respiration is suspended for only about a second. Because most individuals begin the pharyngeal swallow following a respiratory inspiration, they exhale when the swallow is completed. This expiration expels any residual food at the laryngeal entryway, which is blown clear and propelled to the esophagus.

Summary

- In the oral preparation stage, food is introduced into the oral cavity, moved onto the molars for chewing, and mixed with saliva to form a concise bolus between the tongue and hard palate.
- In the oral stage, the bolus is moved back by pressure of movement of the tongue on the hard palate.
- The pharyngeal stage begins when the bolus reaches the faucial pillars. The soft palate and larynx elevate, the vocal folds tightly adduct, the epiglottis depresses, the cricopharyngeal muscle relaxes, and the lower esophageal sphincter opens. Food passes through the valleculae at the base of the tongue, over the epiglottis, and through the piriform sinuses to the esophagus.
- The esophageal stage involves peristaltic movement of the bolus through the esophagus to the lower esophageal sphincter.

Speech Function

Speech production requires execution of an extremely well-organized and well-integrated sequence of neuromotor events. The orbicularis oris is primarily responsible for ensuring a labial seal, but numerous facial muscles insert into it. The lower lip achieves a greater velocity and force than the upper lip, and it does most of the work in lip closure. Extra force is exerted by the mentalis muscle.

The mandible assists the lips, and changes its position for tongue movement. The mandible is an extremely important articulator in its supportive role of carrying the lips, tongue, and teeth to their targets in the maxilla (lips, teeth, alveolar ridge, hard palate), but its adjustments are rather minute in normal speech. In speech, the mandibular elevators and depressors stay in dynamic balance, so that slight modification in muscle activation (and inhibition of antagonists) permits a quick adjustment of the mandible.

The tongue is the most important articulator. It is involved in production of the majority of English phonemes. A summary of tongue movements is presented in Table 4–4.

You can think of the tongue as a group of highly organized (intrinsic) muscles being carried on the "shoulders" of the extrinsic muscles. Much as the muscles of the legs and trunk move your upper body to a position where your arms and head can interact with the environment, the extrinsic muscles set the basic posture of the tongue, whereas the intrinsic muscles have a great deal of responsibility for the microstructure of articulation. The two groups of muscles work together closely to achieve the target articulatory gesture.

Velum (Soft Palate)

Early in the history of our field we found it tempting to treat the velum as a binary element: It was either opened or closed. We have since realized that its function is more complex. The velum is capable of a range of motion and rate of movement that matches the needs of rapid speech and nonspeech functions.

The velum generally is closed for non-nasal speech, and this is the result of contraction of the levator veli palatini, a direct antagonist to the palatoglossus muscle. In speech, opening and closing of the velar port must occur precisely and rapidly, or the result will be hyper- or hyponasality. Failure to open the port turns a 70-ms nasal phoneme into a voiced stop consonant, an unacceptable result. The soft palate opens and closes in coordination with the other articulators, thus preventing nasal resonance on other phonemes (assimilation). In reality, some nasal assimilation is inevitable and acceptable, and in some geographic regions, dialectically appropriate.

Table 4–4. Muscles of Tongue Movement

Movement	Muscle
Elevate tongue tip	Superior longitudinal muscles
Depress tongue tip	Inferior longitudinal muscles
Deviate tongue tip	Simultaneous contraction of either left or right superior and inferior longitudinal muscles for left or right deviation
Relax lateral margin	Posterior genioglossus for protrusion; superior longitudinal for tip elevation; transverse intrinsic pulls sides medially
Narrow tongue	Transverse intrinsic muscles
Deep central groove	Genioglossus depresses tongue body; vertical intrinsic depresses central dorsum
Broad central groove	Moderate genioglossus depresses tongue body; vertical intrinsic depresses dorsum; superior longitudinal elevates margins
Protrude tongue	Posterior genioglossus advances body; vertical muscles narrow tongue; superior and inferior longitudinal balance and point tongue
Retract tongue	Anterior genioglossus retracts into oral cavity; superior and inferior longitudinal muscles shorten tongue; styloglossus retracts into pharyngeal cavity
Elevate posterior tongue	Palatoglossus elevates sides; transverse intrinsic bunches tongue
Depress tongue body	Genioglossus contraction depresses medial tongue; hyoglossus and chondroglossus depress sides if hyoid is fixed by infrahyoid muscles

Production of high-pressure consonants (such as fricatives and stops) requires greater velopharyngeal effort to seal air in the oral cavity. To accomplish this seal, additional help is needed from the tensor veli palatini, superior pharyngeal constrictor, and uvular muscles. Even then, the pressures for speech are far less than those for, say, actions required in playing a wind instrument. Some individuals have difficulty avoiding nasal air escape when playing in the brass section but have perfectly normal speech.

Summary

- Movement of the mandible for speech is slight compared with movement for chewing. In addition, the mandibular posture for speech is one of sustained dynamic tension between antagonists.
- The tongue is an extremely versatile organ, with the extrinsic muscles providing the major movement of the

Mouth Breathing

Chronic mouth breathing is more than an unpleasant habit because it is at the root of facial malformation and hearing loss. Mouth breathing is attributed to hypertrophy of the tonsillar ring, prohibiting adequate nasal respiration. In children with this condition, the adenoids are frequently enlarged, blocking the nasal choanae and also the orifice of the eustachian tube. Inadequate ventilation of the middle ear cavity may result in otitis media (inflammation of the middle ear cavity). Chronic otitis media is often associated with fluid in the middle ear (serous otitis media), a condition resulting in conductive hearing impairment.

The hypertrophy also makes mouth breathing mandatory. During normal nasal respiration, the tongue maintains fairly constant contact with the upper alveolar ridge and hard palate; but with the mouth open constantly for respiration, the tongue exerts little pressure there. Without that pressure, the dental arch narrows and the palate bulges upward to an extreme vault as the facial bones develop. With narrow dental arches, the permanent teeth do not have adequate space, and so they become crowded and prone to caries (decay of bone or tooth). The narrowed maxillae cause the upper lip to pull up, exposing the upper front teeth. The nasal cavity becomes narrow, increasing the probability of later nasal obstruction. The look of "adenoid facies" includes an open mouth, narrow mandible, and dental crowding. Coupled with a persistent conductive hearing loss, mouth breathing presents a sizable (yet generally preventable) deficit to the developing child.

Unilateral Tongue Weakness

One element of the oral-peripheral examination is evaluation of relative tongue strength. When you ask a client to push forcefully with his or her tongue sideways against a resistance, you are interested in identifying whether the client has adequate strength and symmetrical strength. If there appears to be greater strength in one direction than the other, the speech-language pathologist will consider activities to strengthen the musculature. Improving muscle strength will improve tone and muscle control.

body and the intrinsic muscles providing the shaping of the tongue. Muscle spindle and tactile sensors make the tongue quite sensitive to position and the forces placed on it by contact with other articulators.

■ The soft palate must be maintained in a reasonably elevated position for most speech sounds, although it is capable of a range of movements.

Effects of Neuromuscular Disease on Velopharyngeal Function

A deficit associated with the velum can have significant effects on speech. In neuromuscular disorders, such as amyotrophic lateral sclerosis and multiple sclerosis, muscular weakness arises from damage to the myelin sheath of the axons of motor neurons. When the weakness involves the muscles of the velum, the nasal cavity resonance is added to that of the oral cavity for non-nasal sounds. This "anti-resonance," as it is called, pulls energy out of the speech signal in the 1500 to 2500 Hz range, causing a marked loss of clarity in the speech signal. Speech of the affected individual sounds muffled, monotone, and low in vocal intensity.

It is not uncommon for the speech-language pathologist to be the first person approached by an individual with early signs of neuromuscular disease. The velum requires constant elevation for non-nasal sounds and is an early indicator of progressive muscular weakness. An individual may come to the clinician with the complaint that people say his or her speech sounds muffled. Your supervisor's oral-peripheral examination will reveal slow velar activity, and the person may be referred to a physician.

Phonological Development and Motor Control

Certainly the development of a child's phonology is a marvel. It should now be fairly clear that the maturation of the motor speech system governs, in large part, the speech sounds a child is capable of making. The stops (/p,t,k,b,d,g/) are present in the child's repertoire fairly early in development, although their mastery occurs later than their emergence. The reason for this is apparently motoric. A child 2 or 3 years of age is quite capable of the basic "valving" gesture of opening and closing the mouth (/ba/), raising and lowering the tongue on the alveolar ridge (/da/), or near the soft palate (/ga/). However, the controlled production of the stops requires the ability to differentiate labial, mandibular, and lingual movements, and thus mastery of the stops can occur as late as 6 years.

As the child develops greater motor control, he gains the ability to make graded movements with the tongue so that he can sustain one articulator against the other with a constant pressure. The "raspberry" you hear in the preverbal child is very likely the precursor to the fricatives. With graded control of lingual pressure comes the ability to make minute adjustments of an articulatory posture, such as those made with the dorsum of the tongue to differentiate /s/ and s' through width of the tongue groove and tongue tip elevation.

ORGANIZATIONAL PATTERNS OF MASTICATION AND DEGLUTITION

Pressures of Deglutition

You can think of the swallowing process as a series of manipulations of a bolus by muscles, but you can also think of swallowing in terms of manipulation of oral, pharyngeal, and esophageal pressures that in turn move the bolus. During the oral preparation stage, the oral and pharyngeal cavity pressures are equalized with atmospheric pressure, because of the open nasal airway. When entering the oral stage of the swallow, the soft palate tightly closes, separating the oropharynx and nasopharynx, and the tongue begins squeezing the bolus posteriorly. The positive pressure created by the movements of the tongue propels the bolus toward the oropharynx. The tongue makes contact with the posterior oropharynx, transferring the bolus into the pharynx with an additional pressure gradient. The pharyngeal walls compress the bolus, increasing the pressure to prompt it toward the esophagus. Elevation of the larynx creates a relatively lower pressure at the esophageal entryway, and relaxation of the cricopharyngeus further increases the superior-inferior pressure gradient. The laryngeal entryway is tightly clamped to avoid confounding the pressures of deglutition with those of respiration, so that the bolus is naturally drawn to the area of lower pressure, the esophageal entrance. The cricopharyngeus contracts most forcefully during inspiration, prohibiting inflation of the esophagus.

CHAPTER SUMMARY

Movement of the mandible for speech is slight compared with movement for chewing. The mandibular posture for speech is one of sustained dynamic tension between antagonists. The tongue is versatile, with the extrinsic muscles providing the major movement of the body and the intrinsic muscles providing the shaping of the tongue. The soft palate must be maintained in a reasonably elevated position for most speech sounds, although it is capable of a range of movements.

The source-filter theory states that speech is the product of sending an acoustic source, such as the sound produced by the vibrating vocal folds, through the filter of the vocal tract that shapes the output. Sources may be voicing, as in the case of vowels, or the product of turbulence,

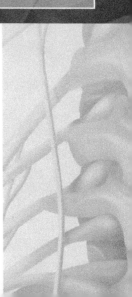

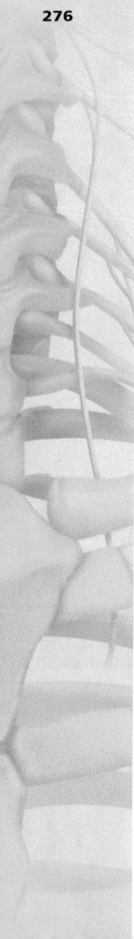

as in fricatives. Articulators may be movable (such as the tongue, lips, pharynx, mandible, and velum) or immobile (such as the teeth, hard palate, and alveolar ridge).

Facial bones and those of the skull work together to produce the structures of articulation. The mandible provides the lower dental arch, alveolar regions, and the resting location for the tongue. The maxillae provide the bulk of the hard palate, alveolar ridge, upper dental arch, and dominant structures of the nasal cavities, and the palatine bones provide the rest of the hard palate and the point of attachment for the soft palate. The midline vomer articulates with the perpendicular plate of ethmoid and the cartilaginous septum to form the nasal septum. The zygomatic bone articulates with the frontal bone and maxillae to form the cheekbone. The small nasal bones form the upper margin of the nasal cavity. The ethmoid bone serves as the core of the skull and face, with the prominent crista galli protruding into the cranium and the perpendicular plate dividing the nasal cavities. The frontal, parietal, temporal, and occipital bones of the skull overlie the lobes of the brain of the same name. The sphenoid bone has a marked presence in the braincase, with the prominent greater and lesser wings of sphenoid lateral to the corpus. The hypophyseal fossa houses the pituitary gland.

Incisors, cuspids, bicuspids, and molars are housed in the alveoli of the maxillae and mandible. Teeth have roots and crowns, and the exposed tooth surface is covered with enamel. Each tooth has medial, lateral, lingual, buccal (or labial), and occlusal surfaces. Clinical eruption of the deciduous arch begins between 6 and 9 months, and eruption of the permanent arch begins at 6 years. Class I occlusion refers to normal orientation of mandible and maxillae. Class II malocclusion refers to a relatively retracted mandible, and Class III malocclusion refers to a relatively protruded mandible. Individual teeth may have aberrant orientations within the alveolus, including torsiversion, labioversion, linguaversion, distoversion, and mesioversion. Inadequately erupted or hypererupted teeth are referred to as infraverted and supraverted, respectively.

The cavities of the articulatory and resonatory system can be envisioned as a series of linked tubes. The vertically directed pharynx comprises the laryngopharynx, oropharynx, and nasopharynx. The nasal cavities arise from the nasopharynx, with the nasal and nasopharyngeal regions entirely separated from the oral cavity by the soft palate. The oral cavity is flanked by the small buccal cavities. The shape and size of the oral cavity is altered through movement of the tongue and mandible, and the nasal cavity may be coupled with the oral and pharyngeal cavities by means of the soft palate. The shape of the pharyngeal cavity is altered by the pharyngeal constrictor muscles, but it is secondarily changed by elevation or depression of the larynx.

Facial muscles are important for articulation that involves the lips. Numerous muscles insert into the orbicularis oris inferior and superior muscles, permitting lip protrusion, closure, retraction, elevation, and depression. The risorius and buccinator muscles retract the lips and support entrapment of air in the oral cavity. The levator labii superioris, zygomatic minor, levator labii superioris alaeque nasi, and levator anguli oris elevate the upper lip, and the depressor labii inferioris depresses the lower lip. The zygomatic major muscle elevates and retracts the corner of the mouth. The depressor labii inferioris pulls the lips down and out. The depressor anguli oris muscle depresses the corner of the mouth, and the mentalis muscle pulls the lower lip out. The platysma depresses the mandible.

The tongue occupies the floor of the mouth, being divided into dorsum, apex (tip), and base. Fine movements are the product of the intrinsic musculature (transverse, vertical, inferior longitudinal and superior longitudinal muscles of the tongue). Larger adjustments of lingual movement require extrinsic muscles. The genioglossus retracts, protrudes, or depresses the tongue, and the hyoglossus and chondro-glossus depress the tongue. The styloglossus and palatoglossus elevate the posterior tongue.

Muscles of mastication include mandibular elevators and depres-sors, as well as muscles to protrude the mandible. The masseter, tempo-ralis, and medial pterygoid muscles elevate the mandible, and the lateral pterygoids protrude it. Mandibular depression is achieved by the mylo-hyoid, geniohyoid, and platysma muscles.

The soft palate, or velum, is attached to the posterior hard palate. The levator veli palatini muscle elevates the soft palate and the musculus uvulae bunches it. The tensor veli palatini tenses and shortens the palate. The soft palate is depressed by the palatoglossus and palatopharyngeus. The superior pharyngeal constrictor assists in gaining velopharyngeal closure, while peristaltic movement of food is facilitated by the middle and inferior pharyngeal constrictors. The cricopharyngeus forms the muscular orifice of the esophagus. The salpingopharyngeus elevates the pharyngeal wall, and the stylopharyngeus assists in elevation of the pharynx.

Mastication and deglutition can be viewed behaviorally or as a system of reflexive responses. The behavioral stages of mastication and deglutition include the oral preparatory, oral, pharyngeal, and esopha-geal stages. In the oral preparation stage, food is introduced into the oral cavity, moved onto the molars for chewing, and mixed with saliva to form a concise bolus between the tongue and the hard palate. In the oral stage, the bolus is moved back toward the oropharynx by the tongue. The pharyngeal stage begins when the bolus reaches the faucial pillars. The soft palate and larynx elevate, and the bolus is propelled through the pharynx to the upper esophageal sphincter, which has re-laxed to receive the material (realize that this is not a true sphincter, in the sense that it is not a "ring" of muscle, but rather a valve that capital-izes on tonic contraction). The epiglottis has dropped to partially cover the laryngeal opening, whereas the intrinsic musculature of the larynx has effected a tight seal to protect the airway. Food passes over the epi-glottis and through the piriform sinuses to the esophagus. The final, esophageal stage involves the peristaltic movement of the bolus through the esophagus.

STUDY QUESTIONS

1. The _____ theory of vowel production states that the voicing source is routed through the vocal tract where it is shaped into the sounds of speech by the articulators.

2. On the accompanying figure, identify the indicated bones and landmarks.

   A. _____ (bone)

   B. _____ (bone)

   C. _____ bone

   D. _____ bone

   E. _____ bone

   F. _____ process

   G. _____ process

   H. _____

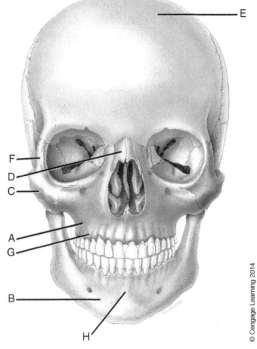

© Cengage Learning 2014

3. On the accompanying figure, identify the indicated bones and landmarks.

A. _____ (bone)

B. _____ bone

C. _____ bone

D. _____

E. _____

F. _____

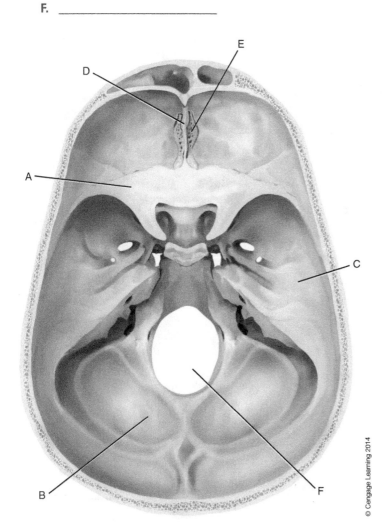

© Cengage Learning 2014

4. On the accompanying figure, identify the indicated bones and landmarks.

A. _____ bone

B. _____ bone

C. _____ (bone)

D. _____ (bone)

E. _____ bone

F. _____ bone

G. _____ bone

H. _____ bone

I. _____

J. _____

K. _____ process

L. _____ process

M. _____ process

N. _____

O. _____ process

P. _____ process

Q. _____

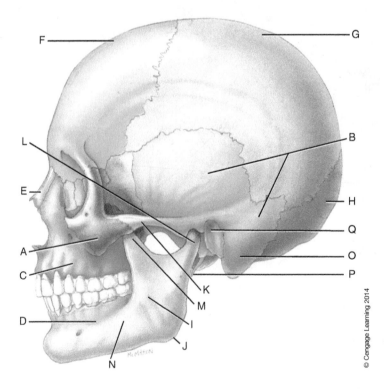

© Cengage Learning 2014

5. On the accompanying figure, identify the indicated structures.

A. _____ process

B. _____ (bone)

C. _____ bone

D. _____

E. _____ foramen

F. _____ suture

G. _____ process

H. _____ plate

I. _____ plate

J. _____ process

K. _____

L. _____

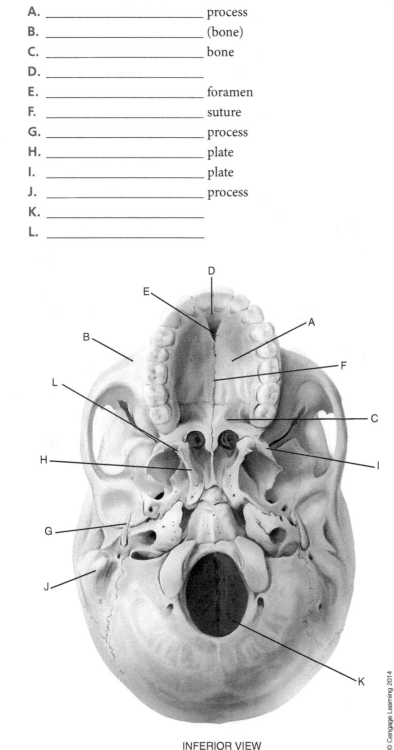

INFERIOR VIEW

© Cengage Learning 2014

6. On the accompanying figure, identify the indicated muscles.

A. _____

B. _____

C. _____

D. _____

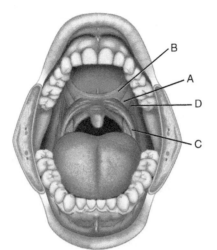

ANTERIOR VIEW

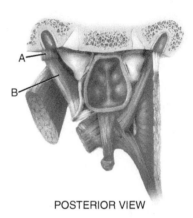

POSTERIOR VIEW

LATERAL VIEW

© Cengage Learning 2014

7. On the accompanying figure, identify the indicated muscles.

A. _____

B. _____

C. _____

D. _____

E. _____

F. _____

G. _____

H. _____

I. _____

J. _____

K. _____

L. _____

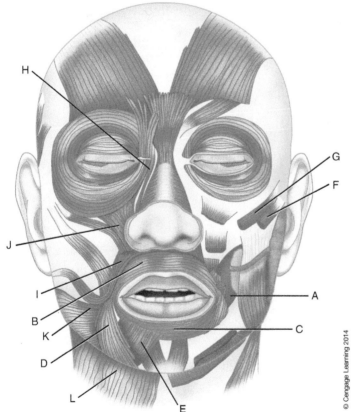

© Cengage Learning 2014

8. On the accompanying figure, identify the indicated muscles.

A. _____

B. _____

C. _____

D. _____

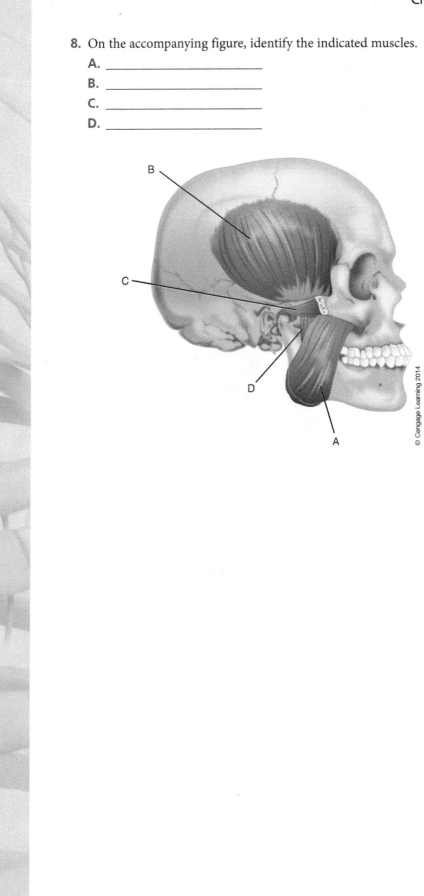

© Cengage Learning 2014

9. On the accompanying figure, identify the indicated muscles.

A. _____

B. _____

C. _____

D. _____

E. _____

F. _____

G. _____

H. _____

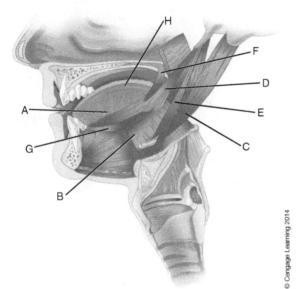

© Cengage Learning 2014

10. On the accompanying figure, identify indicated structures.

A. _____ (bone)

B. _____ process

C. _____ plate

D. _____ plate

E. _____

F. _____ bone

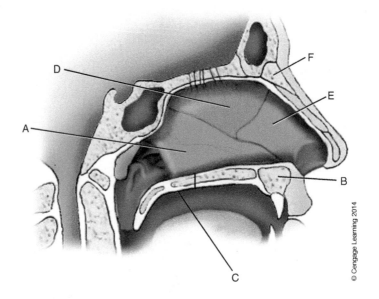

© Cengage Learning 2014

11. _____ refers to the processes involved in food preparation, such as chewing food, moving the food onto the molars, and so forth.

12. _____ refers to swallowing.

13. In the _____ stage of swallowing, food is prepared for swallowing.

14. In the _____ stage of swallowing, mastication ceases, the tongue drops down and pulls posteriorly, and the anterior tongue elevates to the hard palate and squeezes the bolus back toward the faucial pillars.

15. In the _____ stage of swallowing, the bolus contacts the anterior faucial pillars, the soft palate elevates, respiration stops, the vocal folds tightly adduct, the larynx elevates and moves forward, and the cricopharyngeus relaxes as food enters the pharynx.

16. During the _____ stage of swallowing, the bolus is transported through the esophagus.

17. Identify the muscle that best fits the statement. (In some cases more than one muscle fills the bill.)

    A. _____ Elevates tongue tip

    B. _____ Depresses tongue tip

    C. _____ Protrudes tongue

    D. _____ Retracts tongue

    E. _____ Elevates posterior tongue

    F. _____ Narrows tongue

    G. _____ Flattens tongue

    H. _____ Depresses soft palate

    I. _____ Tenses soft palate

    J. _____ Constricts esophageal opening

    K. _____ Constricts upper pharynx

    L. _____ Elevates soft palate

18. Motor control in the body develops from _____ (head/tail) to _____ (head/tail) and from _____ (proximal/distal) to _____ (proximal/distal).

19. Tongue movement depends on the graceful balance of many muscles. Which muscles are involved in elevation of the back of the tongue? As you think of this, ponder the muscles that must work as antagonists to help structures as well.

REFERENCES

Abbs, J. H., & Cole, K. J. (1991). Consideration of bulbar and suprabulbar afferent influences upon speech motor coordination and programming. In Grillner, S., Lindblom, B., Lubker, J., & Persson, A. (Eds.), *Speech motor control* (pp. 159–186). Oxford: Pergamon.

Abrahams, P. H., McMinn, R. M. H., Hutchings, R. T., et al. (2003). *McMinn's color atlas of human anatomy* (5th ed.). Philadelphia: Mosby.

Arvedson, J. C., & Brodsky, L. (2001). *Pediatric swallowing and feeding: Assessment and management*. Clifton Park, NY: Delmar Cengage Learning.

Baken, R. J., & Orlikoff, R. F. (1999). *Clinical measurement of speech and voice* (2nd ed.). San Diego: Singular Publishing Group.

Barlow, S. M., & Netsell, R. (1986). Differential fine force control of the upper and lower lips. *Journal of Speech and Hearing Research, 29,* 163–169.

Barlow, S. M., & Rath, E. M. (1985). Maximum voluntary closing forces in the upper and lower lips of humans. *Journal of Speech and Hearing Research, 28,* 373–376.

Basmajian, J. V. (1975). *Grant's method of anatomy*. Baltimore: Williams & Wilkins.

Bateman, H. E. (1977). *A clinical approach to speech anatomy and physiology*. Springfield, IL: Charles C. Thomas.

Bateman, H. E., & Mason, R. M. (1984). *Applied anatomy and physiology of the speech and hearing mechanism.* Springfield, IL: Charles C. Thomas.

Beck, E. W., Monson, H., & Groer, M. (1982). *Mosby's atlas of functional human anatomy.* St. Louis: Mosby.

Bhatnagar, S. C. (2007). *Neuroscience for the study of communicative disorders* (3rd ed.). Philadelphia, PA: Lippincott, Williams & Wilkins.

Bly, L. (1983). *The components of normal movement during the first year of life and abnormal motor movement.* Chicago: Neuro-Developmental Treatment Association.

Bly, L. (1994). *Motor skills acquisition in the first year.* Tucson, AZ: Therapy Skill Builders.

Buck, L. B. (2000). Smell and taste: The chemical senses. In E. R. Kandel, J. H. Schwartz, & T. M. Jessell (Eds.), *Principles of neural science* (4th ed.). New York: McGraw-Hill.

Bunton, K., & Weismer, G. (1994). Evaluation of a reiterant force-impulse task in the tongue. *Journal of Speech and Hearing Research, 37,* 1020–1031.

Burbank, E., Seikel, J., & Burke, R. (2006). The perception of umami in non-pathological individuals. Poster presented at the Annual Convention of the American Speech-Language Hearing Association.

Chusid, J. G. (1985). *Correlative neuroanatomy and functional neurology* (17th ed.). Los Altos, CA: Lange Medical Publications.

Corbin-Lewis, K., Liss, J. M., & Sciortino, K. L. (2005). *Clinical anatomy and physiology of the swallow mechanism.* Clifton Park, NY: Delmar Cengage Learning.

Cotman, C. W., & McGaugh, J. L. (1980). *Behavioral neuroscience.* New York: Academic Press.

DeNil, L. F., & Abbs, J. H (1991). Influence of speaking rate on the upper lip, lower lip, and jaw peak velocity sequencing during bilabial closing movements. *Journal of the Acoustical Society of America, 89* (2), 845–849.

Duffy, J. R. (1995). *Motor speech disorders.* St. Louis: Mosby.

Ettema, S. L., & Kuehn, D. P. (1994). A quantitative histologic study of the normal human adult soft palate. *Journal of Speech and Hearing Research, 37,* 303–313.

Fairbanks, G. (1954). A theory of the speech mechanism as a servosystem. *Journal of Speech and Hearing Disorders, 19,* 133–139.

Flege, J. E. (1988). Anticipatory and carry-over nasal coarticulation in the speech of children and adults. *Journal of Speech and Hearing Research, 31,* 525–536.

Folkins, J. W., Linville, R. N., Garrett, J. D., & Brown, C. K. (1988). Interactions in the labial musculature during speech. *Journal of Speech and Hearing Research, 31,* 253–264.

Ganong, W. F. (2003). *Review of medical physiology* (21st ed.). New York: McGraw-Hill/Appleton & Lange.

Garcia-Colera, A., & Semjen, A. (1988). Distributed planning of movement sequences. *Journal of Motor Behavior, 20* (3), 341–367.

Gelb, H. (1985). *Clinical management of head, neck and TMJ pain and dysfunction.* Philadelphia: Saunders.

Goffman, L., & Smith, A. (1994). Motor unit territories in the human perioral musculature. *Journal of Speech and Hearing Research, 37,* 975–984.

Gosling, J. A., Harris, P. F., Humpherson, J. R., et al. (1985). *Atlas of human anatomy.* Philadelphia: J. B. Lippincott.

Gracco, V. L. (1988). Timing factors in the coordination of speech movements. *Journal of Neuroscience, 8* (12), 4628–4639.

Gracco, V. L. (1994). Some organizational characteristics of speech movement control. *Journal of Speech and Hearing Research, 37,* 4–27.

Gracco, V. L., & Abbs, J. H. (1989). Sensorimotor characteristics of speech motor sequences. *Experimental Brain Research, 75,* 586–598.

Gray, H., Bannister, L. H., Berry, M. M., & Williams, P. L. (Eds.). (1995). *Gray's anatomy.* London: Churchill Livingstone.

Grobler, N. J. (1977). *Textbook of clinical anatomy* (Vol. 1). Amsterdam: Elsevier Scientific.

Groher, M. E. (1997). *Dysphagia* (3rd ed.). St. Louis: Butterworth-Heinemann.

Hall, P. K., Hardy, J. C., & LaVelle, W. E. (1990). A child with signs of developmental apraxia of speech with whom a palatal lift prosthesis was used to manage palatal dysfunction. *Journal of Speech and Hearing Disorders, 55,* 454–460.

Hauser, G., Daponte, A., & Roberts, M. J. (1989). Palatal rugae. *Journal of Anatomy, 124,* 237–249.

Hellstrand, E. (1981). The neuromuscular system of the tongue. In S. Grillner, B. Lindblom, J. Lubker, & A. Persson (Eds.), *Speech motor control* (pp. 141–157). Oxford: Pergamon.

Horak, M. (1992). The utility of connectionism for motor learning: A reinterpretation of contextual interference in movement schemas. *Journal of Motor Behavior, 24* (1), 58–66.

Jordan, M. I. (1990). Motor learning and the degrees of freedom problem. In M. Jeannerod (Ed.), *Attention and performance XIII: Motor representation and control.* Hillsdale, NJ: Lawrence Erlbaum.

Kahane, J. C., & Folkins, J. F. (1984). *Atlas of speech and hearing anatomy.* Columbus, OH: Charles E. Merrill.

Kandel, E. R., Schwartz, J. H., & Jessell, T. M. (2000). *Principles of neural science* (4th ed.). New York: McGraw-Hill.

Kapetansky, D. I. (1987). *Cleft lip, nose, and palate reconstruction.* Philadelphia: Lippincott.

Kaplan, H. (1960). *Anatomy and physiology of speech.* New York: McGraw-Hill.

Katz, W. F., Kripke, C., & Tallal, P. (1991). Anticipatory coarticulation in the speech of adults and young children: Acoustic, perceptual, and video data. *Journal of Speech and Hearing Research, 34,* 1222–1249.

Kelso, J. A. S., Tuller, B., Vatikiotis-Bateson, E., & Fowler, C. A. (1984). Functionally specific articulatory cooperation following jaw perturbations during speech: Evidence for coordinative structures. *Journal of Experimental Psychology: Perception and Performance, 19,* 812–832.

Kelso, J. A., & Ding, M. (1993). Fluctuations, intermittency, and controllable chaos in biological coordination. In K. M. Newell & D. M. Corcos (Eds.), *Variability and motor control* (pp. 291–316). Champaign, IL: Human Kinetics.

Kent, R. D. (1997). *The speech sciences.* San Diego: Singular Publishing Group.

Kent, R. D., Kent, J. F., & Rosenbek, J. C. (1987). Maximum performance tests of speech production. *Journal of Speech and Hearing Disorders, 52,* 367–387.

Kuehn, D. P., Lemme, M. L., & Baumgartner, J. M. (1989). *Neural bases of speech, hearing, and language.* Boston: Little, Brown.

Kuehn, D. P., Templeton, P. J., & Maynard, J. A. (1990). Muscle spindles in the velopharyngeal musculature of humans. *Journal of Speech and Hearing Research, 33,* 488–493.

Landgren, S., & Olsson, K. A. (1981). Oral mechanoreceptors. In S. Grillner, B. Lindblom, J. Lubker, & A. Persson (Eds.), *Speech motor control* (pp. 129–139). Oxford: Pergamon.

Langley, M. B., & Lombardino, L. J. (1991). *Neurodevelopmental strategies for managing communication disorders in children with severe motor dysfunction.* Austin, TX: Pro-Ed.

Lashley, K. S. (1951). The problem of serial order in behavior. In L. A. Jerrers (Ed.), *Cerebral mechanisms in behavior* (pp. 506–528). New York: Wiley.

Lieberman, P. (1977). *Speech physiology and acoustic phonetics: An introduction.* New York: Macmillan.

Liss, J. M. (1990). Muscle spindles in the human levator veli palatini and palatoglossus muscles. *Journal of Speech and Hearing Research, 33,* 736–746.

Logemann, J. (1998). *Evaluation and treatment of swallowing disorder* (2nd ed.). Austin, TX: Pro-Ed.

Love, R. J., Hagerman, E. L., & Taimi, E. G. (1980). Speech performance, dysphagia, and oral reflexes in cerebral palsy. *Journal of Speech and Hearing Disorders, 45,* 59–75.

McClean, M. (1973). Forward coarticulation of velar movement at marked junctural boundaries. *Journal of Speech and Hearing Research, 16,* 286–296.

McMinn, R. M. H., Hutchings, R. T., & Logan, B. M. (1994). *Color atlas of head and neck anatomy.* London: Mosby-Wolfe.

McNeil, M. R., Weismer, G., Adams, S., & Mulligan, M. (1990). Oral structure nonspeech motor control in normal, dysarthric, aphasic, and apraxic speakers: Isometric force and static position control. *Journal of Speech and Hearing Research, 33,* 255–268.

Minifie, F. (1973). Speech acoustics. In F. D. Minifie, T. J. Hixon, & F. Williams (Eds.), *Normal aspects of speech, hearing, and language* (pp. 11–72). Englewood Cliffs, NJ: Prentice-Hall.

Møller, A. R. (2003). *Sensory systems: Anatomy and physiology.* New York: Academic Press.

Moore, C. A. (1993). Symmetry of mandibular muscle activity as an index of coordinative strategy. *Journal of Speech and Hearing Research, 36,* 1145–1157.

Moore, C. A., Smith, A., & Ringel, R. L. (1988). Task-specific organization of activity in human jaw muscles. *Journal of Speech and Hearing Research, 31,* 670–680.

Moore, K. L. (1988). *The developing human.* Philadelphia: Saunders.

Mountcastle, V. B. (1974). *Medical physiology.* St. Louis: Mosby.

Netsell, R. (1973). Speech physiology. In F. D. Minifie, T. J. Hixon & F. Williams (Eds.), *Normal aspects of speech, hearing, and language* (pp. 134–211). Englewood Cliffs, NJ: Prentice-Hall.

Netsell, R. (1986). *A neurobiologic view of speech production and the dysarthrias.* San Diego: College-Hill.

Netter, F. (1976). *Clinical symposia: Development of the upper respiratory system.* Summit, NJ: CIBA Pharmaceutical Company.

Netter, F. H. (1983). *The CIBA collection of medical illustrations.* Vol. 1. *Nervous system.* Part I. *Anatomy and physiology.* West Caldwell, NJ: CIBA Pharmaceutical Company.

Netter, F. H. (1989). *Atlas of human anatomy.* Summit, NJ: CIBA Pharmaceuticals Division.

Netter, F. H. (1997). *Atlas of human anatomy.* Los Angeles: Icon Learning Systems.

Newman, K. D., & Randolph, J. (1990). Surgical problems of the esophagus in infants and children. In D. C. Sabiston & F. C. Spencer (Eds.), *Surgery of the chest* (5th ed., pp. 815–839). Philadelphia: W. B. Saunders.

Nolte, J. (2002). *The human brain* (5th ed.). St. Louis: Mosby.

Payne, W. S., & Ellis, F. H., Jr. (1984). Esophagus and diaphragmatic hernias. In S. I. Schwartz, G. T. Shires, F. C. Spencer, & E. H. Storer (Eds.), *Principles of surgery* (4th ed., pp. 1063–1112). New York: McGraw-Hill.

Perlman, A. L., Grayhack, J. P., & Booth, B. M. (1992). The relationship of vallecular residue to oral involvement, reduced hyoid elevation, and epiglottic function. *Journal of Speech and Hearing Research, 35,* 734–741.

Perlman, A. L., Luschei, E. S., & DuMond, C. E. (1989). Electrical activity from the superior pharyngeal constrictor during reflexive and nonreflexive tasks. *Journal of Speech and Hearing Research, 32,* 749–754.

Pickett, J. M. (1980). *The sounds of speech communication.* Baltimore: University Park Press.

Rademaker, A. W., Pauloski, B. R., Logemann, J. A., & Shanahan, T. K. (1994). Oropharyngeal swallow efficiency as a representative measure of swallowing function. *Journal of Speech and Hearing Research, 37,* 314–325.

Rohen, J. W., & Yokochi, C. (1993). *Color atlas of anatomy.* New York: Igaku-Shoin.

Rohen, J. W., Yokochi, C., Lutjen-Drecoll, E. L., & Romrell, L. J. (2002). *Color atlas of anatomy: A photographic study of the human body* (5th ed.). Philadelphia: Lippincott, Williams & Wilkins.

Rosenbaum, D. A., Kenny, S. B., & Derr, M. A. (1983). Hierarchical control of rapid movement sequences. *Journal of Experimental Psychology: Human Perception and Performance, 9* (1), 86–102.

Rosenbek, J. C., Robbins, J., Fishback, B., & Levine, R. L. (1991). Effects of thermal application on dysphagia after stroke. *Journal of Speech and Hearing Research, 34,* 1257–1268.

Rosse, C., Gaddum-Rosse, P., & Rosse, G. (1997). *Hollinshead's textbook of anatomy.* Philadelphia: Lippincott-Raven.

Saltzman, E. (1986). Task dynamic coordination of the speech articulators: A preliminary model. *Experimental brain research* (pp. 129–144). Berlin-Heidelberg: Springer-Verlag.

Sawashima, M., & Cooper, F. S. (1977). *Dynamic aspects of speech production.* Tokyo: University of Tokyo Press.

Schmidt, R. A. (1975). A schema theory of discrete motor skill learning. *Psychological Review, 82,* 225–260.

Shaffer, L. H. (1976). Intention and performance. *Psychological Review, 33* (5), 375–393.

Shprintzen, R. J., & Bardach, J. (1995). *Cleft palate speech management.* St. Louis: Mosby.

Shriberg, L. D., & Kent, R. D. (2002). *Clinical phonetics* (3rd ed.). Boston: Allyn & Bacon.

Small, A. M. (1973). Acoustics. In F. D. Minifie, T. J. Hixon, & F. Williams (Eds.), *Normal aspects of speech, hearing, and language.* Englewood Cliffs, NJ: Prentice-Hall.

Smith, A., McFarland, D. H., & Weber, C. M. (1986). Interactions between speech and finger movements: An exploration of the dynamic pattern perspective. *Journal of Speech and Hearing Research, 29,* 471–480.

Snell, R. S. (1978). *Gross anatomy dissector.* Boston: Little, Brown.

Sonies, B. C. (1997). *Dysphagia. A continuum of care.* Gaithersburg, MD: Aspen.

Square-Storer, P., & Roy, E. A. (1989). The apraxias: Commonalities and distinctions. In P. Square-Storer (Ed.), *Acquired apraxia of speech in aphasic adults: Theoretical and clinical issues.* London: Taylor & Francis.

Weber, C. M., & Smith, A. (1987). Reflex responses in human jaw, lip, and tongue muscles elicited by mechanical stimulation. *Journal of Speech and Hearing Research, 30,* 70–79.

Westbury, J. R. (1988). Mandible and hyoid bone movements during speech. *Journal of Speech and Hearing Research, 31,* 405–416.

Wickens, J., Hyland, B., & Anson, G. (1994). Cortical cell assemblies: A possible mechanism for motor programs. *Journal of Motor Behavior, 26* (2), 66–82.

Wohlert, A. B., & Goffman, L. (1994). Human perioral muscle activation patterns. *Journal of Speech and Hearing Research, 37,* 1032–1040.

Zemlin, W. R. (1998). *Speech and hearing science. Anatomy and physiology* (4th ed.). Needham Heights, MA: Allyn & Bacon.

Zickefoose, W. (1989). *Techniques of oral myofunctional therapy.* Sacramento, CA: O.M.T. Materials.

5

Anatomy and Physiology of Hearing

OUTLINE

C. Inner ear
   1. Osseous labyrinth
      a. Osseous semicircular canals
      b. Osseous cochlear canal
      c. Scala vestibuli
      d. Scala tympani
      e. Osseous spiral lamina
      f. Helicotrema
      g. Round window
      h. Oval window
      i. Cochlear aqueduct
   2. Membranous labyrinth
      a. Vestibular organ
      b. Ampulla
      c. Crista ampullaris
      d. Utricle and saccule
   3. Cochlear duct
      a. Between the scala vestibuli and tympani
      b. Reissner's membrane
      c. Basilar membrane
      d. Support cells for Organ of Corti
      e. Organ of Corti
      f. Hair cells, outer and inner
      g. Innervation

II. Auditory Physiology

A. Outer and middle ear functions
   1. Localization
   2. Resonant frequencies
   3. Impedance matching
B. Inner ear function
   1. Cochlear function
      a. Spectral (frequency) and temporal analyses
      b. Movement of fluid in the scala vestibuli
      c. Disturbance at basilar membrane causes
         the traveling wave
      d. Frequency selectivity
      e. Stiffness, thickness, and width of basilar
         membrane
      f. Shearing effect on the cilia of outer hair
         cells
      g. Fluid flow and turbulence of endolymph
         activates inner hair cells
   2. Neural Responses
      a. Low-threshold and high-threshold neurons
      b. Frequency specificity
      c. Characteristic frequency
      d. Tuning curve

3. Auditory pathway responses
   a. Superior olivary complex
   b. Heschl's gyrus: core, belt, parabelt

THE STRUCTURES OF HEARING

Of all the systems of communication, hearing is the single "communication system" that corresponds precisely with the physical system. We use the other physical systems for purposes beyond their intention, but hearing is precisely designed for communication! It is an evolutionarily "old" system, with pretty obvious importance in protection of an organism. Because it has been evolving over so many years, it has become a very graceful and elegant system of communication. Admittedly, humans use hearing as part of a very complex communication process, but the basics of hearing hold for virtually all organisms.

We will talk about the structure of hearing in humans, examining the anatomy of the outer, middle, and inner ears, and will look at the auditory pathway as well. The auditory mechanism is amazingly powerful, considering its small size! The physical structures of the ear are deceptively simple, especially in light of their exquisite function (see Figure 5–1). The ear is an energy transducer, which means that it converts acoustic energy into electrochemical energy.

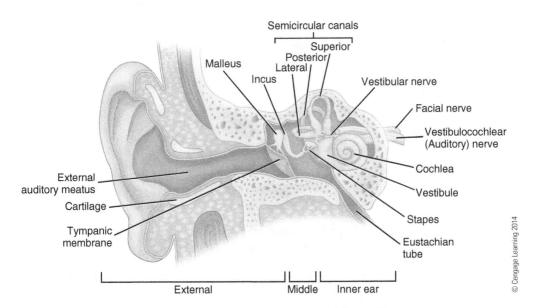

Figure 5–1. Schematic of frontal section revealing outer, middle, and inner ear structures.

Outer Ear

The outer ear is composed of two basic components with which you are quite familiar (Table 5–1). The *pinna* (or auricle) is the prominence we colloquially refer to as the ear, although it serves primarily as a collector of sound to be processed at deeper levels (e.g., the eardrum and cochlea). The structure of the pinna is provided by cartilage (see Figure 5–2 and Table 5–1).

The pinna has several important functions, including aiding localization of sound in space and "capturing" sound energy. The *helix* forms the curled margin of the pinna, and immediately ahead of the helix is the *antihelix*, a similar fold of tissue that marks the entrance to the *concha*. The concha is the entrance to the ear canal, known as the *external auditory meatus* (EAM). A flap of epithelium-covered cartilage known as the *tragus* may have at one time served as a partial cover for the entrance to the *meatus*, or opening. The *lobule* has no cartilage; it is the prominence at the inferior pinna made up of epithelial tissue and fat.

Table 5–1. Landmarks of the Outer Ear

Auricle
Helix
Auricular tubercle (Darwin's tubercle)
Antihelix
Crura
Crura anthelicis
Triangular fossa
Scaphoid fossa
Concha
Cymba conchae
Cavum conchae
Tragus
Intertragic incisure
Antitragus
Lobule

External Auditory Meatus
Cartilaginous meatus
Osseous meatus
Isthmus
Tympanic membrane

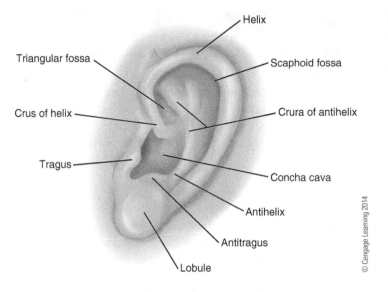

© Cengage Learning 2014

Figure 5–2. Landmarks of the auricle of pinna.

The external auditory meatus is approximately 7 mm in diameter and 2.5 cm long when measured from the depth of the concha, or 4 cm. The lateral one third of the canal is cartilage and is about 8 mm long; the medial two thirds are the bony meatus of the temporal bone. At the end of the EAM is the *tympanic membrane,* or eardrum, a thin trilaminar sheet of tissue that sits at an oblique angle in the EAM. The epithelial cover of the pinna continues into the EAM and serves as the outer layer of the tympanic membrane, to be discussed later.

Because the adult ear canal takes a turn downward, you cannot see the medial end of the canal without some effort. If you were to look into the ear canal, you would see that the outer third of the EAM is lined with hairs, and has cerumen, or ear wax. These are both quite functional additions to the canal because they trap insects and dirt, protecting the medial-most point of the outer ear, the tympanic membrane.

The *tympanic membrane* marks the boundary between the outer and middle ear. It completely separates the two spaces, being an extremely thin three-layered tissue. The epithelial lining of the EAM continues as the external layer of the tympanic membrane, while the lining of the middle ear provides the inner layer. Sandwiched between these two delicate epithelial linings is a layer of fibrous tissue that provides structure for the tympanic membrane.

The tympanic membrane is approximately 55 mm^2 in area and has a number of important landmarks (see Figure 5–3). If you view the tympanic membranes, you will see the *umbo,* which is the most distal point of attachment of the inner tympanic membrane to one of the bones of the middle ear, the *malleus.* The tympanic membrane is particularly taut at this point, and the location inferior and anterior to this

Otitis Externa and Cerumen

The epithelial lining of the pinna and EAM is tightly bound to the cartilage and bone of these structures, which accounts for the pain when the tissue swells. Otitis externa is inflammation of the skin of the external ear. When tissue is inflamed, it responds by edema, or swelling. If the epithelium is tightly bound to its underlying structure, as it is in the EAM and pinna, the swelling increases the tension on the epithelium, making it quite painful.

Otitis externa may result from bacterial infection following trauma or abrasion. Failure to clean probe tips and specula could result in transmission of the infection between clients. Otitis externa can also result from viral infection, including infection with herpes zoster virus. This painful infection may lead to facial paralysis or hearing loss if the facial or vestibulocochlear nerves are involved.

The EAM is invested with cilia and ceruminous glands, largely restricted to the cartilaginous portion of the canal. Cerumen (ear wax) is secreted by the glands into the ear canal, trapping insects and dirt that would otherwise threaten the tympanic membrane. Individuals with overly active ceruminous glands may find that the EAM becomes occluded, and removal of the cerumen may be required. A person's attempts to remove the cerumen with cotton swabs often results in cerumen and dirt being packed against the inferior boundary of the tympanic membrane; the oblique angle forms a perfect "pocket" to catch the matter.

The interested student and budding audiologist or audiology assistant would be well advised to read the descriptions of these and other conditions provided by Martin (1981).

Figure 5–3. Tympanic membrane of the left ear, as viewed from the external auditory meatus.

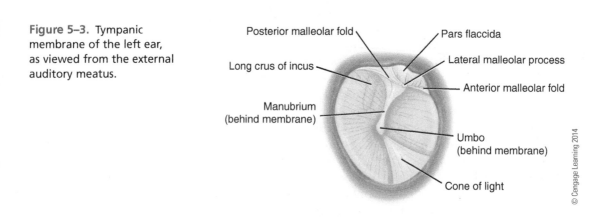

© Cengage Learning 2014

is referred to as the *cone of light*. You may be able to see the handle, or *manubrium*, of the malleus behind the tympanic membrane, appearing as a streak on the membrane.

The tympanic membrane is slightly concave when viewed from the EAM, and the umbo is the most depressed portion of this concavity. Although most of the tympanic membrane is invested with fibrous tissue, the *pars flaccida* is not, and this "flaccid part" can be seen in the superior quadrant of the tympanic membrane. On each side of the pars flaccida is a recess, consisting of the anterior and posterior malleolar folds. These folds and the region at the cone of light are the result of the malleus pushing distally on the membrane, much as if you were to stretch an unfilled balloon and push it from behind. This tight binding between membrane and malleus permits ready transmission of acoustic energy from the tympanic membrane to the ossicular chain. If the tympanic membrane is particularly transparent, you may also be able to see the long process of the incus parallel to the lateral process of malleus. In addition, the *chorda tympani* can sometimes be seen through the superior tympanic membrane.

Summary

- The outer ear is composed of the pinna, the structure that serves primarily as a sound collector, and the external auditory meatus, or ear canal.
- Landmarks of the pinna include the margin of the auricle, the helix, the lobule, and the tragus.

atresia: *Absence.*

stenosis: *Narrowing.*

aplasia: *Lack of development.*

microtia: *Small ear.*

Malformations of the Pinna and EAM

If the pinna is subjected to trauma, as in that inflicted during the "sport" of boxing, the result can be permanent deformation of its structure. Trauma can cause hemorrhaging between the epithelium and cartilage, and if left untreated, the resulting swelling might cause a permanent distortion.

Several congenital conditions can be manifested in the EAM and pinna. Atresia, or congenital absence, of the EAM may signal absence of middle ear structures as well. Stenosis, or narrowing, of the ear canal reduces its ability to transmit sound to the middle ear structures. Aplasia of the pinna occurs when it fails to develop or does not develop completely. If the pinna is abnormally small, it is termed microtia. If something interferes with development, the pinnae may remain set low on the sides of the head.

A number of genetic syndromes cause auricular anomalies. Children affected by branchio-oto-renal syndrome often have cupped ears or microtia in conjunction with disarticulation of the bones of the middle ear and conductive or sensorineural hearing loss. A high proportion of individuals with Down syndrome (trisomy 21) show microtia, have small earlobes and helix malformation, and occasionally have stenosis of the ear canal.

■ The external auditory meatus has both osseous and cartilaginous parts.

■ At the terminus of the external auditory meatus is the tympanic membrane, the structure that separates the outer and middle ear.

Middle Ear

Structure of the Tympanic Membrane

The tympanic membrane is a slightly oval structure, being approximately 10 mm in diameter in the superior-inferior dimension. The anterior-posterior dimension is slightly smaller (about 9 mm in diameter), and the entire membrane is placed in the canal at a 55° angle with the floor. The circumference of the membrane is a fibrocartilaginous ring that fits into the tympanic sulcus, a groove in the temporal bone. The sulcus is incomplete in the superior aspect, accommodating the anterior and posterior malleolar folds.

The tympanic membrane is made up of three layers of tissue: outer, intermediate, and inner. The outer (cuticular) layer is a continuation of the epithelial lining of the EAM and pinna. The intermediate (fibrous) layer is made up of two parts: (1) The superficial layer is composed of fibers that radiate out from the handle of the malleus to the periphery. (2) The deep layer is made up of circular fibers that are found mostly in the periphery of the membrane. The inner (mucous) layer is continuous with the mucosa of the middle ear.

The middle ear is a small but extremely important space occupied by three of the smallest bones of the body. First, let us examine these bones and their attachments, then we will explore their attachments, and then we will explore the landmarks of the cavity itself (Table 5–2).

Ossicles

The bones of the ear, known as the *ossicles*, include the *malleus, incus,* and *stapes* (see Figures 5–4 and 5–5). This ossicular chain of three articulated bones provides the means for transmission of acoustic energy by impinging on the tympanic membrane to the inner ear. The malleus, the largest ossicle, provides the point of attachment with the tympanic membrane.

As you can see in Figure 5–4, the handle, or manubrium, of the malleus is a long process, separated from the head by a thin neck. The anterior and lateral processes provide points of attachment for ligaments. The manubrium attaches to the tympanic membrane along its length, terminating with the lateral process.

The incus (fancied to be shaped like an anvil) provides the intermediate link of the ossicular chain. The body of the

Table 5–2. Landmarks of the Middle Ear

Ossicles
Malleus
    Manubrium (handle)
    Head (caput)
    Lateral process
    Anterior process
    Facet for incus
    Ligaments
        Superior ligament
        Lateral ligament
        Anterior ligament
Incus
    Short process (crus breve)
    Long process (crus longum)
    Lenticular process
    Facet for malleus
    Superior ligament of incus
    Posterior ligament of incus
Stapes
    Head (caput)
    Neck
    Posterior crus (crus posterius)

© Cengage Learning 2014

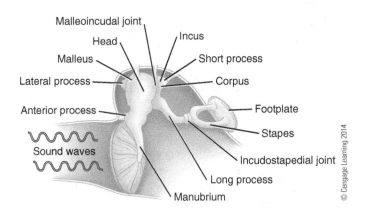

Malleoincudal joint
Head
Malleus
Lateral process
Anterior process
Sound waves
Incus
Short process
Corpus
Footplate
Stapes
Incudostapedial joint
Long process
Manubrium

© Cengage Learning 2014

Figure 5–4. Articulated ossicular chain of the right ear in medial view.

incus articulates with the head of the malleus by means of the malleolar facet in such a way that the long process of the incus is nearly parallel to the long process of the malleus. The long process bends medially, forming the lenticular process with which the stapes articulate.

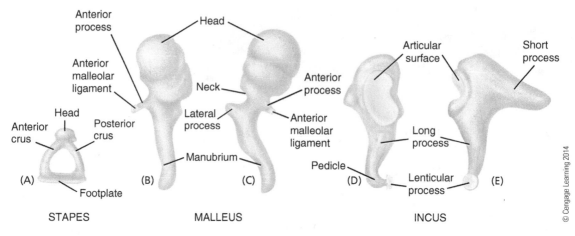

Figure 5–5. Ossicles of the middle ear and their landmarks. (A) Stapes landmarks. (B) Posteromedial view of malleus. (C) Anteromedial view of malleus. (D) Anteromedial view of incus. (E) Posteromedial view of incus.

The stapes, or "stirrup," is the third bone of this chain. The head (caput) of the stapes articulates with the lenticular process of incus, and the neck of the stapes bifurcates to become the crura. The arch formed by the anterior and posterior crura converges on the footplate, or base, of the stapes. The footplate of the stapes rests in the oval window of the temporal bone, held in place by the annular ligament.

Tympanic Muscles

Two important muscles of the middle ear are attached to the ossicles. These are the smallest muscles of the human body.

Stapedius. The *stapedius muscle*, approximately 6 mm long, is embedded in the bone of the posterior wall of the middle ear, with only its tendon emerging from the pyramidal eminence in the middle ear space. The muscle inserts into the posterior neck of stapes, so that when it contracts, the stapes is rotated posteriorly. Innervation of the stapedius is by means of the stapedial branch of the facial nerve (cranial nerve VII).

Tensor Tympani. The *tensor tympani* is approximately 19.5 to 25 mm long, arising from the anterior wall of the middle ear space, superior to the orifice of the eustachian tube. As with the stapedius, only the tendon of the tensor tympani is found in the middle ear space, with the muscle housed in bone. The muscle originates from the cartilaginous part of the eustachian tube, as well as from the greater wing of sphenoid, coursing through the canal for the tensor tympani in the anterior wall of the middle ear. Contraction of this muscle reduces the range of movement of the tympanic membrane by placing indirect tension on it. Indeed, both tensor tympani and stapedius muscles stiffen the middle ear transmission system, thereby reducing transmission of acoustical information in the lower frequencies. Innervation of the tensor tympani is by the trigeminal nerve (cranial nerve V).

Landmarks of Middle Ear

The middle ear space is invested with numerous landmarks of importance in the study of auditory function. Refer to Figure 5–6 for a schematic of the right middle ear, to help follow our discussion.

Medial Wall. On the medial wall (Figure 5–6B) you can see the *oval window* in which the *footplate of the stapes* is embedded, and the *round window*. Between these two is the *promontory*, a bulge created by the basal turn of the cochlea. Immediately above the oval window is the prominence of the *lateral semicircular canal* of the vestibular mechanism.

Examination of the anterior wall reveals the entrance to the eustachian tube, and within that wall the internal carotid artery courses. The canal for the tensor tympani arises from the medial-most aspect of this wall, marked by the trochleariform process.

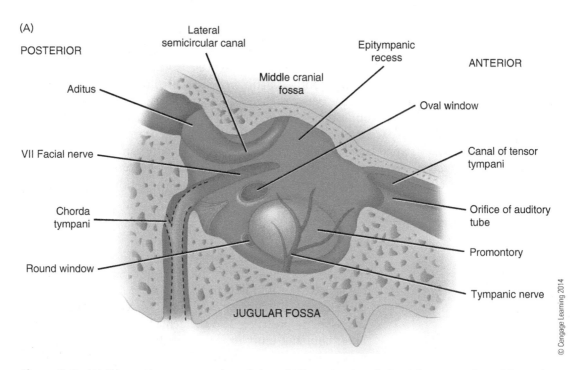

Figure 5–6. (A) Schematic representation of the middle ear cavity of the right ear, as viewed from the external auditory meatus with tympanic membrane and ossicles removed. *(continues)*

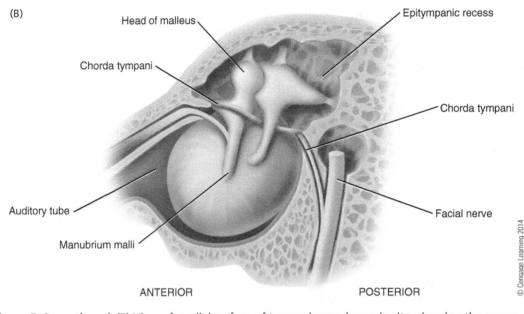

(B)

Head of malleus

Epitympanic recess

Chorda tympani

Chorda tympani

Auditory tube

Facial nerve

Manubrium malli

ANTERIOR   POSTERIOR

© Cengage Learning 2014

Figure 5–6. continued (B) View of medial surface of tympanic membrane in situ, showing the course of the chorda tympani nerve.

Otitis Media with Effusion

Serous (secretory) otitis media is any condition in which fluid accumulates in the middle ear cavity. The typical sequence is as follows. The eustachian tube stops functioning properly, allowing the middle ear space to become anaerobic as tissue within the space absorbs the available oxygen. Parallel to this, the poorly functioning eustachian tube does not allow equalization of pressure between the middle ear space and the environment. In either condition, a relatively negative pressure can ensue in the middle ear space, pulling serous fluid from the blood of the middle ear tissues (termed transudation). The negative air pressure can also stimulate secretion of mucus from the middle ear tissue. This state, termed middle ear effusion, places a barrier to sound transmission in that the movement of the tympanic membrane is greatly inhibited.

The eustachian tube is the sole means of bringing oxygen to the middle ear space (aeration), an important process for maintaining equilibrium between middle ear and atmospheric pressure. The eustachian tube is about 36 mm long, coursing anteriorly and medially on its way to the nasopharynx. The eustachian tube is capable of expanding by pulling the inferior margins away from each other, a function performed by the tensor veli palatine.

Acoustic Reflex

The acoustic reflex (also known as the stapedial reflex) is a staple of the audiologist's diagnostic toolkit. The stapedius muscle applies a force on the footplate of the stapes that reduces the amplitude of the footplate's movement, thereby reducing the sound pressure level reaching the cochlea. It is thought that this is a basic protective mechanism for the cochlea because it is triggered by loud sounds, typically greater than 85 dB SPL (sound pressure level). The acoustic reflex can also include response by the tensor tympani muscle.

The neural circuit for the acoustic reflex is such that stimulation of either ear results in response by both ears, although attenuation of the signal by the ipsilateral ear (the ear closest to the sound) is stronger than the attenuation in the contralateral ear. As outlined by Møller (1983), a stimulus entering the right ear is transduced by the right cochlea, right ventral cochlear nucleus, and right medial superior olive, consecutively. The right medial superior olive communicates with both the right- and left-side nuclei of the facial (VII) and trigeminal (V) nerves, so that the appropriate stimulus triggers a response in stapedius muscles on both left and right sides.

Pressure Equalization Tubes

Placement of pressure equalization (PE) tubes in the tympanic membrane is one of the most common surgical procedures performed in the United States. A PE tube is a small medical device (also known as a tympanostomy tube) that allows air (and fluid) flow between the middle and outer ear areas. A myringotomy (surgical incision in the tympanic membrane) is performed, and the small PE tube is inserted into the incised eardrum. With the PE tube in place, the air pressure between the outer and middle ear is equalized. High negative pressure in the middle ear (relative to the atmospheric pressure) causes intracellular fluid to seep into the middle ear space, filling it with fluid. The PE tube replaces the function of the auditory tube, which may be temporarily dysfunctional due to inflammation secondary to allergies or other conditions. PE tubes greatly reduce the occurrence of otitis media, improve hearing, and improve language and speech development.

On the posterior wall is the prominence of the stapedial pyramid, from which the tendon of stapedius arises en route to the neck of stapes. Within the posterior wall courses the chorda tympani, and the facial nerve (cranial nerve VII) prominence continues on the medial wall.

Summary

- The malleus is the largest of the ossicles and provides the point of attachment with the tympanic membrane.
- The incus provides the intermediate communicating link of the ossicular chain, and the stapes is the third bone of this chain.
- The ossicular chain is held in place by the superior, anterior, and lateral ligaments of malleus and the posterior and superior ligaments of incus.
- The stapedius muscle inserts into the posterior neck of stapes and pulls the stapes posteriorly.
- The tensor tympani muscle inserts into the upper manubrium mallei and pulls the malleus anteromedially.
- Landmarks of the medial wall of the middle ear cavity include the oval window, the round window, the promontory of the cochlea, and the prominence of facial nerve.
- The anterior wall houses the entrance to the eustachian tube, and the posterior wall houses the prominence of the stapedial pyramid.

Inner Ear

The inner ear houses the sensors for balance (the vestibular system) and hearing (the cochlea) (see Table 5–3). The entryway to the cochlea is the *vestibule*. Depicted in Figure 5–7 is the osseous, or bony, labyrinth, representing the cavities (tunnels) in which the inner ear structures (the membranous labyrinth) are housed. The *osseous labyrinth* is made up of the entryway to the labyrinth, the vestibule, *semicircular canals*, and the *osseous cochlear canal*.

Osseous Semicircular Canals

The osseous semicircular canals house the sense organs for movement of the body in space. These consist of the anterior, posterior, and horizontal semicircular canals, each canal's name describing its orientation. You can envision the canals as a series of three rings attached to a ball (the vestibule), and lying behind and above that ball. Each ring is in a plane at right angles to one other ring, so that the interaction of the three permits the brain to code movement in three-dimensional space. The semicircular canals all open onto the vestibule.

The anterior vertical canal is oriented so that it senses movement in the plane roughly perpendicular to the length of the temporal bone. This configuration transduces lateral movement of the head such as rocking your head from one shoulder to the other. The posterior vertical semicircular

Table 5–3. Landmarks of the Inner Ear

Vestibule
- Saccule
- Utricle
- Macula
- Otolithic membrane
- Stereocilia
- Kinocilium
- Ductus reuniens
- Endolymphatic duct

Semicircular Canals
- Lateral semicircular canal
- Anterior vertical semicircular canal
- Posterior vertical semicircular canal
- Ampulla
- Crista ampullaris
- Stereocilia
- Kinocilium

Cochlea
- Scala vestibuli
- Scala tympani
- Scala media (cochlear duct)
    - Reissner's membrane
    - Basilar membrane
    - Spiral ligament
    - Stria vascularis
    - Organ of Corti
        - Inner and outer hair cells
        - Deiters' cells
        - Tunnel of Corti
        - Spiral limbus
        - Inner spiral sulcus
        - Tectorial membrane
        - Reticular lamina
        - Hensen's cells
        - Cells of Claudius
        - Rods of Corti

Osseous Spiral Lamina
- Habenula perforata

Helicotrema

© Cengage Learning 2014

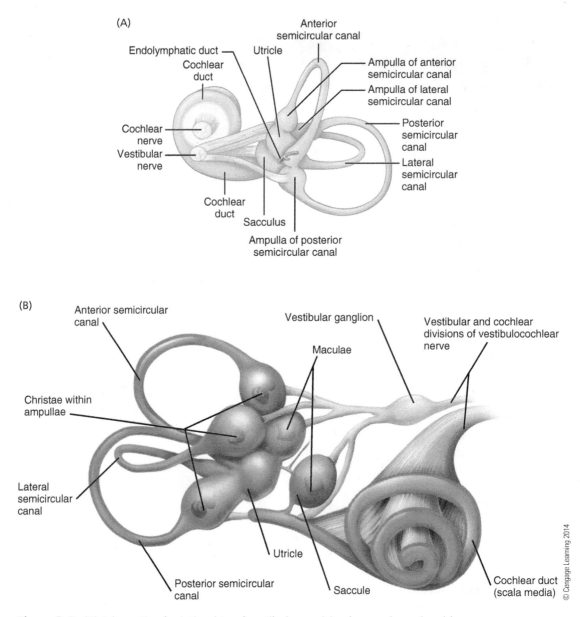

(A)

Endolymphatic duct
Cochlear duct
Utricle
Anterior semicircular canal
Ampulla of anterior semicircular canal
Ampulla of lateral semicircular canal
Posterior semicircular canal
Lateral semicircular canal
Cochlear nerve
Vestibular nerve
Cochlear duct
Sacculus
Ampulla of posterior semicircular canal

(B)

Anterior semicircular canal
Vestibular ganglion
Vestibular and cochlear divisions of vestibulocochlear nerve
Maculae
Christae within ampullae
Lateral semicircular canal
Utricle
Posterior semicircular canal
Saccule
Cochlear duct (scala media)

© Cengage Learning 2014

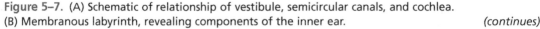

Figure 5–7. (A) Schematic of relationship of vestibule, semicircular canals, and cochlea. (B) Membranous labyrinth, revealing components of the inner ear. *(continues)*

canal is oriented roughly parallel to the length of the temporal bone; it senses movement in the anterior-posterior dimension, as in nodding your head "yes." The lateral horizontal semicircular canal senses movement roughly in the transverse plane of the body, as in shaking your head "no."

Binaural orientation of the two semicircular canals is such that the anterior semicircular canal of one ear is parallel to the posterior canal of the other. The horizontal canals lie in the same plane, but the ampullae are in mirror-image

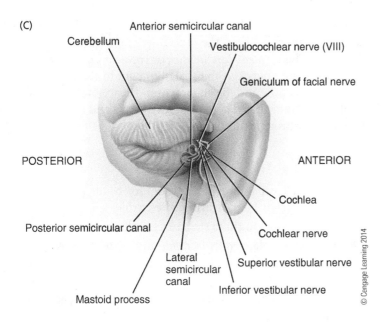

(C)

Anterior semicircular canal

Cerebellum

Vestibulocochlear nerve (VIII)

Geniculum of facial nerve

POSTERIOR

ANTERIOR

Cochlea

Posterior semicircular canal

Cochlear nerve

Lateral semicircular canal

Superior vestibular nerve

Inferior vestibular nerve

Mastoid process

© Cengage Learning 2014

Figure 5–7. continued (C) Orientation of the semicircular canals in the erect human.

locations. As we will see, this horizontal orientation of the canal helps your brain differentiate rotary movement toward the left and right.

Osseous Cochlear Labyrinth

The osseous labyrinth has the appearance of a coiled snail shell. It coils out from a base near the vestibule, wrapping around itself 2¾ times before reaching its apex. The core of the osseous labyrinth, the *modiolus*, is finely perforated bone. Fibers of the vestibulocochlear nerve (cranial nerve VIII) pass through these perforations en route to ganglion cells within the modiolus. The core of the modiolus is continuous with the *internal auditory meatus* of the temporal bone, through which the vestibulocochlear nerve passes.

The labyrinth is partially divided into two chambers, the *scala vestibuli* and the *scala tympani*, by an incomplete bony shelf protruding from the modiolus. This shelf is called the *osseous spiral lamina*. This structure forms the point of attachment for the scala media, which houses the sensory organ for hearing. The osseous spiral lamina becomes progressively smaller as it approaches the apex, such that the space between it and the opposite wall of the labyrinth increases. At the apex, the two chambers formed by the incomplete lamina become hooklike, forming the *helicotrema*, the region through which the scala tympani and scala vestibuli communicate.

The osseous labyrinth has three prominent openings. The *round window (foramen rotundum)* provides communication between the scala tympani and the middle ear.

The oval window, within which the stapes is placed, permits communication between the scala vestibuli and the middle ear space. The *cochlear canaliculus*, or *cochlear aqueduct*, is a minute opening between the scala tympani in the region of the round window and the subarachnoid space of the cranial cavity. The fluid that fills the scala vestibuli and scala tympani passes through this duct.

Summary

- The inner ear houses the sensors for balance (the vestibular system) and hearing (the cochlea).
- The entryway to these structures is the vestibule.
- The osseous labyrinth is made up of the entryway to the labyrinth, the vestibule, semicircular canals, and the osseous cochlear canal.
- The semicircular canals in the inner ear are organs of balance.
- The osseous labyrinth has the appearance of a coiled snail shell.
- The labyrinth is divided into two incomplete chambers, the scala vestibuli and the scala tympani, by an incomplete bony shelf protruding from the modiolus, the osseous spiral lamina.
- The round window provides communication between the scala tympani and the middle ear.
- The oval window permits communication between the scala vestibuli and the middle ear space.
- The cochlear aqueduct connects the upper duct and the subarachnoid space.

Membranous Labyrinth

The structure of the *membranous labyrinth* parallels that of the *bony labyrinth*. First, orient yourself to the oval window, recognizing its link to the stapes of the middle ear. Beneath it, but not quite visible, is the round window. The *vestibule*, or entryway, to the inner ear is a space shared by the sense organ of hearing (the *cochlea*) and the sense organs of balance (the semicircular canals). Let us examine the sensory components of the inner ear (see Figure 5–8).

Vestibular System

The membranous labyrinth can be thought of as a fluid-filled sac that rests in the cavity of the osseous labyrinth. This sac does not completely fill the labyrinth, but rather forms an additional space in the already fluid-filled region. The duct forms only a small portion of the labyrinth and contains *endolymph*, fluid of a slightly different composition.

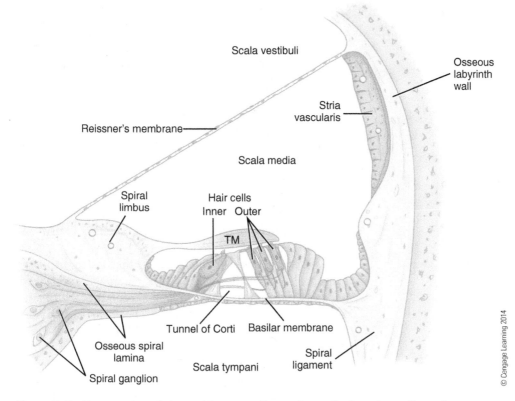

Figure 5–8. Cross section of the cochlea, revealing scala vestibuli, scala media, scala tympani, and tectorial membrane (TM).

In the vestibular system, the membranous labyrinth houses the vestibular organ. Each *ampulla* houses a *crista ampullaris*, which is the receptor organ for movement. From each of the 6000 vestibular receptor cells protrude approximately 50 stereocilia, minute hairs that sense movement in fluid, and one kinocilium. A *cupula* overlays the crista ampullaris such that the cilia are embedded in the cupula.

The *utricle* and *saccule* lie within the vestibule, the housing for the otolithic membrane of the vestibular system. The *otolithic membrane* is a layer of gelatinous material in which the cilia of the hair cells are embedded, and which has the effect of distending the cilia when the fluid is moved (Bhatnagar and Andy, 2002). The *utricular macula* is the sensory organ, which is endowed with hair cells and cilia. It is covered by the otolithic membrane, which is invested with crystals (*otoliths*). The saccule lies near the scala vestibuli in the vestibule, and it is similarly endowed with macula and otolithic membrane. The saccule and utricle communicate by means of the *endolymphatic duct*, which is embedded in the *dura mater*. The saccule communicates with the cochlea by means of the minute *ductus reuniens*.

Cochlear Duct

The membranous labyrinth of the cochlea, the cochlear duct, resides between the scala vestibuli and tympani, making up the intermediate scala media. This structure houses the sensory apparatus for hearing.

A cross section through the region of the scala media reveals its extraordinary structure, as shown in Figure 5–8. The osseous spiral lamina courses across the extent of the osseous labyrinth, forming the major point of attachment for the cochlear duct. Again, looking at Figure 5–8, you can see Reissner's membrane, an extremely thin separation between the perilymph of the scala vestibuli and the endolymph of the scala media. One end is continuous with the stria vascularis, which is highly vascularized tissue that is firmly attached to the spiral ligament.

As you can see in Figure 5–9, the *basilar membrane* forms the "floor" of the scala media, separating the scala media and scala tympani. It is on this membrane that the organ of hearing is found (the organ of Corti). The *organ of Corti* is similar to the vestibular organs. There are four rows of hair cells. The three rows of *outer hair cells (OHC)* are separated from the single row of *inner hair cells (IHC)* by *the tunnel of Corti*, the product of pillar cells of Corti. The *spiral limbus* arises from the *tectorial membrane*, which overlays the hair cells. The outer hair cells are embedded in the tectorial membrane but the inner hair cells do not make physical contact with it.

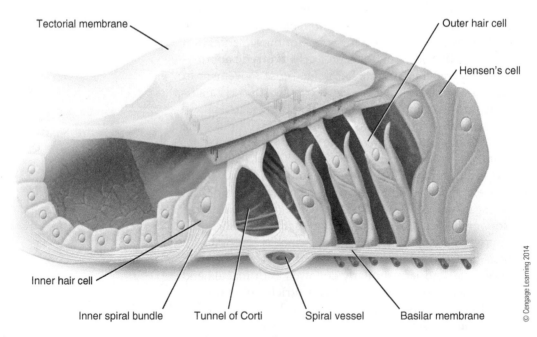

Tectorial membrane

Outer hair cell

Hensen's cell

Inner hair cell

Inner spiral bundle   Tunnel of Corti   Spiral vessel   Basilar membrane

© Cengage Learning 2014

Figure 5–9. Landmarks and structures of the organ of Corti.

Hair Cell Regeneration

Gene therapy is being developed to regenerate hair cells. We have known for a few years that avian hair cells regenerate, but only recently have researchers identified a means for regenerating hair cells in mammals. Izumikawa et al. (2005) genetically modified a cold virus and injected it into guinea pigs. Not only did new hair cells grow, but when the guinea pigs were tested using auditory brainstem responses, it was clear that the hair cells were functioning.

The 3500 inner hair cells form a single row stretching from the base to apex of the cochlear duct. The three rows of outer hair cells (approximately 12,000) broaden to four rows in the apical end.

The hair cells of the cochlea receive both sensory and motor innervation. Clearly afferent information relates to the business of the cochlea (receiving and processing sound), but the motor innervation has a surprising function, discussed in the next section.

Innervation

There is sensory information transmitted through the auditory pathway that relates to vestibular sense and stimulation by sound. There is also motor innervation of the outer hair cells that is inhibitory, reducing the sensory activity caused by hair cell stimulation. The *olivocochlear bundle* comprises about 1600 fibers, consisting of the crossed olivocochlear bundle (COCB) and uncrossed olivocochlear bundle (UCOB). When activated, these fibers reduce the response of the hair cells to sound. That is, they serve to reduce the effects that sound has on the cells they inhibit. It appears that this system helps us to "tune out" irrelevant information in noisy environments.

Summary

- The membranous labyrinth can be thought of as a fluid-filled sac that rests in the cavity of the osseous labyrinth and is filled with endolymph.
- In the vestibular system, the membranous labyrinth houses the vestibular organ.
- The ampulla is the expanded region of the semicircular canals that contains the crista ampullaris. Within the vestibule lie the utricle and saccule.

- The membranous labyrinth of the cochlea resides between the scala vestibuli and tympani, making up the intermediate scala media.
- Reissner's membrane forms the upper boundary of the scala media, and the basilar membrane forms the floor.
- The organ of Corti has four rows of hair cells.
- The outer hair cells are separated from the inner row of hair cells by the tunnel of Corti.
- The upper surface of each hair cell is graced with a series of stereocilia.

AUDITORY PHYSIOLOGY

The auditory mechanism processes the acoustic signal of speech. Auditory stimuli can arrive at the tympanic membrane with an amazingly wide range of sound pressures, from the whisper of a leaf blowing in the breeze to the pressures associated with a jet engine. Likewise, the human auditory mechanism has a frequency range of approximately 10 octaves, spanning 20 Hz to 20,000 Hz. Within these broad requirements are much finer tasks, including differentiating small increments in frequency and intensity.

The field of audiology owes a great deal to the extraordinary scientist, Georg von Békésy, whose work was awarded a Nobel prize. Von Békésy (1960) performed exceedingly intricate measurements on the auditory mechanism, being forced to create tools where none existed. We refer frequently to his work, which defined the function of the middle and inner ears, as we discuss the basic physiological principles involved in transmission of an acoustic stimulus to a form that is interpretable by the brain. The simplified version of the process of hearing includes the following steps: (1) The outer ear collects sound and "shapes" its frequency components somewhat; (2) the middle ear matches the airborne acoustic signal with the fluid medium of the cochlea; (3) the inner ear performs temporal and spectral analysis on the ongoing acoustical signal; (4) the auditory pathway conveys and further processes that signal; and (5) the cerebral cortex interprets the signal.

Outer Ear Function

The outer ear can be seen primarily as a collector of sound. The pinna, with its ridges, grooves, and dished-out regions, is an excellent funnel for information directed toward the head from the front or side, although less effective for sound arising from behind the head.

Noise Pollution

Psychologically, auditory noise is anything that gets in the way of what we want to hear, the signal. Noise is more than a psychological phenomenon, however. Haralabidis et al. (2008) examined the effects of nighttime noise on individuals living near airports in Europe. When a subject heard noise at or above 35 dB HL (hearing level) the systolic blood pressure increased by 6.2 mm Hg and diastolic blood pressure increased by 6.4 mm Hg. The authors found that every 10-dB increase in noise during the night raised the likelihood of a person developing high blood pressure (hypertension) by 14%. The authors note that it is not just airplane noise, but even a loudly snoring partner can have the same effect. Considering that hypertension is one of the most significant predictors of stroke, it would do well to sleep in the quiet!

Indeed, the crevices and crannies of the pinna are functional. Because the human outer ear cannot move as a cat's ear can, it has only a passive effect on the input stimulus. The pinna acts as a "sound funnel," focusing acoustic energy into the external auditory meatus, and the external auditory meatus funnels sound to the tympanic membrane. Both of these structures, however, have shapes that boost the relative strength of the signal through resonance, with the result being relatively enhanced signal intensity between 1500 Hz and 8000 Hz. The components of the pinna contribute a net gain reaching 20 dB at approximately 2000 Hz.

Middle Ear Function

The cochlea is a fluid-filled cavity, and were it not for the presence of the middle ear mechanism, talking to each other would be like trying to talk to someone under water: The sound energy would reflect off the oval window because of the vast differences in the liquid and gaseous media of perilymph and air. Somewhere in our evolution, a mechanism arose to improve our plight.

The middle ear mechanism has evolved to increase the pressure arriving at the cochlea, thereby overcoming the resistance to flow of energy. Resistance to flow of energy is *impedance*, and the middle ear system overcomes a great deal of this resistance through three significant mechanisms. You will recall that sound intensity is a direct function of increase in sound pressure. Because pressure is equal to force divided by area ($P = F/A$), to increase the sound pressure you would have to either increase the force applied or decrease the area over which the force is applied. In reality our middle ear does both of these things, using area benefits and lever benefits.

The tympanic membrane has an area of about 55 mm^2, and the area of the oval window is about 3.2 mm^2, making the tympanic membrane 17 times larger, depending on species size. Sound energy reaching the tympanic membrane is funneled to the much smaller area of the oval window, so there is a gain of 17:1, which translates to an increase of about 25 dB.

The second impedance-matching function is achieved by a lever effect. The length of the manubrium is approximately 9 mm and that of the long process of stapes is about 7 mm, giving an overall gain of about 1:2. The lever effect arising from this gain is nearly 2 dB.

Combined, the area and lever effects result in a signal gain of about 27 dB, from tympanic membrane to cochlea, depending on the stimulus frequency. Again, were the middle ear removed, a signal entering the external auditory meatus would have to be 27 dB more intense to be heard.

A third effect arises from the buckling of the tympanic membrane. As it moves in response to sound, the tympanic membrane buckles somewhat so that the arm of the malleus moves a shorter distance than the surface of the tympanic membrane. This results in a reduction in velocity of the malleus, with an increased force that provides a 4- to 6-dB increase in effective signal.

Summary

- The outer and middle parts of the ear serve as funneling and impedance-matching devices.
- The pinna funnels acoustical information to the external auditory meatus and aids in localization of sound in space.
- The resonant frequencies of the pinna and external auditory meatus are important components of the speech signal, between 1500 Hz and 8000 Hz.
- Resistance to flow of energy is impedance.
- The middle ear mechanism is an impedance-matching device, increasing the pressure of a signal arriving at the cochlea.
- The area ratio between the tympanic membrane and the oval window provides a 25-dB gain.
- The lever advantage of the ossicles provides a 2-dB gain.
- The buckling effect of the tympanic membrane relative to the malleus provides a 4-dB to 6-dB gain.

Inner Ear Function

Vestibular Mechanism

The semicircular canals are uniquely designed to respond to rotatory movement of the body. By virtue of their orientation, each canal is at right angles to one other canal, so that all movements of the head can be mapped by combinations of outputs of the sensory components, the cristae ampullares. As your head rotates, the fluid in the semicircular canals tends to remain in the same location, and the cilia are stimulated by relative movement of the fluid during rotation. The utricle and saccule sense acceleration, rather than rotation, of the head during body or head tilting. Taken together, the vestibular mechanisms provide the major input to the proprioceptive system that provides the sense of one's body in space. This information is integrated with joint sense, muscle spindle afferents, and visual input to form the perception of body position.

Auditory Mechanism: Mechanical Events

The inner ear is responsible for spectral and temporal acoustic analyses of incoming acoustical signals. By spectral analysis we refer to the process of extracting or defining the various frequency components of a given signal.

spectral analysis: *Analysis of a signal that identifies frequency components of that signal.*

Sound causes the tympanic membrane to move, and that movement is translated to the oval window. When the tympanic membrane moves inward or outward, the stapes footplate in the oval window follows. When the stapes compresses the perilymph of the scala vestibuli, Reissner's membrane is distended toward the scala media, and the basilar membrane is distended toward the scala tympani. Because the frequency of a sound is determined by the number of oscillations or vibrations per second, a 100-Hz signal results in the footplate moving inward and outward 100 times per second, and that periodic vibration is translated to the basilar membrane, where it initiates a wave action known as the *traveling wave*.

Georg von Békésy discovered that when high-frequency sounds impinge on the inner ear, they cause vibration of the basilar membrane closer to the vestibule, the basal end of the cochlea. Low-frequency sounds result in a long traveling wave that reaches toward the apex, covering a greater distance along the basilar membrane. In this way, the traveling wave separates out the frequency components of complex sounds because high-frequency sounds are processed in basal regions, whereas low-frequency sounds are processed nearer the apex. When a sound has both high- and low-frequency components, those components are separated out and processed at their respective portions of the basilar membrane. The traveling wave moves along the basilar membrane, growing and swelling as it travels, until it reaches a point of maximum displacement.

Excitation of the hair cells occurs as the result of the traveling wave's effect on the basilar membrane. The cilia of the outer hair cells are embedded in the tectorial membrane, and as the traveling wave moves along the basilar membrane, the hair cells are displaced relative to the tectorial membrane. This produces a shearing action that is greatest at the point of maximum perturbation of the basilar membrane.

Summary

- The inner ear is responsible for spectral (frequency) and temporal acoustic analyses of incoming acoustical signals.
- Movement of the tympanic membrane is translated into analogous movement of the stapes footplate and the fluid in the scala vestibuli.
- Compression in the fluid of the scala vestibuli is translated directly to the basilar membrane, and the disturbance at the basilar membrane initiates the traveling wave.
- The cochlea is arranged so that high-frequency sounds are resolved at the base and low-frequency sounds are processed at the apex.

Neural Responses

There are two basic types of eighth cranial nerve neuron: low spontaneous rate (high-threshold) and high spontaneous rate (low-threshold) fibers. High-threshold neurons require a higher level of stimulation to fire, respond to the higher end of our auditory range of signal intensity, and have little or no random background firing noise. (Background "neural noise" is caused by random firing of neurons in the absence of stimulation and is a widespread phenomenon in the nervous system.) Low-threshold fibers, on the other hand, respond at very low signal intensities and display random firing even when no stimulus is present. Thus, it appears that the low-threshold neurons may be a mechanism for hearing sound at near-threshold levels, whereas high-threshold fibers may pick up where the low-threshold fibers stop, as the signal increases.

Because neurons are all-or-none devices, every unit response is equal to the next in intensity and duration. Thus, the only way neurons can provide differential response is in rate of firing. When an eighth nerve fiber responds to tonal stimulation, there is an initial burst of strong activity followed by a decline to a plateau of discharge over the duration of the tone. When the tone is terminated, the response of the fiber drops below baseline levels, rising up the baseline "noise" level after recovery. This fairly straightforward post-stimulus time histogram has provided us with very important verification of the *frequency specificity*, the ability of the cochlea to differentiate spectral components of a signal.

Researchers who study auditory perceptual abilities as they relate to the physical mechanism (*psychoacousticians*) have found that, in general, humans can discriminate change in frequency of signals of about 2%. Figure 5–10 shows a tuning curve for a single unit recording. A tuning curve is basically a composite of the responses of a single fiber at each frequency of presentation. For instance, researchers placed an electrode on a neuron and presented different frequencies of stimulation. They then recorded the stimulus intensity at which the neuron began to fire in response to the stimulus (its threshold) and plotted that intensity. In Figure 5–10, you can see that the fiber was most sensitive to the 10,000-Hz signal. This is its *characteristic frequency*, or *CF*. As the signal frequency decreased to 8000 Hz, the signal had to be of greater intensity to cause the neuron to fire. The signal at 5000 Hz had to be 60 dB stronger than that at the CF for that neuron.

This tuning curve is a measure of neural specificity in one sense, but probably is as much a measure of basilar membrane response. The electrode is, in effect, measuring the activity at one point on the basilar membrane (10,000 Hz, near the base), and activity farther up the cochlea toward the apex has less and less effect on the neuron we are recording. The sharper the tuning curve is, the greater is the frequency specificity of the basilar membrane. Indeed, when Khanna and Leonard (1982) compared the tuning curves of the basilar membrane and the auditory nerve, they found that the two curves were quite similar. That is, the basilar membrane is a very finely tuned filter capable of fine differentiation.

What happens when the stimulation to the cochlea is more complex than a simple sinusoidal tone? For instance, if a tone complex including 500 Hz, 1000 Hz, 1500 Hz, and 2000 Hz were presented to the ear, how would the cochlea and eighth nerve respond? Essentially, the nerve fibers with characteristic frequencies of the stimulus components (500 Hz, 1000 Hz, etc.) will respond, whereas fibers with CF at other frequencies (510 Hz, 511 Hz, 512 Hz, etc.) will take much more stimulation to fire. We judiciously avoided 505 Hz in our list of off-stimulus CF because that difference is probably not discriminable. That is, the cochlea generally cannot differentiate smaller than 1% change of its CF (i.e., 5 Hz in this situation), so the fibers at 502 Hz would respond the same as those at 500 Hz. To the brain, these two frequencies are indiscriminable.

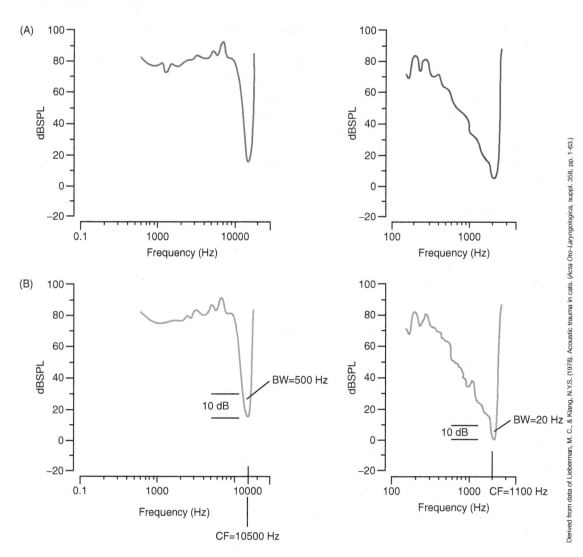

Figure 5–10. Plot of tuning curves from two different cranial nerve VIII fibers, representing characteristic frequencies of 10,500 Hz (left) and 1000 Hz (right). Note that the tuning curve on the left looks sharper.

Derived from data of Lieberman, M. C., & Kiang, N.Y.S. (1978). Acoustic trauma in cats. (*Acta Oto-Laryngologica*, suppl. 358, pp. 1–63.)

As the intensity of stimulation increases, rate of firing increases, up to a point. Because neurons are limited by the refractory period, they typically cannot fire more than once per millisecond. The dynamic range for intensity that can be encoded in rate of firing is in the order of 30 to 40 dB, far too low for encoding of intensity. We are capable of differentiating a much greater range of intensities than this. Recall that different neurons have different thresholds of response (low- and high-threshold neurons). Apparently, intensity is coded by using both types of neuron: Low-threshold neurons can process low-intensity signals and high-threshold neurons carry the load of higher intensity sound.

Recall that we mentioned the motor system of the auditory mechanism earlier, stating that it helps to reduce the response of some hair cells. When this system of nerve fibers, called the *crossed olivocochlear bundle (COCB)* and *uncrossed olivocochlear bundle (UOCB)*, is stimulated, the firing rate of neurons innervated by them is reduced dramatically. This has the effect of reducing response to unwanted information, perhaps permitting the nervous system to "focus" on a desired signal while damping the response to noise. The motor system also appears to have a role in frequency discrimination.

Summary

- There are two basic types of eighth cranial nerve neuron, and specific techniques have been developed to assess their functions.
- High-threshold neurons require a higher intensity and encompass the higher end of our auditory range of signal intensity.
- Low-threshold fibers respond at very low signal levels and display random firing even when no stimulus is present.
- Low-threshold neurons may process near-threshold sounds, whereas high-threshold fibers process higher level sounds.
- Frequency specificity is the ability of the cochlea to differentiate the spectral components of a signal.
- The characteristic, or best, frequency of a neuron is the frequency to which it responds best.
- A tuning curve is a composite of the responses of a single fiber at each frequency of presentation.
- The sharper the tuning curve is, the greater is the frequency specificity of the basilar membrane.
- As the intensity of stimulation increases, rate of firing increases.
- When the crossed olivocochlear and uncrossed olivocochlear bundles are stimulated, the firing rate of neurons innervated by them is reduced dramatically.

AUDITORY PATHWAY RESPONSES: ANATOMY AND FUNCTION

The cochlea and eighth cranial nerve represent only the first stage of information extraction of the auditory signal. Temporal and tonotopically arrayed information is passed to progressively higher centers for further extraction of information (see Figure 5–11). Researchers have identified a wide variety of responses at every level of the auditory pathway, indicating very detailed information processing by the auditory nervous system, but let us focus on only one aspect of that processing.

The *superior olivary complex (SOC)* has the primary responsibility for localization of sound in space. It receives information from both ears and compares that information to determine the origination of the sound in space.

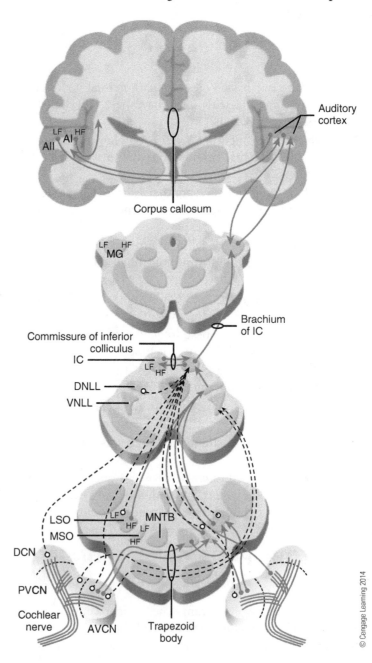

Figure 5–11. Course of the vestibulocochlear nerve (eighth cranial nerve) and auditory pathway.
Note: AI = primary auditory reception area ; AII = higher order auditory processing; LF = low frequency; HF = high frequency; IC = Inferior Colliculus; DNLL = Dorsal Nucleus of Lateral Lemniscus; VNLL = Ventral Nucleus of Lateral Lemniscus; DCN = Dorsal Cochlear Nucleus; PVCN = Posteroventral Cochlear Nucleus; AVCN = Anteroventral Cochlear Nucleus; MNTB = Medial Nucleus of Trapezoid Body; LSO = Lateral Superior Olive; MSO = Medial Superior Olive.

One portion of the SOC (the lateral superior olive, or "S segment") compares the intensity between the two ears to identify the location of high-frequency sounds. The *medial superior olive (MSO)* compares the time patterns of low-frequency sounds to identify the locations based on phase differences between the two signals.

The cerebral cortex receives input primarily from the contralateral ear via the thalamus (specifically, the medial geniculate body, or MGB). The cerebral cortex then proceeds to make sense of this acoustical information.

Information is received at Heschl's gyrus in the cerebral cortex, which we typically state as being located in the superior aspect of the temporal lobe, at the Sylvian fissure. Heschl's gyrus is actually located on the superior surface of the superior temporal gyrus as if it were tucked into the lateral sulcus, and can barely be seen in the lateral view of the cerebrum. There may be more than one area that is functionally or physiologically equivalent to Heschl's gyrus in each temporal lobe.

Kaas and Hackett (2000) have helped us to see that the auditory cortex consists of zones of processing, including a medially placed core (classically Heschl's gyrus), a more distal belt, and a surrounding parabelt. The core is the primary receptive area, surrounded by a belt that processes auditory information in a more specific fashion, identifying features and even clarifying whether the input belongs to your species or not! Many of these areas on the belt have tonotopic arrangement similar to Heschl's gyrus. The parabelt is a zone of further processing before information is sent to the frontal and parietal lobes for processing. It's worth noting that the planum temporale, the region immediately posterior to Heschl's gyrus, is nearly 10 times larger in the left (dominant) hemisphere than in the right hemisphere, and appears to be specialized for rapidly changing stimuli such as those that occur in speech. We'll discuss this critical difference when we talk about hemispheric specialization (Chapter 6).

Summary

- Temporal and tonotopically arrayed information is passed to progressively higher centers for further extraction of information.
- The superior olivary complex (SOC) is the primary site of localization of sound in space.
- The medial geniculate body (MGB) is a relay of the thalamus.
- The cortex completes the analysis of the auditory signal that is accomplished by the auditory pathway.

CHAPTER SUMMARY

The outer ear is composed of the pinna and the external auditory meatus. Landmarks of the pinna include the margin of the auricle, the helix, and the auricular tubercle on the helix. The external auditory meatus has both osseous and cartilaginous parts: The cartilaginous portion makes up one third of the ear canal, while the other two thirds are housed in bone. At the terminus of the external auditory meatus is the tympanic membrane, the structure that separates the outer and middle ears.

The middle ear cavity houses the middle ear ossicles. The malleus is the largest ossicle, providing the point of attachment with the tympanic membrane. The incus provides the intermediate communicating link of the ossicular chain, and the stapes is the third bone of this chain. The ossicular chain is held in place by a series of important ligaments. The stapedius muscle inserts into the posterior neck of stapes and pulls the stapes posteriorly, and the tensor tympani muscle inserts into the upper manubrium mallei, pulling the malleus anteromedially. Landmarks of the medial wall of the middle ear cavity include the oval window, the round window, the promontory of the cochlea, and the prominence of the facial nerve. The anterior wall houses the entrance to the eustachian tube, and the posterior wall houses the prominence of the stapedial pyramid.

The inner ear contains the sense mechanism for balance (the vestibular system) and hearing (the cochlea). The entryway to these structures is the vestibule. The osseous labyrinth is made up of the entryway to the labyrinth, the vestibule, semicircular canals, and the osseous cochlear canal. It has the appearance of a coiled snail shell, and it is divided into two incomplete chambers, the scala vestibuli and the scala tympani, by an incomplete bony shelf protruding from the modiolus, the osseous spiral lamina. The round window provides communication between the scala tympani and the middle ear. The oval window permits communication between the scala vestibuli and the middle ear space. The cochlear aqueduct connects the upper duct and the subarachnoid space.

The membranous labyrinth is an endolymph-filled sac that rests within the cavity of the osseous labyrinth. In the vestibular system, the membranous labyrinth contains the vestibular organ. The ampulla is the expanded region of the semicircular canals and contains the crista ampullaris. Within the vestibule lie the utricle and saccule. The membranous labyrinth of the cochlea resides between the scala vestibuli and scala tympani, making up the intermediate scala media. Reissner's membrane forms the distal boundary of the scala media, and the basilar membrane forms the proximal boundary. The organ of Corti has four rows of hair cells resting on a bed of Deiters' cells for support. The outer hair cells are separated from the row of inner hair cells by the tunnel of Corti. The upper surface of each hair cell is graced with a series of stereocilia. Each inner hair cell innervates as many as ten eighth nerve fibers, while each outer hair cell shares its innervation with 10 other outer hair cells, all being innervated by the same eighth nerve fiber.

The outer and middle ears serve as funneling and impedance-matching devices. The pinna funnels acoustical information to the external auditory meatus and aids in localization of sound in space. Resistance to flow of energy is termed impedance. The middle ear mechanism is an impedance-matching device, increasing the pressure of a signal arriving at the cochlea. The area ratio between the tympanic membrane and the oval window provides a significant gain in output over input, and the lever advantage of the ossicles provides a smaller gain.

The inner ear is responsible for performing spectral (frequency) and temporal acoustic analyses of incoming acoustical signals. Movement of the tympanic membrane is translated into parallel movement of the stapes footplate and the fluid in the scala vestibuli. Movement of the fluid of the scala vestibuli is translated directly to the basilar membrane, and the disturbance at the basilar membrane causes the initiation of the traveling wave. The cochlea has a tonotopic arrangement, with high-frequency sounds resolved at the base and low-frequency sounds processed toward the apex. The point of maximum displacement of the basilar membrane determines the frequency information transmitted to the brain. The traveling wave quickly damps after reaching its point of maximum displacement. The frequency analysis ability of the basilar membrane is determined by graded stiffness, thickness, and width. The basilar membrane is stiffer, thinner, and more narrow at the base than apex. Excitation of the outer hair cells occurs primarily as the result of a shearing effect on the cilia. Excitation of the inner hair cells is produced by the effect of fluid flow and turbulence of endolymph.

There are two basic types of eighth nerve neuron. High-threshold neurons require a higher intensity and encompass the higher end of our auditory range of signal intensity. Low-threshold fibers respond at very low signals and display random firing even when there is no stimulus. Low-threshold neurons may process near-threshold sounds, whereas high-threshold fibers process higher level sounds. Frequency specificity is the ability of the cochlea to differentiate spectral components of a signal. A tuning curve is a composite of the responses of a single fiber at each frequency of presentation. The sharper the tuning curve is, the greater is the frequency specificity of the basilar membrane.

STUDY QUESTIONS

1. The _____ of the outer ear is important for localization of sound in space.

2. Resistance to flow of energy is called _____.

3. The area ratio between the tympanic membrane and the oval window provides a _____ dB gain, and the lever advantage gives a _____ dB gain.

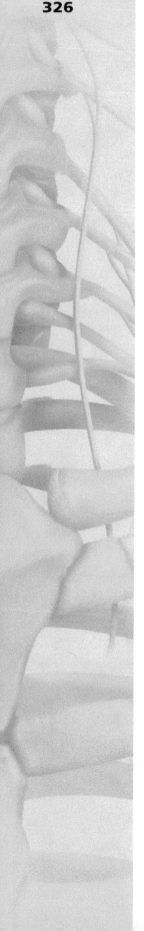

4. The cochlea performs both _____ analysis and _____ analysis.

5. Compression in the fluid of the scala vestibuli is translated directly to the basilar membrane, and the disturbance at the basilar membrane causes the initiation of a _____ wave.

6. High-frequency sounds are resolved at the base of the cochlea, with progressively lower sounds processed at progressively higher positions on the cochlea. This array is called _____.

7. The frequency analysis ability of the basilar membrane is determined by graded_____, _____, and _____.

8. At the apex, the basilar membrane is _____(thinner/thicker) than at the base.

9. At the apex, the basilar membrane is _____(wider/narrower) than at the base.

10. T / F _____ The cilia of the outer hair cells are embedded in the tectorial membrane.

11. T / F _____ The cilia of the inner hair cells are embedded in the tectorial membrane.

12. _____ neurons require a higher intensity and encompass the higher end of our auditory range of signal intensity, whereas _____ neurons respond at very low signal levels and display random firing even when there is no stimulus.

13. _____ refers to the ability of the cochlea to differentiate spectral components of a signal.

14. The _____ frequency of a neuron is the frequency to which it responds best.

15. Tuning curves are composites of the responses of a single fiber at each frequency of presentation. The sharper the tuning curve is, the greater is the _____ of the basilar membrane.

16. Rate of firing of neurons increases as the _____ increases.

17. Stimulation of the _____ bundle and the _____ bundle reduces the firing rate of neurons innervated by them.

18. The _____ meatus is a conduit for sound reaching the tympanic membrane.

19. The _____ meatus is a conduit for the eighth cranial nerve fibers coursing to the brainstem.

20. The tympanic membrane (or eardrum) is made up of _____ layers of tissue.

21. The outer layer of the tympanic membrane is continuous with the _____.

22. The _____ layer of the tympanic membrane is made up primarily of radiating fibers.

23. The _____ is a landmark produced by the most distal part of the manubrium mallei.

24. The _____ is the bone of the middle ear directly attached to the tympanic membrane.

25. The _____ is the bone of the middle ear directly communicating with the oval window.

26. The _____ of the malleus attaches to the tympanic membrane.

27. The _____ of the stapes articulates with the oval window.

28. The _____ muscle pulls the stapes posteriorly.

29. The _____ muscle pulls the malleus anteromedially.

30. The entryway to the cochlea and vestibular system is via the space known as the _____.

31. The _____ is the system of cavities within bone that houses the membranous labyrinth.

32. The scala _____ and scala _____ are incomplete spaces in the osseous labyrinth.

33. The _____ window provides communication between the scala tympani and the middle ear.

34. The _____ window permits communication between the scala vestibuli and the middle ear space.

35. The _____ is a fluid-filled sac attached to the walls of the osseous labyrinth and is filled with endolymph.

36. The _____ membrane separates the scala vestibuli and the scala media; the _____ membrane separates the scala media from the scala tympani.

37. There is/are _____ row(s) of outer hair cells and _____ row(s) of inner hair cells.

38. The hair cells are innervated by the _____ nerve.

39. Microsurgery procedures have advanced rapidly in recent years, permitting re-articulation of ossicles that have become disarticulated. Considering how well protected the ossicles are, what could cause them to become disarticulated?

40. Comparative anatomy provides insight into function. What differences in the cochlea would you predict when comparing the cochlea of a human with that of a mammal that used ultra-high-frequency sound to echo-locate, such as a fruit bat? What differences would you predict that you would find when comparing an elephant's cochlea with that of a human?

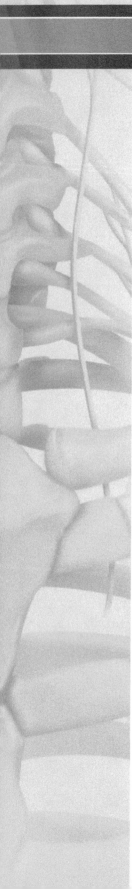

REFERENCES

Altschuler, R. A., Bobbin, R. P., & Hoffman, D. W. (1986). *Neurology of hearing: The cochlea.* New York: Raven.

Anson, B. J., & Donaldson, J. R. (1973). *Surgical anatomy of the temporal bone and ear.* Philadelphia: W. B. Saunders.

Belin, P., & Zatorre, R. J. (2005). Voice processing in human auditory cortex. In R. Konig, P. Heil, E. Budinger, & H. Scheich (Eds.). *The auditory cortex* (pp. 163–180). Mahwah, NJ: Lawrence Erlbaum Associates, Publishers.

Bhatnagar, S. C., & Andy, O. J. (2002). *Neuroscience for the study of communicative disorders* (2nd ed.). Baltimore: Williams & Wilkins.

Budinger, E. (2005). Introduction: Auditory cortical fields and their functions. In R. Konig, P. Heil, E. Budinger, & H. Scheich (Eds.). *The auditory cortex* (pp. 3–6). Mahwah, NJ: Lawrence Erlbaum Associates, Publishers.

Carpenter, M. B. (1991). *Core text of neuroanatomy* (4th ed.). Baltimore: Williams & Wilkins.

Cazals, Y., Demany, L., & Horner, K. (1991). *Auditory physiology and perception.* Oxford: Pergamon.

Chusid, J. G. (1985). *Correlative neuroanatomy and functional neurology* (17th ed.). Los Altos, CA: Lange Medical Publications.

Cianfrone, G., & Grandori, F. (1985). Cochlear mechanics and otoacoustic emissions. *Scandinavian Audiology (Suppl. 25).*

Clarke, S., Adriani, M., & Tardif, E. (2005)."What" and "where" in human audition: Evidence from anatomical, activation, and lesion studies. In R. Konig, P. Heil, E. Budinger, & Scheich, H. (Eds.). *The auditory cortex* (pp. 77–94). Mahwah, NJ: Lawrence Erlbaum Associates, Publishers.

Dallos, P. (1973). *The auditory periphery.* New York: Academic.

Dallos, P., Billone, M. C., Durrant, J. D., et al. (1972). Cochlear inner and outer hair cells: Functional differences. *Science, 177,* 356–358.

Davis, H. (1958). Transmission and transduction in the cochlea. *Laryngoscope, 68,* 359–382.

Duifhuis, H., Horst, J. W., van Dijk, P., & van Netten, S. M. (1993). *Biophysics of hair cell sensory systems.* Singapore: World Scientific.

Durrant, J. D., & Lovrinic, J. H. (1995). *Bases of hearing science.* Baltimore: Williams & Wilkins.

Engstrom, H., Ades, H. W., & Andersson, A. (1966). *Structural pattern of the organ of corti.* Baltimore: Williams & Wilkins.

Gardner, E., Gray, D. J., & O'Rahilly, R. (1986). *Anatomy: A regional study of human structure* (5th ed.). Philadelphia: W. B. Saunders.

Gelfand, S. A. (2001). *Essentials of audiology* (2nd ed.). New York: Thieme Medical.

Gollisch, T., & Meister, M. (2008). Rapid neural coding in the retina with relative spike latencies. *Science, 319,* 1108–1111.

Gray, H., Bannister, L. H., Berry, M. M., & Williams, P. L. (Eds.) (1995). *Gray's anatomy.* London: Churchill Livingstone.

Green, D. (1976). *An introduction to hearing.* Hillsdale, NJ: Lawrence Erlbaum.

Gulick, W. L. (1971). *Hearing physiology and psychophysics.* New York: Oxford University Press.

Haralabidis AS, Dimakopoulou K, Vigna-Taglianti F, Giampaolo M, Borgini A, Dudley ML, Pershagen G, Bluhm G, Houthuijs D, Babisch W, Velonakis M, Katsouyanni K, Jarup L, HYENA Consortium (2008). Acute Effects of Night-Time Noise Exposure on Blood Pressure in Populations Living Near Airports. *European Heart Journal, 29,* 658–664.

Henson, O. W. (1974). Comparative anatomy of the middle ear. In H. Autrum, R. Jung, W. R. Loewenstein, et al. (Eds.), *Handbook of sensory physiology* (pp. 40–110). New York: Springer-Verlag.

Izumikawa, M., Minoda, R., Kawamoto, K., et al. (2005). Auditory hair cell replacement and hearing improvement by Atoh1 gene therapy in deaf mammals. *Nature Medicine, 11,* 271–276.

Javel, E. (1986). Basic response properties of auditory nerve fibers. In R. A. Altschuler, R. P. Bobbin, & D. W. Hoffman (Eds.), *Neurobiology of hearing: The cochlea* (pp. 213–245). New York: Raven.

Kaas, J. H., & Hackett, T. A. (2000). Subdivisions of auditory cortex and processing streams in primates. *Proceedings of the National Academy of Sciences USA, 97*(22), 11793–11799.

Kaas, J. H., & Hackett, T. A. (2005). Subdivisions and connections of the auditory cortex in primates: A working model. In R. Konig, P. Heil, E. Budinger, & H. Scheich (Eds.), *The auditory cortex* (pp. 7–26). Mahwah, NJ: Lawrence Erlbaum Associates, Publishers.

Kandel, E. R., Schwartz, J. H., & Jessell, T. M. (2000). *Principles of neural science* (4th ed.). New York: McGraw Hill.

Khanna, S. M., & Leonard, D. G. B. (1982). Basilar membrane tuning in the cochlea. *Science, 215,* 305–306.

Kiang, N. Y-S. (1965). *Discharge patterns of single fibers in the cat's auditory nerve.* Cambridge, MA: M.I.T. Press.

Kiang, N. Y-S., Liberman, M. C., Sewell, W. F., & Guinan, J. J. (1986). Single unit clues to cochlear mechanisms. *Hearing Research, 22,* 171–182.

Konig, R., Heil, P., Budinger, E., & Scheich, H. (2005). *The auditory cortex.* Mahwah, NJ: Lawrence Erlbaum Associates, Publishers.

Kuehn, D. P., Lemme, M. L., & Baumgartner, J. M. (1991). *Neural bases of speech, hearing, and language.* Boston: Little, Brown.

Lewis, E. R., Leverenz, E. L., & Bialek, W. S. (1985). *The vertebrate inner ear.* Boca Raton, FL: CRC Press.

Lim, D. J. (1980). Cochlear anatomy related to cochlear micromechanics: A review. *Journal of the Acoustical Society of America, 67*(5), 1686–1695.

Martin, F. N. (1981). *Medical audiology.* Englewood Cliffs, NJ: Prentice-Hall.

Martin, F., & Clark, J. G. (2006). *Elements of audiology: A learning aid with cases.* Boston: Allyn & Bacon.

Minifie, F. (1973). Speech acoustics. In F. D. Minifie, T. J. Hixon, & F. Williams (Eds.), *Normal aspects of speech, hearing, and language* (pp. 11–72). Englewood Cliffs, NJ: Prentice-Hall.

Minifie, F. D., Hixon, T. J., & Williams, F. (Eds.). (1992). *Normal aspects of speech, hearing, and language.* Englewood Cliffs, NJ: Prentice-Hall.

Møller, A. R. (1973). *Basic mechanisms of hearing.* New York: Academic.

Møller, A. R. (1983). *Auditory physiology.* New York: Academic.

Møller, A. R. (2003). *Sensory systems: Anatomy and physiology.* New York: Academic Press.

Møller, A. (2006). *Neural plasticity and disorders of the nervous system.* Boston: Cambridge University Press.

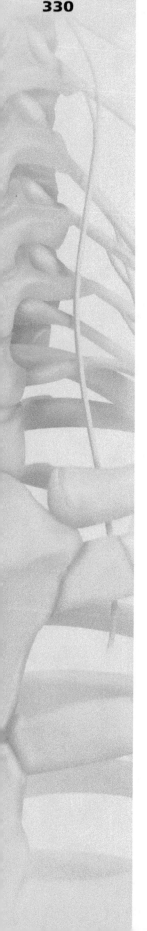

Møller, A. R. (2003). *Sensory systems: Anatomy and physiology.* New York: Academic Press.

Moroson, P., Rademacher, J., Palomero-Gallagher, N., & Zilles, K. (2005). Anatomical organization of the human auditory cortex: Cytoarchitecture and transmitter receptors. In R. Konig, P. Heil, E. Budinger, & H. Scheich (Eds.). *The auditory cortex* (pp. 27–50). Mahwah, NJ: Lawrence Erlbaum Associates, Publishers.

Musiek, F. E., & Baran, J. A. (2006). *The auditory system: Anatomy, physiology, and clinical correlates.* Glenview, IL: Allyn & Bacon.

Netter, F. H. (1989). *Atlas of human anatomy.* Summit, NJ: CIBA Pharmaceuticals Division.

Parkins, C. W., & Anderson, S. W. (1983). Cochlear prostheses: An international symposium. *Annals of the New York Academy of Sciences, 405.*

Petkov, C. I., Kayser, C., Steudel, T., et al. (2008). A voice region in the monkey brain. *Nature Neuroscience 11*, 367–374.

Pickles, J. O. (1988). *An introduction to the physiology of hearing* (2nd ed.). London: Academic.

Rhode, W. W. (1985). The use of intracellular techniques in the study of the cochlear nucleus. *Journal of the Acoustical Society of America, 78*, 320–327.

Rosse, C., Gaddum-Rosse, P., & Rosse, G. (1997). *Hollinshead's textbook of anatomy.* Philadelphia: Lippincott-Raven.

Ryan, A., & Dallos, P. (1976). Physiology of the inner ear. In J. L. Northern (Ed.), *Hearing disorders* (pp. 89–101). Boston: Little, Brown.

Shaw, E. A. G. (1974). The external ear. In W. D. Keidel & W. D. Neff (Eds.), *Handbook of sensory physiology* (pp. 455–490). New York: Springer-Verlag.

Spoendlin, H. (1978). The afferent innervation of the cochlea. In R. F. Naunton & C. Fernandez (Eds.), *Evoked electrical activity in the auditory nervous system.* New York: Academic.

Syka, J., & Masterton, R. B. (1988). *Auditory pathway structure and function.* New York: Plenum.

Tobias, J. V., & Schubert, E. D. (1983). *Hearing research and theory* (Vol. 2). New York: Academic.

Tonndorf, J. (1958). The hydrodynamic origin of aural harmonics in the cochlea. *Annals of Otology, 67*, 754–774.

Tonndorf, J. (1960). Shearing motion in scala media of cochlear models. *Journal of the Acoustical Society of America, 32*(5), 238–244.

Von Békésy, G. (1960). *Experiments in hearing.* New York: McGraw-Hill.

Wever, E. G., & Bray, C. W. (1930). Action currents in the auditory nerve in response to acoustical stimulation. *Proceedings of the National Academy of Science, 16*, 344–350.

Wilson, J. P., & Kemp, D. T. (1989). *Cochlear mechanisms: Structure, function, and models.* New York: Plenum.

Winans, S. S., Gilman, S., Manter, J. T., & Gatz, A. J. (2002). *Manter and Gatz's essentials of clinical neuroanatomy and neurophysiology* (10th ed.). Philadelphia: Davis.

Yost, W. A. (2000). *Fundamentals of hearing: An introduction* (4th ed). New York: Academic.

Zemlin, W. R. (1998). *Speech and hearing science. Anatomy and physiology* (4th ed.). Needham Heights, MA: Allyn & Bacon.

6

Neuroanatomy and Neurophysiology

OUTLINE

I. **Anatomy of the Central and Peripheral Nervous Systems**
   - A. Functional divisions of the nervous system
     1. The autonomic nervous system (ANS)
        a. Sympathetic system
        b. Parasympathetic system
     2. The somatic system controls the conscious and voluntary bodily functions
        a. Pyramidal system
        b. Extrapyramidal system
   - B. Anatomic divisions of the nervous system
     1. The central nervous system (CNS) includes the brain (cerebrum, cerebellum, subcortical structures, and brainstem) and spinal cord
     2. The peripheral nervous system (PNS) includes 12 pairs of cranial nerves and 31 pairs of spinal nerves, as well as the sensory receptors
   - C. Meningeal linings
   - D. Cerebral cortex
     1. Two hemispheres connected by corpus callosum
     2. Gyri and sulci
     3. Frontal lobe
     4. Parietal lobe

4. Absolute refractory period
5. Resting membrane potential
B. Propagation
   1. Saltatory conduction
   2. Temporal summation
   3. Convergence and divergence
C. Muscle function
D. Higher neural functioning
   1. Cerebrum
      a. Primary reception for somatic sense, primary motor area, primary auditory cortex, and primary region of visual reception
      b. Higher-order areas
      c. Association areas
   2. Prefrontal area
   3. Temporal-occipital-parietal association area
   4. Limbic association area
E. Hemispheric specialization
   1. Left hemisphere processes language and speech
   2. Right hemisphere processes holistic information
F. Motor control of speech
   1. Precentral gyrus
   2. Motor strip
   3. Premotor regions
   4. DIVA model of neuromotor control
   5. Sensation and reflexes

There is nothing in nature as awe inspiring as the nervous system. Although humans have been studying the brain for thousands of years (there is evidence that the Pueblo Indians of prehistoric New Mexico performed surgical procedures on the skull), we have only begun to understand this very complex system. There are at least 100 billion nerve cells in the nervous system, and each of them may communicate directly with as many as 2000 other neurons, providing at least 1 trillion points of communication. The brain is the control center and processor for all of the functions of communication and life. It is at the very core of communication.

The structure and function of the nervous system are extraordinarily complex, but you should always remember that the nervous system is designed to protect, nourish, and maintain the body. Its most basic function is to protect us from harm, and it does this by monitoring our sensations for conditions that may be problematic (e.g., I feel heat when I touch fire) and removing us from those conditions (I'll retract my hand if it feels like it's getting burned). Our bodily needs include nutrition, and our sensory systems are going to make sure that those needs are met, in either simple (grabbing a handful of chips) or complex (planning to go out to dinner in Paris) ways. Our basic biological needs will tend to trump our other decisions, so that pain, pleasure, hunger, and fear can overwhelm logic if we aren't carefully alert and cognitively aware. We are very complex creatures, and we are endowed with amazing motor, sensory, and cognitive abilities. The function of the brain is arguably the most complex process in nature, and humans have the most complex brain of all species, to the best of our knowledge.

ANATOMY OF THE CENTRAL AND PERIPHERAL NERVOUS SYSTEMS

Even though it is an understatement to say that the central nervous system is extremely complex, it may be a comfort to realize that there is a common denominator to all of the structures of the nervous system: All structures are made of neurons.

Neurons

neurons (nerve cells): *Tissue specialized for communication.*

glia (glial cells): *Nervous system tissue that provides support and nutrients within the nervous system.*

soma: *The cell body of a neuron.*

dendrite: *The component of a neuron that generally receives input from another neuron or sensor.*

axon: *The terminal point of a neuron, through which information passes.*

Neurons, also known as nerve cells, are the communicating elements of the nervous system. Glia, also known as glial cells, are structural and nutrient-bearing cells that support the neurons. Neurons are the functional building blocks of the nervous system and are unique among tissue types.

While different types of neurons have different structures, there are some commonalities. Most neurons have a soma (cell body), a dendrite (receiver of information), which transmits information toward the soma, and an axon, which transmits information away from the soma (see Figure 6–1). We will discuss the function of the neurons later in this chapter.

Neuron Landmarks

If a neuron has many dendrites, it is often referred to as a dendritic tree because it looks "bushy." Most neurons have only one axon. The *axon hillock* is the junction of the axon and soma. Many axons are covered with a white fatty wrapping called the *myelin sheath*. Myelin speeds up neural conduction. Myelin is segmented, and the areas between

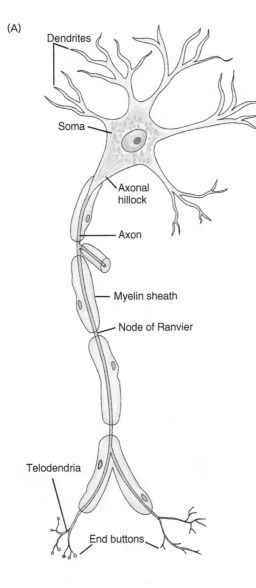

(A)

Dendrites

Soma

Axonal hillock

Axon

Myelin sheath

Node of Ranvier

Telodendria

End buttons

© Cengage Learning 2014

Figure 6–1. (A) Schematic of basic elements of a neuron.

(continues)

the myelinated segments are known as *nodes of Ranvier* (see Table 6–1). At the end of the axon are the *telodendria*, which are long, thin projections. At the tips of the telodendria are *terminal end boutons* (buttons), and inside the boutons are *synaptic vesicles*. Synaptic vesicles contain special chemicals called *neurotransmitters*. There are many types of neurotransmitters, and they facilitate synaptic transmission. Neurotransmitters are released into the gap between two neurons, referred to as the presynaptic and postsynaptic neurons to reflect their position in relation to the synapse. This gap, also known as the *synaptic cleft*, causes the next neuron in the chain to be activated or inhibited from acting. Groups of gray cell bodies are referred to as *gray matter*; *white matter* refers to myelin.

(B)

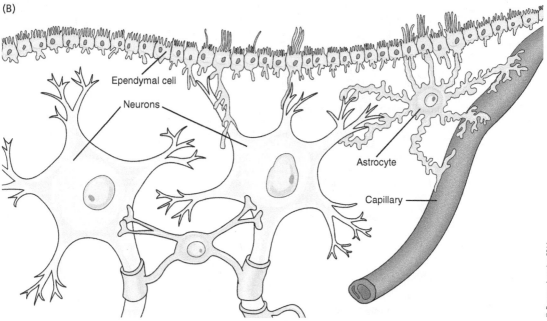

Figure 6–1. continued (B) The astrocyte is a glial cell that supports transport of nutrients to the neuron while shielding it from toxins via the blood-brain barrier.

Table 6–1. Basic Components of the Neuron

Component	Function
Dendrite	Receptor region
Soma	Contains metabolic organelles
Axon	Transmits information from neuron
Hillock	Generator site for action potential
Myelin sheath	Insulates axons
Schwann cells	Forms myelin in peripheral nervous system
Oligodendrocytes	Forms myelin in central nervous system
Nodes of Ranvier	Permit saltatory conduction
Telodendria	Processes from axon
Terminal end boutons	Contain synaptic vesicles
Neurotransmitter	Facilitates synapse
Synaptic cleft	Region between pre- and postsynaptic neurons

© Cengage Learning 2014

Glial Cells

There are many more glial cells than neurons. They provide support and nutrients to neurons and make up the myelin sheath. Different types of glia have different functions. *Astrocytes* provide the primary support for neurons, help suspend neurons, and transport nutrients from a capillary supply to the neuron. They also provide the important blood-brain barrier, a filter system that prohibits some toxins from passing from the brain's blood supply (*cerebrovascular system*) to neurons, and have recently been implicated in long-term memory function.

Oligodendrocytes are glia that make up the myelin in the central nervous system, and *Schwann cells* are glia that make up the myelin in the peripheral nervous system. Microglia perform the housekeeping process that scavenges dead (**necrotic**) tissue that is found after damage (**lesion**) in the nervous system. Astrocytes then form scars around this dead tissue, isolating it from the rest of the brain.

necrotic tissue: *Dead tissue.*

lesion: *Damage to tissue.*

Summary

- The nervous system is a complex, hierarchical structure made of neurons.
- Neurons communicate through synapses by means of neurotransmitter substance, and the postsynaptic neuron may be excited or inhibited by the transmitting neuron.
- Glial cells make up the myelin sheath and provide support for neurons.

FUNCTIONAL VIEW: AUTONOMIC AND SOMATIC NERVOUS SYSTEMS

A functional view of the nervous system categorizes the brain into autonomic and somatic nervous systems. The **autonomic nervous system (ANS)** governs involuntary activities of the visceral muscles (or viscera), including glandular secretions, heart function, digestive function, and so forth. You have little control over what happens to that triple chili cheeseburger as you digest it, although you may occasionally be aware of the digestive process.

The ANS can be divided into two subsystems, the sympathetic and the parasympathetic nervous systems. The **sympathetic nervous system** responds to stimulation by expending energy, and the **parasympathetic nervous system**, or craniosacral system, reduces the sympathetic

autonomic nervous system: *The division of the central nervous system that is responsible for involuntary functions.*

sympathetic nervous system: *The component of the autonomic nervous system responsible for body system responses that prepare the body to cope with stressful situations by increasing states of physiological vigilance and preparedness for muscular action.*

parasympathetic nervous system: *The component of the autonomic nervous system responsible for body system responses that reverse autonomic responses, thereby preserving energy.*

Hematoma

A hematoma is a pooling of blood, typically caused by breakage of a blood vessel. Subdural hematoma involves intracranial bleeding beneath the dura mater of the brain, caused by rupture of cortical arteries or veins, usually the result of trauma to the head. Pressure from the pooling blood displaces the brain, shifting and compressing the brainstem, forcing the temporal lobe under the tentorium cerebelli, and compressing cerebral arteries. This critically dangerous condition may not be immediately recognized because it may take several hours before pooling blood compresses the brain sufficiently to produce symptoms such as reduced consciousness, hemiparesis, or pupillary dilation. Epidural hematoma, a hematoma above the dura mater, may result in a person's being initially lucid but displaying progressively decreasing levels of consciousness, reflecting compression of the brain.

Hematomas are characterized by location of insult. Frontal epidural hematomas are caused by blows to the frontal bone and may result in personality changes. Posterior fossa epidural hematomas are caused by blows to the back of the head, resulting in visual and coordination deficits.

response. When you have had a significant scare, such as a near collision in an automobile, your body's sympathetic responses include vasoconstriction (constriction of blood vessels), increase in blood pressure, dilation of pupils, cardiac acceleration, sweating, and "goose bumps." You may be less aware of the parasympathetic system response that is responsible for counteracting the effects of sympathetic response, such as slowing of the heart rate, reduction of blood pressure, and pupillary constriction.

somatic nervous system: *The subdivision of the nervous system responsible for voluntary motor function and nonvisceral sensation.*

The **somatic nervous system** (voluntary component) is very important to the discipline of speech-language pathology. The somatic system controls the conscious and voluntary bodily functions, including control of all skeletal (somatic) muscles. The central nervous system's control of muscles arises mostly from the precentral region of the cerebral cortex. Neural impulses are conveyed through descending motor tracts of the brainstem and spinal cord. Cranial nerves of the brainstem and spinal nerves of the spinal cord are activated and cause muscles to contract. Likewise, the sensory component of the somatic nervous system monitors information about the function of the skeletal muscles, their environment, and other "nonvisceral" activities.

direct (pyramidal) motor system: *The motor system under voluntary control.*

indirect (extrapyramidal) motor system: *The motor system that provides background support for the direct motor system.*

The motor component of the somatic system can be divided into pyramidal and extrapyramidal systems. The **direct**, or **pyramidal**, **motor system** is responsible for initiating voluntary motor acts. The **indirect**, or **extrapyramidal**, motor system also is responsible for the background tone and movement that supports the primary acts.

Sensation is an essential part of communication. Without sensation, a perfectly functioning brain would be worthless as a communicating system. Likewise, because communication requires some sort of muscular activity, the absence of motor activity would signal the end of communication. Fortunately, the large number of sensors in the human body permits us to use various pathways for receiving communication and for passing information to another person. We are rarely completely cut off from communication with others. Let us now examine the components of this system.

ANATOMICAL VIEW: CENTRAL AND PERIPHERAL NERVOUS SYSTEMS

Anatomically, the nervous system can be divided into the central nervous system and peripheral nervous system (see Table 6–2). The central nervous system (CNS) includes the brain (cerebrum, cerebellum, subcortical structures, brainstem) and spinal cord. The peripheral nervous system (PNS) includes 12 pairs of *cranial nerves* and 31 pairs of *spinal nerves*, as well as the sensory receptors. All of the CNS components are housed in bone (skull or vertebral column), but most of the PNS components are outside bone. We will spend a great deal of time with this organizational structure as we discuss the anatomy of the nervous system.

central nervous system (CNS): *The division of the nervous system that contains the brain and spinal cord.*

peripheral nervous system (PNS): *The division of the nervous system that contains cranial and spinal nerves.*

Table 6–2. Divisions of the Nervous System from Anatomical and Physiological Perspectives

Anatomical Divisions of Nervous System

Central Nervous System: Cerebrum, cerebellum, brainstem, spinal cord, thalamus, subthalamus, basal ganglia, etc.

Peripheral Nervous System: Spinal nerves, cranial nerves, sensors

Functional Divisions of Nervous System

Autonomic Nervous System: Involuntary bodily function

    Sympathetic nervous system: Expends energy (e.g., vasoconstriction when frightened)

    Parasympathetic nervous system: Conserves energy (e.g., vasodilation upon removal of fearful stimulation)

Somatic Nervous System: Voluntary bodily function

ANATOMY OF THE CEREBRAL CORTEX

The *cerebral cortex*, or *cerebrum*, is the largest structure of the nervous system, weighs approximately 3 pounds, and contains billions of neurons. The cerebrum is divided into left and right hemispheres. In exploring the cerebral cortex we will start at the outside and work toward the center.

Meningeal Linings

Brain structures of the CNS are surrounded by a three-layer *meningeal lining* that protects neurons. Three meningeal linings cover the brain. The *dura mater* is the tough outer meningeal lining. The *arachnoid mater* is the middle meningeal lining through which many blood vessels for the brain pass. The inner lining is the *pia mater*, which is a thin, filmy covering that follows the contour of the brain. The major arteries and veins serving the surface of the brain course within this layer. Together the meningeal linings provide an excellent means of nurturing and protecting the CNS structures.

Landmarks of the Cerebral Cortex

The cerebral cortex is divided into two hemispheres or roughly equal halves of the brain (see Figure 6–2). The term *cortex*

An Ounce of Prevention

If you choose to work in a trauma center, a significant portion of your caseload will arise from traumatic brain injury (TBI). TBI is a leading cause of death of individuals younger than 24 years old, with motor vehicle accidents far exceeding all other causes (falls, assaults, sport, firearms). The addition of safety belts to automobiles has reduced death in automobile accidents caused by TBI by nearly 50%. Unfortunately, use of alcohol is related to reduced seatbelt use and increased death due to head injury during accidents. Mandatory use of helmets has reduced the frequency of TBI in motorcycle accidents by 20–50% and up to 85% in bicycle accidents.

Gunshot wounds to the head result in most deaths attributable to firearms, and handguns are involved in more than 60% of homicides. More than 40,000 people in the United States are killed by firearms annually. While laws that restrict access to firearms are being hotly debated as a constitutional issue, trigger lock systems could greatly reduce the carnage that occurs in the United States, where nearly 50% of households have firearms. You can refer to MacKay and colleagues (1997) for an extremely thorough review of causes and treatment of TBI.

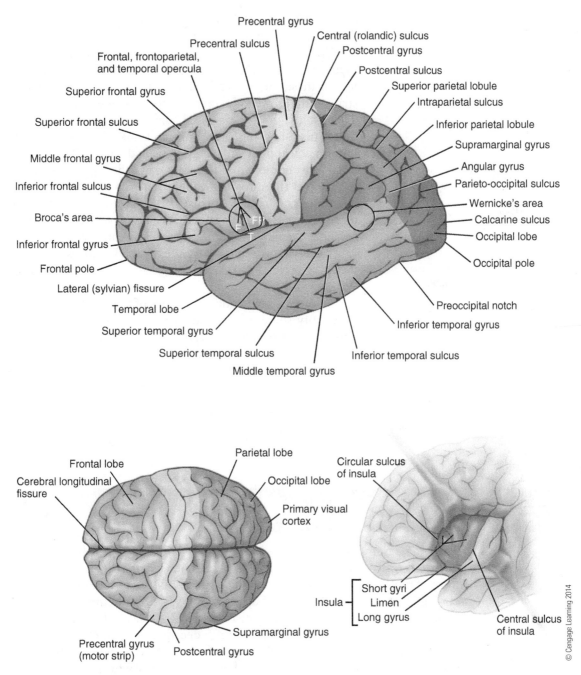

Figure 6–2. Major landmarks of the cerebrum as seen from above and from the side. Note that the insular cortex (insula, bottom left) is typically hidden from view.

actually means "bark," referring to the bark or outer surface of a tree, and the cerebral cortex is the outer surface of the brain.

The surface of the brain is quite convoluted (see Figure 6–3). Early in development, the cerebral cortex has few of these furrows and bulges, but as brain growth outstrips skull growth, the cerebral cortex doubles in on itself. The result is greatly increased surface area, translating into more "neural horsepower." You can think of the surface as a topographical map with mountains and valleys. The mountains (convolutions) in this case are called **gyri** (singular, gyrus) and the infolding valleys that separate the gyri are called **sulci** (singular, sulcus). If the groove is deeper and more pronounced, it is a **fissure**. These gyri, sulci, and fissures are the major landmarks of the cerebral cortex.

gyri: *Outfolding of tissue on the cerebral or cerebellar cortex.*

sulci: *Minor infolding of tissue on the cerebral or cerebellar cortex.*

fissure: *Significant infolding or complete separation of two structures of the cerebral or cerebellar cortex.*

We divide the cerebral cortex into five lobes. Four of them are reasonably easy to recognize, but the other one is less obvious.

Before we differentiate the lobes of the brain, it will help to identify some major landmarks. The *lateral fissure*, also known as the *sylvian fissure*, divides the temporal lobe from the frontal and anterior parietal lobes. The *central sulcus* separates the frontal and parietal lobes.

Frontal Lobe

The *frontal lobe* is the largest lobe, making up one third of the cortex (see Figure 6–3). This lobe controls the planning,

Amyotrophic Lateral Sclerosis

There are a number of conditions that cause degeneration of the brain function. Amyotrophic lateral sclerosis (ALS, Lou Gehrig's disease), a form of motor neuron disease, is a progressive condition of unknown etiology that causes destruction of upper and lower motor neurons. The typical course is 2 to 5 years from date of diagnosis to death. People typically develop ALS in their fourth or fifth decade of life, and they experience initial weakness in a limb, with fatigue and cramping. As the disease progresses, limb function is lost, although sensory function typically is retained. Motor symptoms indicate both upper and lower motor neuron degeneration, which sometimes produces alternating spasticity and flaccidity. In the later stages of the disease, the person experiences difficulty with respiration, requiring alteration of posture to accommodate reduced ability to work against gravity. The individual eventually experiences dysphagia and paralysis of muscles of speech while retaining full cognitive function. For a very moving account of the effects of the disease, read *Tuesdays with Morrie*, by Mitch Albom.

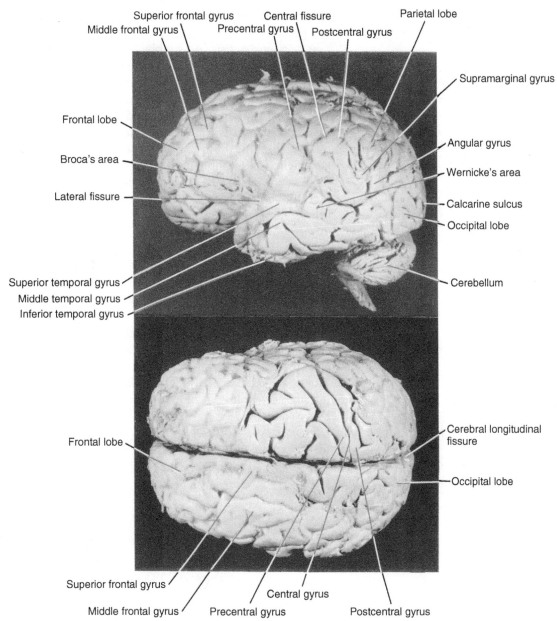

Figure 6–3. Lateral (upper) and superior (lower) views of cerebral cortex. Note that the pia mater can be seen in portions of both photographs.

initiation, and inhibition of voluntary motions, as well as thought processes.

The *pars opercularis*, or simply the *frontal operculum* (see Figure 6–2), is on the surface of the inferior frontal lobe that overlies one of the "hidden lobes," the *insular lobe*. The frontal operculum is commonly referred to as **Broca's area**, which is classically referred to as Brodmann areas 44 and 45. This is an extremely important region for speech motor planning within the dominant hemisphere. The anterior portion of the frontal lobe, particularly the area just above the eyes, is associated with memory, emotion, motor inhibition, and thought processes.

Another important landmark of the frontal lobe is the *precentral gyrus*, or *motor strip*, which is the site of initiation of voluntary motor movement. Anterior to the motor strip is the *premotor region*, generally involved in motor planning (see Figure 6–2). Axons from the motor strip make up the corticospinal and corticobulbar tracts, the major motor tracts of voluntary movement.

Different regions of the motor strip serve different regions of the body (see Figure 6–4). The face, head, and laryngeal regions are on the far lateral edge, while leg, thigh, and thorax are represented on the more medial surface of the superior cortex. If you compare this with the location of Broca's area on the side view of the hemisphere in Figure 6–5, you will see that these two regions are in close proximity. The area for motor function for the speech mechanisms (larynx,

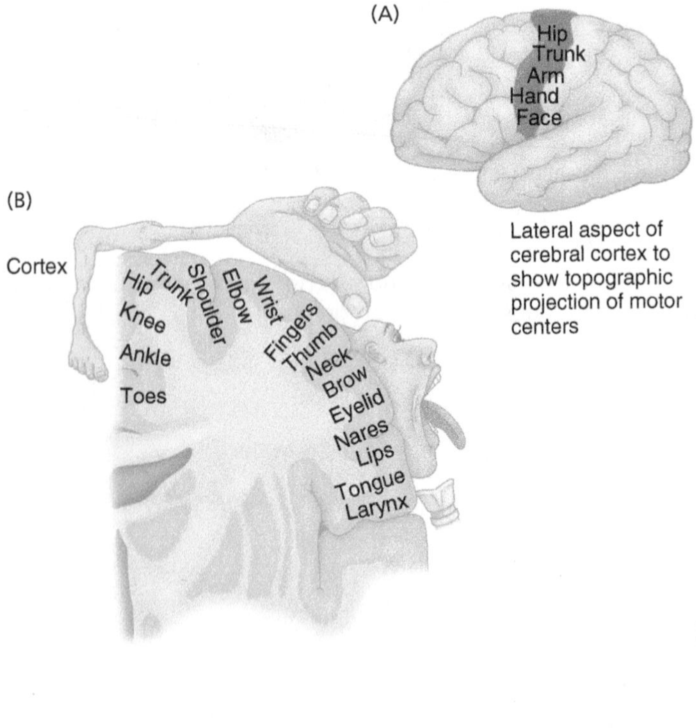

Broca's area: *The region of the third frontal convolution of the dominant hemisphere responsible for speech motor planning.*

(A)

Hip
Trunk
Arm
Hand
Face

Lateral aspect of cerebral cortex to show topographic projection of motor centers

(B)

Cortex

Hip
Trunk
Knee
Shoulder
Elbow
Wrist
Fingers
Thumb
Neck
Brow
Eyelid
Nares
Lips
Tongue
Larynx
Ankle
Toes

Figure 6–4. (A) Right hemisphere, displaying regions of motor strip governing activation of specific muscle groups. (B) Homunculus revealing areas of representation on the motor strip. Note that this represents a frontal section through the cerebral cortex. Size of structure drawn represents the degree of neural representation of the given structure (i.e., neural density).

© Cengage Learning 2014

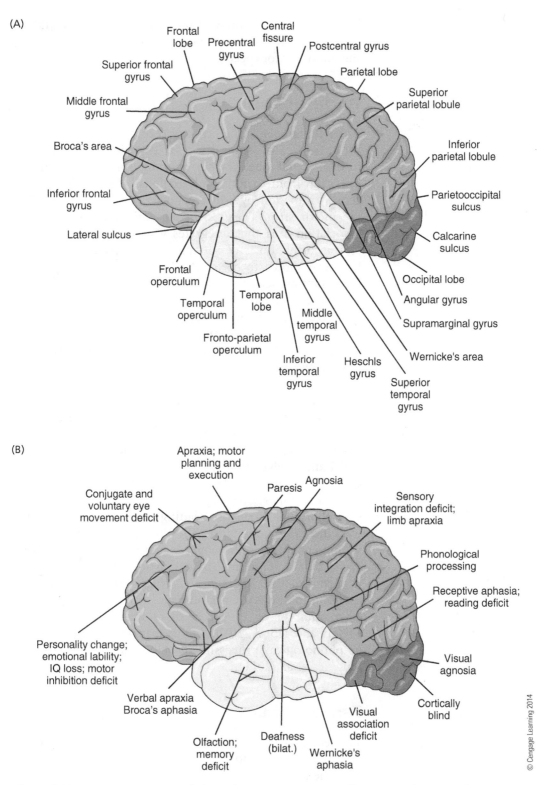

Figure 6–5. (A) Landmarks of the left cerebral hemisphere. (B) Effects upon function of lesion at different cerebral locations.

lips, facial muscles, muscles of mastication) is immediately adjacent to Broca's area, the region responsible for planning the motor act for speech.

Parietal Lobe

The *parietal lobe* is the primary reception site for somatic (body) sense. All senses that reach consciousness terminate in the parietal lobe. The *postcentral* gyrus receives somatic sensation from various body regions. The distribution of sensory function by body region is quite close to that of the motor strip. The *inferior parietal lobule* is a cortical association area that integrates visual information, auditory information, and somatic sense. The *angular gyrus* has been shown to be involved in a number of critically important associative functions. It lies to the posterior of Wernicke's area (a critical language center), and receives input from visual and auditory centers, as well as somatosensory information from the parietal lobe, and is involved in mathematical calculation as well as being a contributor to cognitive function.

Dysgraphia (difficulty writing language), dyslexia (difficulty reading language), and semantic processing deficits can arise from lesions to the left angular gyrus, but this area is also implicated in a person's knowledge of who is completing an action. That is to say, there is evidence that knowing that I am involved in a specific motor act may involve circuitry of the right angular gyrus (Farrer et al., 2007).

The angular gyrus apparently collaborates with the supramarginal gyrus in reading and rhyming activity, with increased activity in children, perhaps reflecting development of the phonology during that period (Church et al., 2008). It is thus important for comprehension of written material. The *supramarginal gyrus* is involved in spatiomotor tasks in nonhumans identifying if physical orientation of an object is functionally correct (Bach, Peelen, and Tipper, 2010), but appears intimately involved in phonological processing developmentally in humans (Sugiura et al., 2011).

Temporal Lobe

The *temporal lobe* is the site of auditory reception and is important for auditory and receptive language processing. The *superior temporal gyrus* is of great importance in both speech-language pathology and audiology. The upper surface of the superior temporal lobe is *Heschl's gyrus*, the location of the brain to which all auditory information is projected. The posterior portion of the superior temporal gyrus is *Wernicke's area*. This area is responsible for processing receptive language within the dominant hemisphere. Damage to this site results in profound disturbances of language ability.

Occipital Lobe

The *occipital lobe* is the region responsible for receiving visual stimulation, as well as some of the higher level visual processing. The regions surrounding the *calcarine sulcus* are the primary reception areas for visual information.

Insular Lobe

The *insular lobe* (insula) is beneath the region of the cerebrum known as the operculum. To see the insular lobe, one would have to pull the temporal lobe laterally and lift the frontal and parietal opercula. Upon doing that, you would see the circular sulcus, which surrounds the insula. The insula is directly involved in **gustation** (sense of taste) and motor planning for speech.

gustation: *Sense of taste.*

Summary

- The gyri and sulci of the hemisphere provide important landmarks for lobes and other regions of the cerebral cortex.
- The anterior-most region is the frontal lobe, the site of most voluntary motor activation and the important speech region known as Broca's area.
- Adjacent to the frontal lobe is the parietal lobe, the region of somatic sensory reception.
- The temporal lobe is the prominent lateral lobe separated from the parietal and frontal lobes by the lateral (sylvian) fissure.
- The temporal lobe is the site of auditory reception and Wernicke's area.
- The occipital lobe is the most posterior of the regions and is the site of visual input to the cerebrum.
- The insular lobe lies deep in the lateral sulcus and is revealed by deflecting the temporal lobe.
- The operculum overlies the insula.

Alcohol and the Brain

Alcohol is a toxin to neural tissue, hence the name *intoxication*. Alcohol use is widespread throughout the world and in all cultures, as are the effects of alcohol on the brain. Acute alcohol intoxication results in the disabling of the hippocampus, which effectively removes the ability to learn or memorize, including the ability to learn from aversive responses. Thus, attempting to discuss meaningful information with an intoxicated person is a futile activity. Chronic alcohol use has a more sinister effect. The frontal lobes of individuals who chronically abuse alcohol deteriorate, reducing the patient's ability to make cognitive judgments and process information. Alcohol consumption over time results in liver damage (sclerosis of the liver) that causes the body to be unable to metabolize vitamin B_1 (thiamine).

A vitamin B deficiency results in reduced neural function of neurons and glial cells, as well as the inability to process iron, which in turn results in the reduced oxygen-carrying capacity of blood. The result is permanent brain damage due to the chronic anemic condition. Finally, individuals who chronically abuse alcohol and who are genetically predisposed to Alzheimer's disease develop the disease at twice the rate of the average population. Finally, thiamine deficiency ultimately results in Wernicke-Korsakoff syndrome, a permanent dementia characterized by confusion, confabulation, memory loss, inability to encode new memory, and various motor signs such as nystagmus and ataxia.

Myelinated Fibers

The gray matter of the cortex is made up mostly of neuron bodies, while the white matter of the brain represents myelinated axon fibers. These fibers make up the communication link among the neurons; without them there would be no neural function. In diseases that cause demyelination of the fibers, dysfunction of the areas served is virtually guaranteed. There are three basic types of fiber: projection, association, and commissural.

Projection Fibers

The tracts running to and from the cortex to the brainstem and the spinal cord are made up of projection fibers. Projection fibers connect the cortex with distant locations.

Association Fibers

Association fibers provide communication between regions of the same hemisphere. *Short association fibers* connect neurons of one gyrus to the next, traversing the sulcus

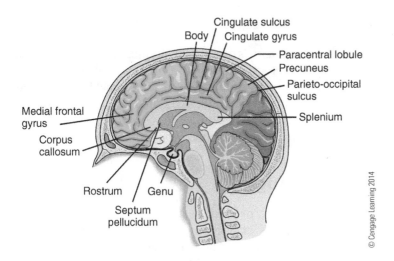

Figure 6–6. Medial surface of the cerebral cortex.

between them. *Long association fibers* interconnect the lobes of the brain in the same hemisphere. The *arcuate fasciculus* is one group of association fibers that permits the superior and middle frontal gyri to communicate with the temporal, parietal, and occipital lobes. A lesion of the arcuate fasciculus can result in conduction aphasia, in which expressive and receptive language remain essentially intact, but the individual remains unable to repeat information presented auditorily.

Commissural Fibers

Commissural fibers run from one location on a hemisphere to the corresponding location on the other hemisphere, such as from the supramarginal gyrus of the left parietal lobe to the supramarginal gyrus of the right parietal lobe. Viewing a sagittal section of the brain reveals the *corpus callosum* (literally, "large body"). It is the large structure immediately inferior to the cerebral gray matter (see Figure 6–6). The corpus callosum is the "information superhighway" of the brain. It provides communication concerning sensation and memory among the diverse regions of the two hemispheres by means of myelinated fibers. Any information arising in the left postcentral gyrus can be potentially shared by the right postcentral gyrus so that each hemisphere "knows" what the other one knows.

ANATOMY OF THE SUBCORTEX

Although the following structures are extremely important, an extensive discussion of them is beyond the scope of this introductory view of neuroanatomy.

Limbic System

The *limbic system* is not an anatomically distinct region, but a system of structures with functional relationships associated with motivation, sex drive, emotional behavior, and affect. The limbic system includes the *uncus* (formed by the *amygdala*), *parahippocampal gyrus, cingulate gyrus, olfactory bulb* and *tract*, and the *hippocampal formation*.

Basal Ganglia

The *basal ganglia*, or *basal nuclei*, are a group of cell bodies related to control of background movement and initiation of movement patterns. The basal ganglia structures are the *caudate nucleus* (including head, body, and tail), the *putamen*, and the *globus pallidus*. Some consider the *amygdaloid body*, or *amygdala*, to be part of the basal ganglia, but it is generally included with the limbic system (see Figure 6–7).

Diencephalic Structures

The *diencephalon* includes the thalamus, hypothalamus, and subthalamus. The *thalamus* is the largest structure of the diencephalon and is the final, common relay for sensory information directed toward the cerebral cortex. The *hypothalamus* provides the organizational structure for the limbic system to regulate reproductive behavior and physiology, the perception of need for food and water, perception of satiation, control of digestive processes, and metabolic functions including maintenance of water balance and body temperature. The *subthalamus* modulates all output of the basal ganglia.

Figure 6–7. The basal ganglia consist of the caudate nucleus, amygdala, globus pallidus, and putamen. The basal ganglia are shown in relation to the other subcortical structures, including the diencephalic thalamus and hypothalamus, as well as the red nucleus and substantia nigra.

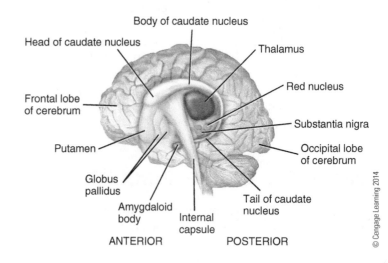

© Cengage Learning 2014

Summary

- The operculum overlies the structures of the limbic system and includes the cingulate gyrus, amygdala, parahippocampal gyrus, and other deep structures.
- The corpus callosum provides direct communication between components of the left and right cerebral hemispheres.
- The basal ganglia are subcortical structures involved in control of movement, and the hippocampal formation of the inferior temporal lobe is implicated in memory function.
- The thalamus of the diencephalon is the final relay for somatic sensation directed toward the cerebrum and other diencephalic structures.
- The subthalamus interacts with the globus pallidus to control movement, and the hypothalamus controls many bodily functions and desires.
- The regions of the cerebral cortex are connected by a complex network of projection fibers, which connect the cortex with other structures; association fibers, which connect regions of the same hemisphere; and commissural fibers, which provide communication between corresponding regions of the two hemispheres.

CEREBROVASCULAR SYSTEM

Although the brain makes up only 2% of body weight, it consumes 20% of the oxygen transported by the vascular system to meet the high metabolic requirements of nervous tissue. The vascular system of the brain (the cerebrovascular system) maintains the constant circulation required by the nervous system. Disruption of this supply for a few seconds will begin cellular changes in neurons, and longer vascular deprivation has devastating effects.

cerebrovascular system: *The vascular supply of the central and peripheral nervous systems.*

The vascular supply of the brain originates in the carotid and vertebral arteries, both of which branch from the aorta. There are some major divisions of the cerebrovascular supply that we should point out (see Figure 6–8). The *anterior cerebral artery* supplies the medial surfaces of the frontal and parietal lobes, the corpus callosum, the basal ganglia, and the anterior limb of the internal capsule. The *middle cerebral artery* provides blood to the lateral surface of the hemispheres, including the temporal lobe, motor strip, Wernicke's area, sensory reception regions, and association areas. The *superior cerebellar* and *anterior inferior cerebellar arteries* serve the cerebellum. The *basilar artery* serves the brainstem structures. The *posterior cerebral artery* serves the

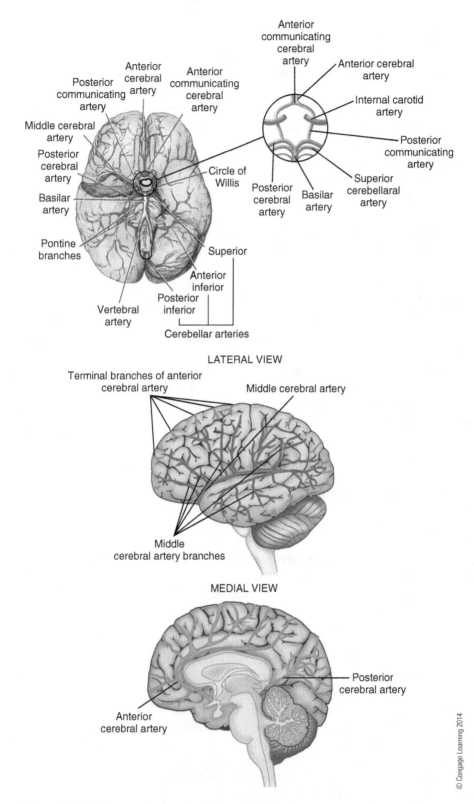

Figure 6–8. Major vascular supply of the cerebral cortex.

inferior temporal and occipital lobes, the medial occipital lobe and primary visual cortex, upper midbrain, diencephalon, and cerebellum.

Circle of Willis

The circle of Willis is a series of anastomoses, or points of communication between arteries, that completely encircles the optic chiasm. It helps equalize locally high or low blood pressure and promotes equal distribution of blood.

anastomoses: *Points of communication among arteries.*

Summary

- The anterior cerebral arteries serve the medial surfaces of the brain, while the middle cerebral artery serves the lateral cortex, including the temporal lobe, motor strip, Wernicke's area, and much of the parietal lobe.
- The superior and anterior inferior cerebellar arteries serve the cerebellum, and the posterior inferior cerebellar artery arises from the vertebral artery.
- The basilar artery divides to become the posterior cerebral arteries, serving the inferior temporal and occipital lobes, upper midbrain, and diencephalon.
- The circle of Willis is a series of communicating arteries that provides redundant pathways for blood flow to regions of the cerebral cortex, equalizing pressure and flow of blood.

CEREBELLUM

The cerebellum is the largest component of the hindbrain, immediately inferior to the posterior cerebral cortex. The cerebellum coordinates motor commands with sensory inputs to control movement, and it communicates with the brainstem, spinal cord, and cerebral cortex by means of superior, middle, and inferior cerebellar peduncles (see Figure 6–9).

Cerebellar Function

The cerebellum is a vital "silent partner" in integration of body movement with the internal and external environment of the body. Although it is incapable of initiating movement, it is intimately related to control of rate and range of movement, as well as the force with which that movement is executed.

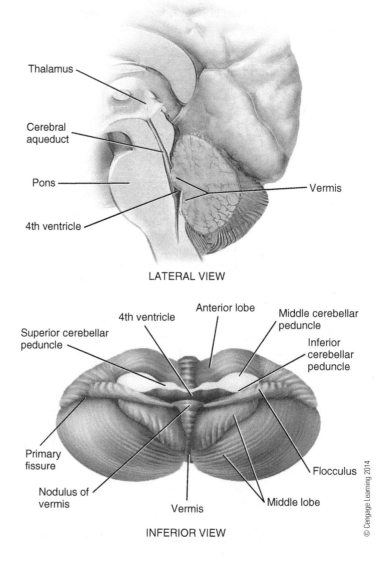

Figure 6–9. Cerebellum as seen in sagittal section and from beneath.

Considering the precise nature of speech production, it should come as no surprise that the cerebellum is an important structure for motor speech control. The cerebellum has information about the state of the entire body, including muscle length, tension, joint position, and movement characteristics. The cerebellum integrates this information with the motor plan for speech, so that your respiratory, phonatory and articulatory mechanisms are not only coordinated but also precisely regulated. When the cerebellum fails, speech becomes discoordinated and inconsistent, resulting in what is termed ataxia of speech.

Summary

- The cerebellum is an important structure for motor function.
- Information about the state of the muscles and structures of the body is integrated with the motor plan to provide smooth execution of movement.

ANATOMY OF THE BRAINSTEM

The brainstem consists of the *medulla oblongata, pons*, and *midbrain*. The brainstem reflects an intermediate stage of organization between the simple reflexive responses at the level of the spinal cord and the exquisitely complex responses generated by the cerebral cortex. Cranial nerves and their nuclei arise from the brainstem, and basic bodily functions for life are maintained here. It will help to refer to Figures 6–10 through 6–13 during the discussion of the brainstem.

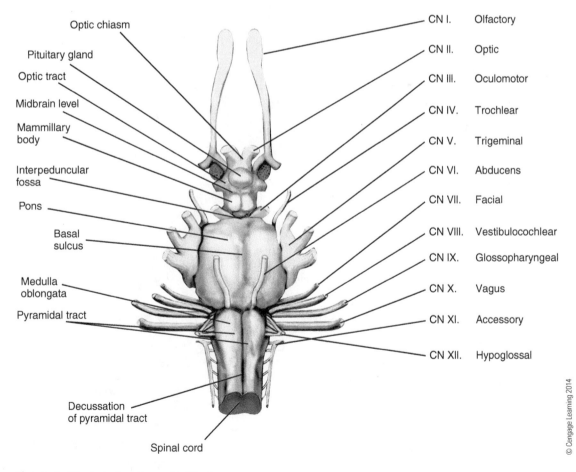

Figure 6–10. Anterior view of brainstem.

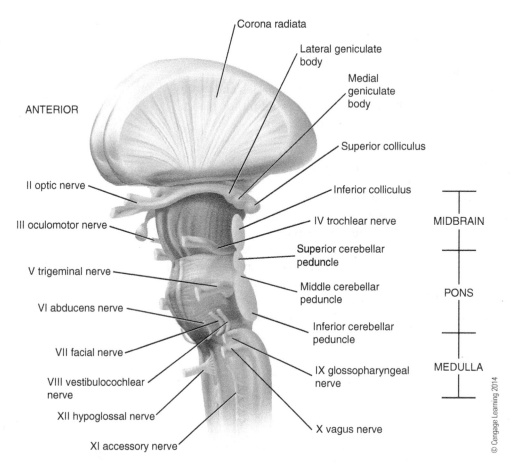

Figure 6–11. Lateral view of brainstem.

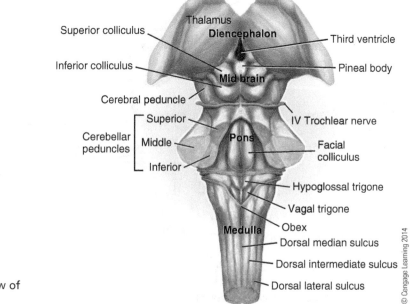

Figure 6–12. Posterior view of
brainstem.

356

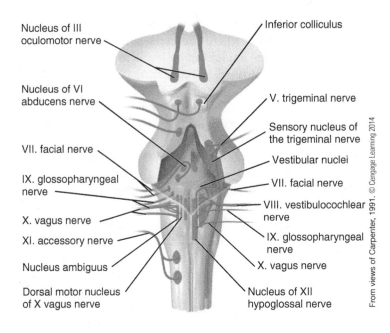

Nucleus of III oculomotor nerve

Inferior colliculus

Nucleus of VI abducens nerve

V. trigeminal nerve

Sensory nucleus of the trigeminal nerve

VII. facial nerve

Vestibular nuclei

IX. glossopharyngeal nerve

VII. facial nerve

X. vagus nerve

VIII. vestibulocochlear nerve

XI. accessory nerve

IX. glossopharyngeal nerve

Nucleus ambiguus

X. vagus nerve

Dorsal motor nucleus of X vagus nerve

Nucleus of XII hypoglossal nerve

From views of Carpenter, 1991. © Cengage Learning 2014

Figure 6–13. Posterior view of brainstem revealing orientation of major nuclei and cranial nerves supplied by those nuclei.

Brainstem Landmarks

Medulla Oblongata

The *medulla oblongata*, or *medulla*, is the inferior-most segment of the brainstem. It looks like an enlargement of the upper spinal cord, and is about 2.5 cm long and 1 cm in diameter. This is a small but mighty structure; damage to the medulla is imminently life threatening.

If you look at the *pyramidal decussation* (see Figure 6–10), you will see the point in the medulla at which fibers of the corticospinal tract cross from one side to the other. That is, most of the axons carrying the motor command from the left hemisphere cross to the right side of the medulla to continue down through the spinal cord on the right side. The significance of this will not be lost on you if you remember meeting an individual with left hemisphere stroke who had right-side hemiparesis. That is, unilateral paralysis signals a neuropathology on the side opposite the lesion. The point of decussation marks the lower border of the medulla, roughly at the level of the foramen magnum of the skull.

Pons and Midbrain

The pons is above the medulla, serving as the bridge between medulla and midbrain, as well as to the cerebellum. The pons is the site of four cranial nerve nuclei, and is the critical bridge between the brainstem and the cerebellum. For those of us in the fields of speech-language pathology and audiology, the pons is the point at which cranial nerve (CN) VIII (vestibulocochlear nerve) enters the brainstem, marking the first stop of the auditory pathway after the cochlea. For the audiologist, the point where the cerebellum and pons join (the cerebellopontine angle) can be home to a cerebellopontine angle tumor, which will affect hearing (CN VIII, vestibulocochlear nerve), facial muscles (CN VII, facial nerve), and muscles of mastication (CN V, trigeminal nerve). The pons is also home to the olivary complex, which is an important part of the auditory pathway associated with localization of sound in space and noise reduction at the level of the cochlea.

The superior-most structure of the brainstem is the midbrain. The midbrain contains the important cerebral peduncles that provide communication between lower pathways and the cerebrum. The midbrain is also the point of origin for cranial nerves III and IV.

The reticular formation is the midposterior "core" of the brainstem, housing some of the phylogenetically oldest structures of the brainstem. It contains nuclei responsible for inspiration, expiration, chewing, and swallowing. It also contains the reticular activating system (RAS), which works with the thalamus to keep the cerebrum conscious.

Summary

- The brainstem is divided into medulla, pons, and midbrain. It is more highly organized than the spinal cord, mediating higher level body functions such as vestibular responses.

- The medulla contains the important pyramidal decussation, the point at which the motor commands originating in one hemisphere of the cerebral cortex cross to serve the opposite side of the body. Cranial nerves IX, X, XI, and XII emerge at the level of the medulla, and the inferior cerebellar peduncle arises there. The fourth ventricle enlargement is a prominent brainstem landmark in cross section. The pons contains the superior and middle cerebellar peduncles, as well as four cranial nerve (V, VI, VII, and VIII) nuclei.

- The midbrain contains the important cerebral peduncles and is the point of origin for cranial nerves III and IV.

- The reticular formation is a phylogenetically old set of nuclei essential for life function, including respiration, mastication, deglutition, and consciousness.

Cranial Nerves

A working knowledge of the cranial nerves is important for speech and hearing professionals because most of these nerves affect speech production and reception (see Tables 6–3 and 6–4).

Table 6–3. Cranial Nerves

Classes of Cranial Nerves

Abbreviation	Class	Description
GSA	General Somatic Afferent	Related to pain, temperature, mechanical stimulation of somatic structures (skin, muscle, joints)
GVA	General Visceral Afferent	From receptors in visceral structures (e.g., digestive tract)
GVE	General Visceral Efferent	Autonomic efferent fibers
GSE	General Somatic Efferent	Innervates skeletal (striated) muscle
SSA	Special Somatic Afferent	Special senses—sight, hearing, equilibrium
SVA	Special Visceral Afferent	Special senses of smell, taste
SVE	Special Visceral Efferent	Innervation of muscle of branchial arch origin: larynx, pharynx, face

© Cengage Learning 2014

Cranial Nerve Classification

Cranial nerves are referred to by name, number, or both. By convention, roman numerals are used when discussing cranial nerves, and the number represents inverse height in the brainstem. Cranial nerves I through IV are at the level of the midbrain, V through VIII are pons level, and IX through XII are in the medulla. Nerves can be efferent (motor), afferent (sensory), or mixed efferent/afferent.

Although all of the cranial nerves are important, not all of them are relevant to speech-language pathology or audiology. Therefore we will only lightly cover nonessential cranial nerves, focusing instead on those that will be critical for your career.

The *olfactory nerve* mediates the sense of smell and the *optic nerve* (CN II) mediates the sense of vision. The *oculomotor nerve* (CN III) innervates all but two of the muscles responsible for eye movement, and the *trochlear* (CN III) and *abducens* (CN III) *nerves* innervate the other eye muscles.

Damage to the Olfactory Nerve (CN I)

The most common trauma resulting in *anosmia* (loss of sense of smell and taste) is an injury involving frontal impact. This often causes damage to the sensory apparatus itself, especially as a result of shearing forces applied to the olfactory nerve at the cribriform plate.

Table 6–4. Cranial Nerves, Sources, and Functions

Nerve	Class	Function	Source
I. Olfactory	SVA	Sense of smell	Mitral cells of olfactory bulb
II. Optic	SSA	Vision	Rod and cone receptor cells synapse with bipolar interneurons, which synapse with multipolar ganglionic neuron; optic nerve is axon of multipolar ganglionic neurons; nerve becomes myelinated after exit from eye socket and entrance into cranium; left and right nerves decussate at chiasm and project as optic tract to lateral geniculate body; projects to occipital cortex via optic radiations; left nasal nerve portion and right temporal nerve portion join after chiasm; left temporal nerve portion and right nasal aspect of nerve join after chiasm; visual field result is that left nasal and right temporal visual fields (right portion of image) project to left cerebral cortex; left temporal and right nasal visual fields (left portion of image) project to right cerebral cortex
III. Oculomotor	GSE	All extrinsic ocular muscles except superior oblique and lateral rectus	Oculomotor nucleus
	GVE	Light and accommodation reflexes	Edinger-Westphal nucleus
IV. Trochlear	GSE	Superior oblique muscle of eye (turns eye down when eye is adducted)	Trochlear nuclei

(continues)

Nerve	Class	Function	Source
V. Trigeminal	**GSA**	Exteroceptive afferent for pain, thermal, tactile from face, forehead, mucous membrane of mouth and nose, teeth, cranial dura; proprioceptive (deep pressure, kinesthesis) from teeth, gums, temporomandibular joint, stretch receptors of mastication	Sensory nucleus of trigeminal nerve
	SVE	To muscles of mastication, tensor tympani, tensor veli palatini	Motor nucleus of trigeminal nerve
		Trigeminal Nerve Branches	
	Ophthalmic branch	Sensory only	
	GSA	From cornea, iris, upper eyelid, front of scalp	
	Maxillary branch	Sensory only	
	GSA	From lower eyelid, nose, palate, upper jaw	
	Mandibular branch	Sensory and motor	
	GSA	From lower jaw and teeth, mucosa, cheeks, temporomandibular joint, anterior two thirds of tongue	
	SVE	To muscles of mastication (internal and external pterygoid, temporalis, masseter), tensor tympani	
VI. Abducens	**GSE**	Lateral rectus muscle for ocular abduction	Abducens nucleus
VII. Facial	**SVE**	To facial muscles of expression, platysma, buccinator	Nucleus of nerve VII
	SVA	Taste, anterior two thirds of tongue	Solitary nucleus

(continues)

Table 6–4. Cranial Nerves, Sources, and Functions *(continued)*

Nerve	Class	Function	Source
	GSA	Cutaneous sense of external auditory meatus and skin of ear	Trigeminal nuclei
	GVE	Lacrimal gland (tears); mucous membrane of mouth and nose	Superior salivatory and lacrimal nuclei
VIII. Vestibulocochlear	SSA	Vestibular and cochlear sensation	
	Cochlear (auditory) portion	Sensors are hair cells; cell bodies in spiral ganglion; axons are VIII nerve, auditory portion; low-frequency (apical) fibers terminate at ventral cochlear nucleus (VCN) and high-frequency fibers (basal) terminate at dorsal cochlear nucleus (DCN); transfer of auditory sensation to central nervous system	Spiral ganglion
	Vestibular portion	From semicircular canals, utricle, saccule; project to vestibular nuclei of medulla and subsequently to all levels of brainstem, spinal cord, cerebellum, thalamus, and cerebral cortex; maintenance of extensor tone, anti-gravity responses, balance, sense of position in space; coordinated eye/head movement through projection to III oculomotor, IV trochlear, VI abducens cranial nerves;	Vestibular ganglion
IX. Glossopharyngeal	GVA	Somatic (tactile, thermal, pain sense) from posterior one third of tongue, tonsils, upper pharynx, eustachian tube, mastoid cells	Solitary nucleus

(continues)

Nerve	Class	Function	Source
	SVA	Taste, posterior one third of tongue	Inferior salivatory nucleus
	GSA	Somatic sense of external auditory meatus and skin of ear	Trigeminal nuclei
	SVE	Innervation of stylopharyngeus, superior pharyngeal constrictor	Inferior salivatory nucleus
	GVE	Parotid gland	Inferior salivatory nucleus
X. Vagus	GSA	Cutaneous sense from external auditory meatus	Trigeminal nuclei
	GVA	Sensory from pharynx, larynx, trachea, esophagus, viscera of thorax, abdomen	Solitary nucleus
	SVA	Taste buds near epiglottis and valleculae	Solitary nucleus
	GVE	To parasympathetic ganglia, thorax, and abdomen	Dorsal motor nucleus of nerve X
	SVE	Striated muscle of larynx and pharynx	Nucleus ambiguus
XI. Accessory	SVE, Cranial portion	Joins with X vagus nerve to form recurrent laryngeal nerve to innervate intrinsic muscles of larynx	
	Spinal portion	Innervates sternocleidomastoid and trapezius	Cranial portion: Nucleus ambiguus of medulla
	SVE	Spinal portion: Anterior horn of C1 through C5 spinal nerves; unite and ascend; enter skull via foramen magnum; exit with vagus at jugular foramen	
XII. Hypoglossal	GSE	Muscles of tongue	Nucleus of hypoglossal nerve
	Clinical note	Lesion of lower motor neuron produces ipsilateral damage (tongue deviates to side of damage)	

In more detail, following are the cranial nerves that affect speech and hearing. Motor cranial nerves are activated by means of the corticobulbar tract, a motor pathway from the cerebrum to the brainstem. Individual cranial nerve motor nuclei reside in the brainstem.

Trigeminal Nerve (CN V). The trigeminal nerve is an extremely important nerve for speech production because it provides motor supply to the muscles of mastication and transmits sensory information from the face. The trigeminal divides into the ophthalmic, the maxillary, and the mandibular branches (see Figure 6–14).

The *ophthalmic branch* is the small, superior nerve of the trigeminal. It is entirely afferent (sensory) and transmits information from the skin of the upper face, forehead, scalp, cornea, iris, upper eyelid, conjunctiva, nasal cavity mucous membrane, and lacrimal gland.

The *maxillary nerve* is also only afferent. It transmits information from the lower eyelid, skin on the sides of the nose, upper jaw, teeth, lips, mucosal lining of buccal and nasal cavities, maxillary sinuses, and nasopharynx.

The *mandibular branch* is both afferent and efferent (motor). This largest branch of the trigeminal nerve exits the skull via the *foramen ovale of sphenoid* and divides into a number of branching nerves. The afferent component conducts sensory information from a region roughly

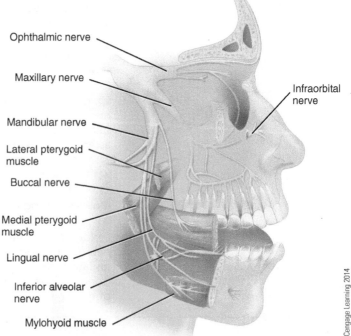

Ophthalmic nerve

Maxillary nerve

Infraorbital nerve

Mandibular nerve

Lateral pterygoid muscle

Buccal nerve

Medial pterygoid muscle

Lingual nerve

Inferior alveolar nerve

Mylohyoid muscle

© Cengage Learning 2014

Figure 6–14. Ophthalmic, maxillary, and mandibular branches of the V trigeminal nerve.

Lesions of the Trigeminal Nerve

The trigeminal nerve has both motor and sensory components, and all trigeminal nerves can be affected by lesions. With a lesion of the cerebral cortex in the area innervating the muscles of mastication you may see increased jaw jerk reflex (elicited by pulling down on the passively opened mandible). Damage to the trigeminal nerve itself results in atrophy (wasting) and weakness on the affected side. When your client closes his or her mouth, the jaw will deviate toward the side of the lesion as a result of the action of the intact internal pterygoid muscle. The jaw will hang open with bilateral lower motor neuron damage, which has an extreme effect on speech. The tensor veli palatine muscle is also innervated by the trigeminal nerve, and weakness or paralysis may result in hypernasality because of this muscle's role in maintaining the velopharyngeal sphincter.

Damage to the sensory component of the CN V results in loss of tactile sensation for the anterior two thirds of the tongue, loss of the corneal blink reflex, and alteration of sensation at the orifice of the eustachian tube, external auditory meatus, and tympanic membrane, teeth, and gums. Sensation of the forehead, upper face, and nose region are lost with ophthalmic branch lesion, and the sensation to the skin region roughly lateral to the zygomatic arch and over the maxilla is lost with maxillary branch lesion. Damage to the mandibular branch affects sensation from the side of the face down to the mandible. Trigeminal neuralgia (tic douloureux) may also arise from damage to cranial nerve V. The result is a severe and sharp shooting pain along the course of the nerve, which may be restricted to areas served by only one of the branches.

encompassing the mandible, including the skin, lower teeth, gums and lower lip, a portion of the skin and mucosal lining of the cheek, external auditory meatus and auricle, temporomandibular joint, and the region of the temporal bone. It also transmits kinesthetic and proprioceptive sense of muscles of mastication. The lingual nerve conducts somatic sensation from the anterior two thirds of the mucous membrane of the tongue and floor of the mouth.

The efferent component of the mandibular branch serves the muscles of mastication (masseter, temporalis, lateral and medial pterygoids), as well as the tensor veli palatine and tensor tympani of the middle ear.

Facial Nerve (CN VII). The facial nerve supplies motor innervation to the facial muscles of expression and tear glands, as well as sense of taste for a portion of the tongue (see Figure 6–15). The facial nerve also transmits the sense of taste (gustation) from the anterior two thirds of the tongue.

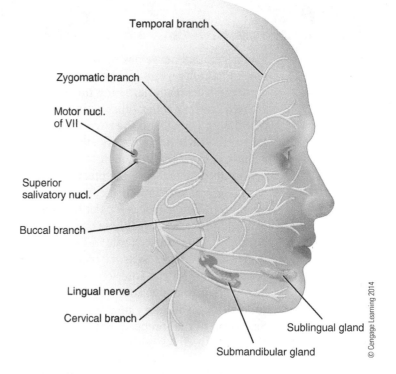

Temporal branch

Zygomatic branch

Motor nucl. of VII

Superior salivatory nucl.

Buccal branch

Lingual nerve

Cervical branch

Sublingual gland

Submandibular gland

© Cengage Learning 2014

Figure 6–15. General course of VII facial nerve.

Vestibulocochlear Nerve (CN VIII). This nerve, also known as the auditory nerve, is extremely important in both speech-language pathology and audiology because it mediates both auditory information and sense of movement in space. The nerve consists of both sensory and motor components. The sensory portion mediates information concerning hearing and balance, while the motor component appears to assist in selectively damping output of hair cells (see Figure 6–16).

Glossopharyngeal Nerve (CN IX). The glossopharyngeal nerve serves both sensory and motor functions of the stylopharyngeus muscle and the superior constrictor muscle. The nerve mediates sensation from taste receptors of the posterior one third of the tongue and a portion of the soft palate.

Vagus Nerve (CN X). The motor component of the vagus provides motor innervation of many smooth muscles but, more important, for speech and swallowing, the striated muscles of the larynx used for phonation and protection of the airway are innervated by the recurrent laryngeal nerve and superior laryngeal nerve of the vagus.

The sensory component of the vagus nerve delivers pain, touch, and temperature sense from the skin covering the eardrum, posterior auricle, and external auditory meatus.

Lesions of the Facial Nerve

Lesions of the facial nerve can significantly affect articulatory function. Because the upper motor neuron supply to the upper face is bilateral, unilateral cortical damage does not result in upper face paralysis. It may, however, paralyze all facial muscles below the eyes. Even then, muscles of facial expression (*mimetic muscles*) may be contracted involuntarily in response to emotional stimuli because these motor gestures are initiated at regions of the brain that differ from those that affect speech.

Damage directly to cranial nerve VII causes upper- and lower-face paralysis on the side of the lesion. This may involve the inability to close the eyelid and results in muscle sagging, loss of tone, and reduction in wrinkling around the lip, nose, and forehead. When the individual attempts to smile, the affected corners of the mouth will be drawn toward the unaffected side. The person may drool because of loss of the ability to hold back saliva with the lips, and the cheeks may puff out during expiration due to a flaccid buccinator.

Bell's palsy (*palsy* means "paralysis") may result from any compression of the seventh cranial nerve or even from cold weather. It results in paralysis of facial musculature, which remits in most cases within a few months.

Damage to the facial nerve following penetrating facial or cranial trauma is quite common. Both damage to the middle ear and skull fractures of the temporal bone result in facial nerve damage. Most fractures of the temporal bone occur along the long axis of the temporal bone, although facial paralysis is much more likely if the fracture is transverse (see MacKay et al., 1997).

Accessory Nerve (CN XI). The accessory nerve provides motor innervation directly to the sternocleidomastoid and trapezius muscles and works in conjunction with the vagus nerve to innervate the intrinsic muscles of the larynx, pharynx, and soft palate (see Figure 6–17).

Hypoglossal Nerve (CN XII). This nerve provides the innervation to motor function of the tongue.

Summary

- Cranial nerves are sensory, motor, or mixed sensorimotor.
- The olfactory nerve (CN I) transmits the sense of smell, and the II optic nerve communicates visual information to the brain.
- The oculomotor (CN III), trochlear (CN IV), and abducens (CN VI) nerves provide innervation for eye movements.

Figure 6–16. The auditory pathway, showing the nuclei of the brainstem involved in audition. AVCN, anteroventral cochlear nucleus; IC, inferior colliculus; LSO, lateral superior olive; MSO, medial superior olive; MTB, medial nucleus of trapezoid body; NLL, nucleus of lateral lemniscus; PVCN, posteroventral cochlear nucleus.

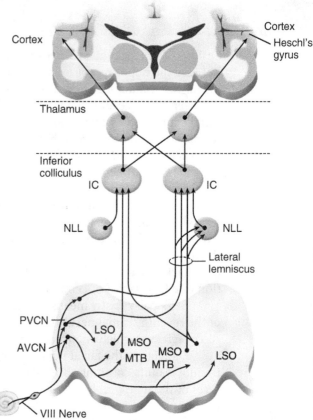

Adapted from Pickles, 1982. © Cengage Learning 2014

Lesions of the Vestibulocochlear Nerve

Damage to cranial nerve VIII results in ipsilateral hearing loss reflecting the degree of trauma. Damage to this nerve can arise from a number of causes, including physical trauma (skull fracture), tumor growth compressing the nerve, and vascular incident.

Traumatic injury to the vestibulocochlear nerve is usually caused by a fracture of the temporal bone or a penetrating injury, such as a gunshot wound. If the fracture is along the long axis of the temporal bone, it often results in sensorineural loss and vertigo without eighth nerve compression or apparent damage to the labyrinth. If the fracture is in the transverse dimension, the seventh and eighth cranial nerves may well be sheared or compressed. Vertigo and nystagmus in head injury often occur when the head position is changed. In absence of evidence of physical damage to the labyrinth, it is hypothesized that the vertigo and nystagmus arise from disturbance of calcium particles used in the sensory mechanisms of the vestibular system. Fortunately, most trauma-induced vertigo remits over time (see MacKay et al., 1997).

Lesions of the Glossopharyngeal Nerve

The glossopharyngeal nerve works in concert with the vagus nerve (CN X), making its independent function difficult to determine. Damage to the ninth cranial nerve results in paralysis of the stylopharyngeus muscle and may result in loss of general sensation (anesthesia) for the posterior one third of the tongue and pharynx, although the vagus nerve may support these functions as well. The cooperative innervation with the vagus nerve results in little effect on the pharyngeal constrictors, although reduced sensation of the auricle and middle ear may indicate ninth nerve damage. Damage to the glossopharyngeal nerve may also cause reduced or absent gag reflex, although absence of the reflex does not guarantee that a lesion exists.

Lesions of the Vagus Nerve

The vagus nerve is the most extensive of the cranial nerves, presenting an important constellation of clinical manifestations. Damage to the pharyngeal branch results in deficit in swallowing, potential loss of the gag reflex through interaction with the glossopharyngeal nerve, and hypernasality due to weakness of the velopharyngeal sphincter (all velopharyngeal muscles are innervated by the vagus nerve with the exception of the tensor veli palatine, which is innervated by the trigeminal nerve). Unilateral pharyngeal branch damage results in failure to elevate the soft palate on the involved side (asymmetrical elevation), producing hypernasality. Bilateral lesion produces absent or reduced (but symmetrical) movement of the soft palate producing hypernasality, nasal regurgitation, dysphagia, and paralysis of the pharyngeal musculature.

Lesions of the superior laryngeal nerve may result in loss of sensation of the upper larynx mucous membrane and stretch receptors, as well as paralysis of the cricothyroid muscle. Recurrent laryngeal nerve (RLN) damage produces either unilateral or bilateral flaccid vocal fold paralysis. Besides affecting voice, this condition puts the individual at risk for aspiration pneumonia because of his or her inability to close the airway during swallow.

- The trigeminal nerve (CN V) innervates muscles of mastication and the tensor veli palatini and communicates sensation from the face, mouth, teeth, mucosal lining, and tongue to the brain.
- The facial nerve (CN VII) innervates muscles of facial expression, and the sensory component transmits taste from the anterior two thirds of the tongue.

Lesions of the Accessory Nerve

Lesion of the accessory nerve may have an effect on the trapezius and sternocleidomastoid muscles. Unilateral lesion affecting the sternocleidomastoid results in the person's being unable to turn his or her head away from the side of the lesion. (The left sternocleidomastoid rotates the head toward the right side when contracted.) Lesions resulting in paralysis of the trapezius result in restricted ability to elevate the arm or drooping shoulder on the side of the lesion.

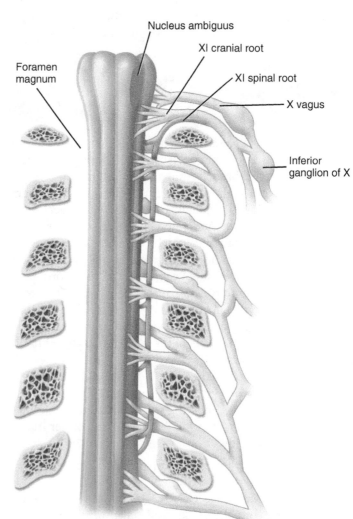

Figure 6–17. Spinal accessory nerve origins.

- The vestibulocochlear nerve (CN VIII) mediates auditory and vestibular sensation.
- The glossopharyngeal nerve (CN IX) transmits information from the posterior tongue taste receptors, as well as somatic sense from the tongue, fauces, pharynx, and eustachian tube. The stylopharyngeus and superior pharyngeal constrictor muscles receive motor innervation via this nerve.
- The vagus nerve (CN X) is extremely important for autonomic function as well as somatic motor innervation. Somatic sensation of pain, touch, and temperature from the region of the eardrum is mediated by the vagus, as well as pain from pharynx, larynx, esophagus, and many other regions. The recurrent laryngeal nerve and superior laryngeal nerves supply motor innervation for the intrinsic muscles of the larynx.
- The accessory nerve (CN XI) innervates the sternocleidomastoid and trapezius muscles, and collaborates with the vagus nerve in activation of palatal, laryngeal, and pharyngeal muscles.
- The hypoglossal nerve (CN XII) innervates the muscles of the tongue with the exception of the palatoglossus.

Spinal Cord

The spinal cord comprises tracts and nuclei. The 31 pairs of spinal nerves serve the limbs and trunk. Sensory nerves have cell bodies in dorsal root ganglia, and motor neuron bodies lie within the spinal cord. Upper motor neurons have their cell bodies above the segment at which the spinal nerve originates. Lower motor neurons are the final neurons in the efferent chain. Efferent tracts, such as the corticospinal tract, transmit information from the brain to the spinal nerves. Afferent tracts, such as the spinothalamic tract, transmit information concerning the physical state of the limbs and trunk to higher brain centers.

NEUROPHYSIOLOGY

Although extraordinary advances over the past 30 years have vastly expanded our understanding of the workings of the brain, we still have a great deal to learn. We will approach our discussion of nervous system function from the "bottom up," looking first at the simplest responses of the system (communication between neurons) and working our way up to the all-important functions of the cerebral cortex.

The Neuron

Neuron Function

Neurons can be stimulated to send a signal out through the axon, which is how information passes from one neuron to another. When a neuron is stimulated, it can send out a response that either excites the next neuron (*excitatory response*) or inhibits the next neuron (*inhibitory*). Excitation causes an increase in activity, and inhibition causes a reduction in activity. This arrangement lets neurons have very different effects on other neurons.

Synapse

When a neuron is sufficiently stimulated its axon discharges a neurotransmitter into the synaptic cleft, or area between its end bouton and the connecting neuron. The neurotransmitter is a lot like the key to your door. The specific neurotransmitter released into the synaptic cleft is the one to which the adjacent neuron responds. If some other type of neurotransmitter makes its way into that synaptic region, it will have no effect on the adjacent neuron. This "lock-and-key" arrangement lets neurons have specific effects on some neurons while not affecting others.

When a neurotransmitter is released into the synaptic cleft, it stimulates receptor sites on the next neuron. Ion channels in the next neuron's membrane open up and allow ions to enter, and this leads to a discharge, or "firing," of that neuron as well. That firing of a neuron is the action potential (see Figure 6–18).

An *action potential* (AP) is a change in electrical potential that occurs when the cell membrane of a neuron is stimulated adequately to permit ions (molecules that are either positively or negatively charged) to pass through the cell wall. When a neuron is stimulated, sodium ion (Na^+) "gates" open up and allow sodium ions to flood the intracellular space. This makes the inside of the neuron more positively charged than the area outside the neuron for a brief time. This is termed *depolarization*. For about half of 1 millisecond (0.5 ms), no amount of stimulation of that region of the membrane will cause it to depolarize again; this time is the absolute refractory period. The absolute refractory period is the time during which the cell membrane cannot be stimulated to depolarize. During the absolute refractory period, potassium ions (K^+) flow into the neuron. The sodium and potassium are actively removed by a protein known as the sodium-potassium pump.

For an action potential to be generated, the membrane channels have to open up. Portions of the cell membrane may be depolarized, but other parts of the membrane will not be depolarized until a critical threshold has been reached.

absolute refractory period: *The time during depolarization when the cell membrane cannot be stimulated to depolarize again.*

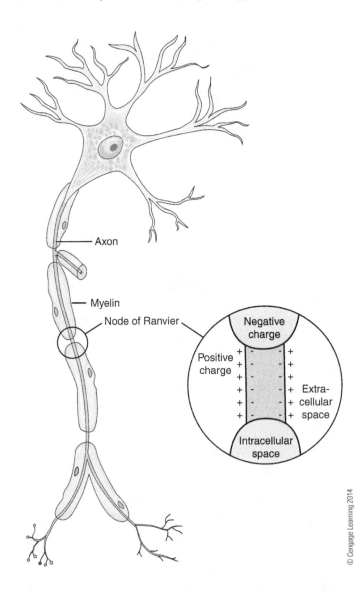

Axon

Myelin

Node of Ranvier

Negative charge

Positive charge

Extra-cellular space

Intracellular space

© Cengage Learning 2014

Figure 6–18. A quiescent neuron, showing equilibrium of membrane potential.

Myasthenia Gravis

Myasthenia gravis is a neuromuscular disease whose primary effect is on the neuromuscular junction. It appears that an individual's autoimmune system develops an immune response to the neurotransmitter receptor of the neuromuscular junction, building antibodies that block the receptor. Blocked receptors are unable to respond to neurotransmitter substance so that as the disease progresses, greater numbers of receptors become blocked and increasingly fewer ion channels can be activated to depolarize a neuron. As was discussed previously, myasthenia gravis causes a person to have extreme fatigue and weakness, but it is treatable.

resting membrane potential (RMP): *The condition of a neuron at rest, in which it is polarized and ready to discharge.*

There have to be sufficient numbers of opened channels for an action potential to be generated. If there are not sufficient numbers, then the membrane returns to the resting membrane potential (RMP), which is the state it was in before being stimulated.

This whole cycle from RMP to AP and back to RMP takes about 1 ms in most neurons, and this is a defining time period. This means that a neuron may respond every 1/1000 of a second, or 1000 times per second. Even if it is stimulated 2000 times per second, it will not be able to respond any faster.

Propagation

propagation: *The spreading effect of wave action; in neural responses, the communication of information through the nervous system.*

An action potential would do no good at all if it did not pass information to the next neuron or to a muscle fiber. Propagation refers to the spreading effect of wave action, much as the wave generated by throwing a rock in a pond spreads out from the stone's point of contact with the water. The depolarization is propagated along the neuron membrane in a wave of depolarization. When the membrane undergoing the local depolarization reaches the critical limit, ions flow rapidly across the membrane. The adjacent membrane contains voltage-sensitive protein channels, which are channels that open when there is a voltage change in their vicinity. The current flow from the first depolarization stimulates regions next to it to depolarize as well. In this manner, the depolarization spreads along the membrane, ultimately reaching the terminal of the axon.

The neuron responds in an all-or-nothing manner. That is, it either depolarizes or it does not. If it fails to depolarize, no action potential is generated and no information is conveyed. If the threshold for depolarization is reached, an action potential will be produced, and information will be transmitted. The neuron acts like a light switch in this sense, and the only variation in information is in the frequency with which the neuron is "turned on," referred to as *spike rate* or *rate of discharge*.

Propagation of the action potential is facilitated by axon diameter and myelin. Axons with larger diameters propagate at a much higher rate than those with smaller fibers, and presence of myelin also speeds propagation. Figure 6–19 shows how myelin is laid down on the axon in "donuts" with nodes of exposed membrane between them. Voltage-sensitive ion channels reside in those nodes.

saltatory conduction: *The process in a neural response in which information in the axon passes from node to node, thereby greatly increasing conduction speed.*

The membrane becomes depolarized at one node, and the effect of that depolarization is felt at the next node, where the membrane depolarizes as well. The propagating action potential is "passed" from node to node, and this jumping is referred to as saltatory conduction. Clearly, many precious milliseconds can be saved by skipping from node to node in long fibers.

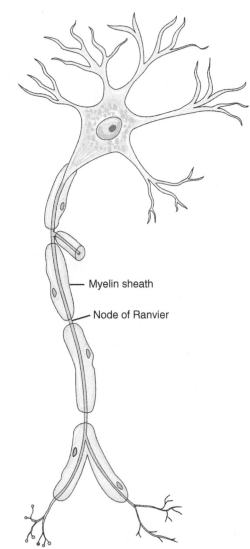

© Cengage Learning 2014

— Myelin sheath

— Node of Ranvier

Figure 6–19. Myelin sheath and nodes of Ranvier.

When the impulse reaches the terminal point on the axon, a highly specialized process begins. The synaptic vesicles in the terminal end buttons contain a neurotransmitter substance that permits communication between the two neurons. As mentioned earlier, a neurotransmitter is a substance released from the terminal end button of an axon that causes either excitation or inhibition of another neuron or excitation of a muscle fiber. When the action potential reaches the terminal point, the vesicles are stimulated to migrate to the membrane wall where they will dump their neurotransmitter through the membrane into the synaptic cleft (see Figure 6–20).

The neurotransmitter travels across the cleft very quickly (100 microseconds [μs]) and is dumped into the cleft to activate receptor proteins on the postsynaptic neuron. Presence of neurotransmitter in the cleft triggers ion channels

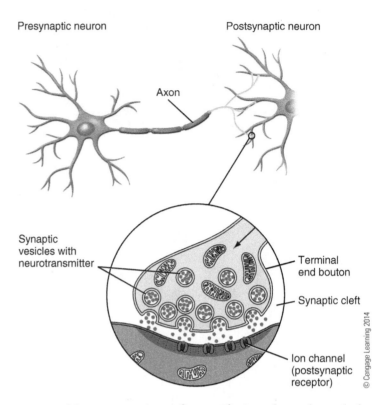

Presynaptic neuron
Postsynaptic neuron

Axon

Synaptic
vesicles with
neurotransmitter

Terminal
end bouton

Synaptic cleft

Ion channel
(postsynaptic
receptor)

© Cengage Learning 2014

Figure 6–20. Expanded view of synapse between two neurons.

to open. Neurotransmitters fit specific ion channels, and if a given neurotransmitter does not match a receptor channel protein, the postsynaptic neuron will not fire. That is, the neurotransmitter is a "key" and the receptor is a "lock": If the key does not fit, the gate will not open.

The neurotransmitter may have either an excitatory or an inhibitory effect on the neuron. Excitatory effects increase the probability that a neuron will depolarize, whereas inhibition decreases that probability. Excitatory stimulation generates an *excitatory postsynaptic potential (EPSP)*, whereas inhibitory synapses produce *inhibitory postsynaptic potentials (IPSPs)*. Excitation causes depolarization, whereas inhibition causes hyperpolarization, greatly elevating the threshold of firing (making it difficult or impossible for the neuron to fire).

The EPSP actually begins as a *micropotential*, depolarizing the membrane by about only 3 mV. If there is a sufficient number of miniature EPSP depolarizations, the sum of their depolarization will reach the critical threshold and an action potential will be generated, as before. If you imagine a very large teeter-totter with an adult on one end, it would take a large number of children to counteract the effect of that one adult. If there are sufficient numbers of children on the teeter-totter, the adult will rise in the air. If a sufficient number of synapses are activated, there will be an action potential. Likewise, there can be **temporal summation**, in which a smaller number of regions depolarize virtually simultaneously.

temporal summation: *The quality of some neurons wherein the neuron requires virtually simultaneous inputs from other neurons before it can be stimulated to depolarize.*

Single neurons may take input from thousands of other neurons to produce a single response, a process called convergence. In this configuration, a mass of information is distilled into a single response. In contrast, divergence occurs when the axon of one neuron makes synapse with many thousands of other neurons. Its single piece of information is transmitted to many other neurons.

convergence: *The neural process in which outputs of many neurons contribute to the depolarization of a single neuron.*

divergence: *The neural process in which one neuron passes information to many other neurons.*

Summary

- Communication between neurons of the nervous system occurs at the synapse.
- Neurotransmitter passing through the synaptic cleft either excites or inhibits the postsynaptic neuron.
- If a neuron is excited sufficiently, an action potential will be generated.
- Stimulation of a neuron membrane to depolarize causes exchange of ions between the extracellular and intracellular spaces, and the ion movement results in a large and predictable change in voltage across the membrane.
- The resting membrane potential is the electrical potential measurable prior to excitation.
- The absolute refractory period after excitation is an interval during which the neuron cannot be excited to fire, whereas it can fire during the relative refractory period, given adequate stimulation.
- Because an action potential always results in the same neural response, the neuron is capable of representing differences in input only through rate of response.
- Myelinated fibers conduct the wave of depolarization more rapidly than demyelinated fibers, primarily due to saltatory conduction.
- Temporal summation is the quality of some neurons wherein the neuron requires virtually simultaneous inputs from other neurons before it can be stimulated to depolarize.
- Single neurons can take input from thousands of other neurons to produce a single response, a process called convergence.
- Divergence occurs when the axon of one neuron makes synapse with many thousands of other neurons.

Muscle Function

Activation of muscle requires that a nerve make contact with the muscle fiber. The neuromuscular junction (point where neuron and muscle connect) looks a lot like a synapse

neuromuscular junction: *The point of synapse between muscle fiber and motor fiber.*

between two neurons. The basic unit of skeletal muscle control is the motor unit, consisting of the motor neuron, its axon, and the muscle fibers it innervates.

Figure 6–21 shows a neuromuscular junction, looking very much like a synapse. In this case, however, there is a terminal end plate on the axon, with a synaptic cleft as before. The neurotransmitter, acetylcholine, is dumped into the active zone, and a *miniature end plate potential (MEPP)* will be generated. If there are sufficient numbers of MEPPs, a muscle action potential will be generated. This is directly analogous to neuron-to-neuron synapse in that it takes many activated regions to excite a muscle fiber. When the MEPP is generated, the muscle fiber twitches, and the whole muscle contracts.

Muscle Control

When the MEPP is generated, the muscle fiber responds in all-or-none fashion and the muscle twitches. Muscles come in all sizes, from the massive to the minute. In addition, muscles must perform vastly different functions, ranging from gross, slow movement to quick, precise action. How do we manage this?

The answer to this question lies largely in allocation of resources. For fine movement, only a limited number of muscle fibers need to be recruited for movement, because you are not trying to move as much mass. In contrast, heavy lifting requires recruitment of many muscle fibers. You

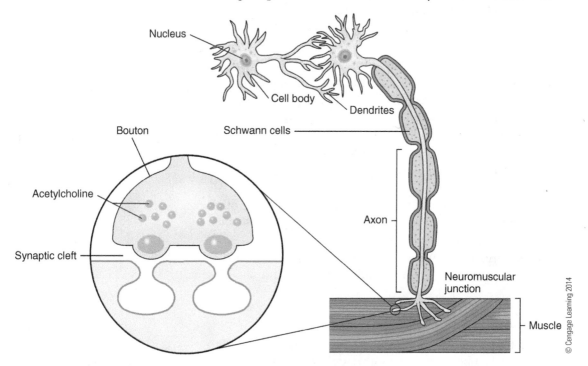

Figure 6–21. Neuromuscular junction between neuron and muscle fiber.

can think of the tasks involved in speech for examples of this, as well. The relatively large genioglossus makes up the bulk of the tongue, but is not nearly as precise as the tip of the tongue. The genioglossus is responsible for moving the tongue around within the oral cavity, but the tip is responsible for the fine movement associated with lingual fricatives.

Summary

- Neuromuscular junctions operate similarly to neuron-to-neuron synapses, except the result is muscle movement.
- Muscle innervation patterns help differentiate fine and gross motor control.

Higher Functioning

We have been discussing responses that occur at the lowest levels of the nervous system and often do not even reach consciousness. Although it is essential for your brain to know what your tongue muscles are doing, it is obvious that there is more to speech than movement of muscles. Saper, Iverson, and Frackowiak (2000) provided a framework for talking about how we receive, integrate, and act on information at the level of the cortex. They viewed cortical regions as being either primary sensory input areas (or motor output areas), higher-order integration areas, or association areas. In this model, sensory information from the body that is received by the thalamus is relayed to one of the sensory reception areas on the cortex, and is processed in higher-order integration regions. Ultimately it is combined in one of the three association areas, allowing the highest level processes to occur. The three association areas included the temporal-occipital-parietal association area (around Wernicke's area), the frontal association area (including Broca's area), and the limbic association area (including limbic structures as well as the cingulate gyrus). This hierarchical processing model allowed information to be distributed across the cortex, but also aggregated in regions where it is critical (i.e., the association areas). Let's look briefly at afferent inputs, and then at these three levels of processing.

In this text, we take a regional approach to function of the cerebral cortex. Our discussion focuses on functional regions and association pathways of the brain and interconnections among regions. The cortex appears to be organized around regions of primary activity for a given area, including the *primary receptive area* for somatic sense, primary motor area, primary auditory cortex, and primary region of

The Great Debate

A lively debate concerning localization of function within the brain has been going on for well over 100 years. On the one hand, *localizationists* (or "materialists" as they were called in the 1860s) held that given sufficiently sensitive tools, specific functions could be localized to specific brain regions. The opposing view, held by "spiritualists," was that it was degrading to think that the human body (much less the brain) could be so mechanically dissected, and that functions such as language or mathematics could not be isolated to a single brain region. Perhaps the first localizationist was Joseph Gall, who also proposed that a properly knowledgeable individual could identify specific cognitive traits of an individual by reading the bumps on that person's head (phrenology) (Kandel, 1991).

Phrenology did not retain many followers, but one admirer of Gall, Paul Broca, was the first to identify the region responsible for expressive language within the dominant hemisphere of the brain (Kandel, 1991). Others provided counterevidence, including people with acquired language deficits that clearly arose from damage to another region distal from the area identified by Broca. Such notables as Sigmund Freud refuted the notion of localization of function, saying that although some specific locations for basic processes might be found, that still did not explain complex cognitive function.

Wernicke entered the battle, clearly identifying a language center within the temporal lobe distinct from that identified by Broca. Indeed, as the twentieth century dawned, localization of function was demonstrated through ablation studies of the occipital and temporal lobes of dogs, eliminating visual and auditory recognition, respectively. Researchers found that they could stimulate specific locales of a dog's cerebrum and cause single, replicable movements of the limbs.

Although such notable researchers as Karl Lashley, an American psychologist who studied memory in the early twentieth century, countered the growing body of evidence, research that examined brain-damaged soldiers during the First and Second World Wars revealed a great deal of "regional" consistency of symptoms, and these findings led us into the study and treatment of acquired language disorders.

Although it is clear that regions of the cerebral cortex, such as the motor strip, are highly specialized for specific functions, other regions of the cortex are less well defined. To further confound things, the developing brain is plastic. The brains of infants who receive trauma are more likely to overcome damage to function than are the brains of adults who receive the same trauma. This and other evidence led to *theories of equipotentiality*, which state that the brain functions as a whole. One could strike a balance with the notion of *regional equipotentiality*. There seems to be a functional unity by regions, but the degree of functional loss to an individual who has received trauma also is related to the total volume of damaged tissue.

visual reception. Adjacent to these are higher-order areas of processing. That is, there are secondary, tertiary, and even quaternary areas of higher-order processing adjacent to the primary receptive areas for sensation. (There also are higher-order areas of processing for motor function, as we will see.) Beyond the higher-order areas of processing are *association areas* where the most complex form of cognitive processing occurs. We receive information from our senses at primary reception areas (Heschl's gyrus for audition; calcarine sulcas for vision; somatosensory cortex of the parietal lobe for body sense) and we extract the information received and put it together with other information associated with the modality at higher-order areas of processing. These higher-order association areas are typically adjacent or close to the primary receptive area. This information is then passed to one of the three association areas for the highest level of cognitive processing.

Afferent Inputs

The motor strip receives input from the thalamus, sensory cortex, and premotor area. There is also heavy sensory input to this motor region, underscoring the notion that control of movement is strongly influenced by information about the ongoing state and position of the musculature. Some muscle stretch sensors (muscle spindles) send information to the motor strip, and spinal reflexes are modified and controlled, at least in part, by activity from this region.

The premotor region is involved in preparation for movement, anticipation of movement, and organization of skilled movement. It receives somatic sensory information from the parietal lobe, as well as sensory information from the thalamus, and projects its output to the motor strip. Afferent parietal information to the supplementary motor area also supports its involvement in active planning and rehearsal of the motor act, as well as decision making about movement. Broca's area (regions of the frontal lobe) uses parietal lobe information to perform a high-level planning function for movement of the speech articulators for speech function.

Sensory Reception Areas

We have spoken of these areas in different contexts, but they are the primary sensory reception areas of the cortex, including Heschl's gyrus for audition, the calcarine sulcus for vision, and the postcentral gyrus for somatosensory information. We will add the efferent component now, which is the precentral gyrus or motor strip. These represent the entrance to the cortex (for sensory information) or the last point before exiting the cortex (for efferent information).

Lead Exposure

We have known for many years that lead exposure is bad for children. Excessive exposure to lead causes permanent brain damage, resulting in mental retardation, learning disability, attention deficit, and memory problems.

Recently, however, researchers have found an even more insidious route for lead effects. Basha et al. (2005) found that when infant monkeys were given milk with low levels of lead, at 23 years of age they developed the plaques associated with Alzheimer's disease. If the monkeys had the genetic markers for Alzheimer's susceptibility, they were twice as likely to develop the plaques.

Higher-order Processing Areas. Sensory information arising at the primary sensory reception regions is projected to areas more distant from the sensory region for further processing. These areas are responsible for extracting critical features of the signal, such as rate, frequency, and fluctuation.

Association Areas. The association areas provide the highest order of information processing of the cerebral cortex. It appears that higher-order integration areas extract detailed information from the signal input to the primary areas, whereas association areas permit that information to flow among the various processing sites, effectively connecting modalities. These regions are involved in intellect, cognitive functions, memory, and language.

There are three major association areas: the temporal-occipital-parietal association cortex, the limbic association cortex, and the prefrontal association cortex. The *temporal-occipital-parietal (TOP)* region is of the utmost importance to speech-language pathologists and speech-language pathology assistants because it includes the areas associated with language. This region includes portions of the temporal, parietal, and occipital lobes. It receives input from auditory, visual, and somatosensory regions, permitting the integration of this information into language function.

The *limbic association area* includes regions of the parahippocampal gyrus and temporal pole (temporal lobe), cingulate gyri (parietal and frontal lobes), and orbital surfaces (inferior frontal lobe). The limbic system is involved with motivation, emotion, and memory, making it an ideal association area. Clearly, memory function is served by reception of information from diverse sensory inputs.

The *prefrontal association area* is involved with integration of information in preparation for the motor act, as well as higher-level cognitive processes. The premotor regions, consisting of the premotor gyrus and supplemental motor area, appear to be vital to initiation of motor activity, whereas the prefrontal region anterior to these regions is involved in the motor plan. The premotor region receives input from the primary sensory reception areas, or low-order processing regions, while the prefrontal regions derive their input from the higher-order regions. Premotor and prefrontal regions project to the motor strip, permitting both low-order and abstract sensory perceptions to influence the motor act. Broca's area, the frontal operculum, and the insula also are involved in motor programming. These regions share qualities with both the prefrontal association region and the premotor gyrus because damage to them results in deficits of both motor planning and higher-level language, including word retrieval problems.

In addition to this, the *orbitofrontal region* (the region on the underbelly of the cerebrum that overlays the orbit region) is involved in limbic system function, as well as motor planning memory associated with delayed execution.

Summary

- The complexity of higher functions of the brain is reflected in the inability to assign precise locations for specific functions.
- General regions, such as Wernicke's area, can be ascribed broad function, and this view facilitates examination of brain function and dysfunction.
- A broad view of brain function classifies regions of the cerebrum as primary, higher-order, and association regions.
- Primary sensory and motor regions include the primary reception area for somatic sense, primary motor area, primary auditory cortex, and primary region of visual reception.
- Adjacent to these areas are higher-order areas of processing, apparently responsible for extracting features of the stimulus.
- Association areas are the regions of highest cognitive processing, integrating sensory information with memory.
- The prefrontal area appears to be involved in higher function related to motor output (such as inhibition of motor function and the ability to change motor responses), whereas the temporal-occipital-parietal association area is involved in language function.
- The limbic association area integrates information relating to affect, motivation, and emotion.

Hemispheric Specialization

Despite the gross similarities between the two cerebral hemispheres, the brain is functionally asymmetrical, and the basic processing differences between the two cerebral hemispheres are of extreme importance to speech-language pathology assistants.

If you write with your right hand, you probably have functional dominance for language and speech in the left hemisphere. Motor pathways decussate as they descend, and auditory pathways decussate in ascension, the result being that your right hand and right ear are dominated by activities of the left hemisphere.

The two hemispheres continually work in concert, being connected via the corpus callosum. Virtually all right-handed individuals have coordination of language function in the left hemisphere, while 30% of left-handers either have their language function in the right hemisphere or have it shared by the two hemispheres. The "dominant hemisphere" for language is the left hemisphere for 90% of the population.

The left hemisphere is specialized for analysis. It takes brief, concise information, analyzes it, categorizes it, and moves on to the next task. It is specialized for processing rapidly changing information (e.g., formant transitions, stop consonant bursts) and information that requires dissection and careful, detailed examination.

In contrast, the right hemisphere is specialized to see the big picture. When presented with a visual image of a group of people sitting in desks, watching a person in front, the right hemisphere will interpret that as a meeting of some sort, and use other cues (chalkboard versus altar) to define the situation as a classroom or church setting. If the left hemisphere were confronted with the same information, it would dutifully list each of the components (person in chair, person at front, desk, chalkboard) but would not identify the situation as a classroom.

The right hemisphere processes emotion much more readily than the left, and that makes sense given the information we use to encode emotion. Intonation contours of speech are long and change relatively slowly, and the right hemisphere processes that very well. Therefore, if you were listening to a person who was depressed and who was speaking slowly with a monotone voice, your right hemisphere would note that something was wrong. The left hemisphere would miss this information entirely, and a person with a lesion of the right hemisphere might be labeled "insensitive" or "apragmatic" because of this deficit. The right hemisphere takes the details of the face (eyes wide open or squinting, mouth in smile or frown, forehead furrowed or eyebrows lifted) and interprets these details as a cohesive unit. The left hemisphere would simply note and list the elements of the face without interpreting their meaning as a group. The right hemisphere can recognize faces, but the left hemisphere is weak in that area because recognition requires putting the various parts of the face together into a "whole" identity.

The right hemisphere also has the significant responsibility of providing alternative definitions. When the left hemisphere is presented with the statement, "One swallow doesn't make a summer," it interprets the sentence literally, without regard to metaphor. It is the right hemisphere's responsibility to provide alternative meanings to words, so the meaning fits the context. A person with right-hemisphere damage may not be able to interpret the saying above as meaning, "one sign of something doesn't mean that thing is present," or the even more abstract warning, "wait until you are sure of something before you act."

How have we come to these conclusions? A large body of work is developing based on studies of people with specific left- or right-hemisphere lesions, and the problems they have help us to understand how the two hemispheres operate. For many years, we assumed the right hemisphere was the linguistic lightweight of the cerebral cortex, but we have come to respect it for its ability to help us gain meaning from context and for its depth of word meaning. The left hemisphere performs very well on tasks of demanding precise knowledge and application of syntax, morphology, and phonology, but falls on its face (figuratively) when confronted with the need to make sense of context.

Summary

- The hemispheres of the brain display clear functional differences.
- The left hemisphere in most individuals is dominant for language and speech, processes brief duration stimuli, and performs detailed analysis.
- The right hemisphere, in contrast, appears to process information in a more holistic fashion, processing spatial and tonal information.
- Face recognition appears to be a right-hemisphere function.

Motor Control of Speech

The production of speech is an extraordinarily complex process. The idea, or cognitive input, for speech arises from the anterior frontal lobe and appears to be encoded linguistically at Broca's area, which is a segment of the premotor region.

Synaptic Pruning

A normal and natural process, called synaptic pruning, involves elimination of synapses that are no longer needed. This pruning, which results in a massive loss of synapses, axons, and neurons, occurs at three significant points in a person's life: prenatally, during childhood, and at puberty. All of these prunings occur as a direct result of experience. You may have heard the statement "use it or lose it." This is the starkest manifestation of it, because literally if you do not use a synapse, you will lose it. This is not bad, mind you, because if you never pruned back on connections in your brain, your thought processes would be overwhelmed by the noise of those residual connections. As it is, the process of learning (experiencing stimuli) causes synapses to increase in strength, and the process of deprivation (not experiencing stimuli) causes synapses to die off. This is an elegant process that supports memory and learning, and keeps our brain from becoming overwhelmed.

Neuroscience has long held that the blood-brain barrier, arising from the protective function of astrocytes, kept the immune system from operating within the brain. Research by Chun and Schatz (1999) has shown that not only are there identity markers for neural tissues (major histocompatibility complex [MHC] markers) within the brain, but it now appears that these MHC markers team up with a molecule (C1q) secreted by neurons to prune synapses that are not needed. Astrocytes secrete thrombospondin to support development of synapses. The C1q marks the synapses as "junk," and macrophages collect and dispose of them.

This synaptic pruning poses some interesting and intriguing questions about neurogenic disorders. It is possible that aberrant C1q function is at the root of demyelinating diseases such as amyotrophic lateral sclerosis or multiple sclerosis. Indeed, individuals who have early signs of Alzheimer's dementia have already lost over half of their synapses, and the C1q molecule is present in overwhelming numbers. Similarly, it is hypothesized that children with autism may have excessive numbers of synapses, as demonstrated by increased cerebral volume. One research group (Belmonte et al., 2004) posited that maternal infection during prenatal development may trigger an immune dysfunction in the brain of the fetus that may later result in inadequate synaptic pruning. One of the long-held observations about autism is the extraordinary response of the individual to sensory overload, and this would be supported by the pruning hypothesis.

The phonological code seems to develop deep to Broca's area in the insula, and the ability to inhibit or initiate speech is regulated by the basal ganglia and supplementary motor area. When the "idea" has been encoded into phonetic elements, the motor plan is developed in the premotor region, and that plan is conveyed to the motor strip for execution.

The premotor region and motor strip receive significant input about body condition from the thalamus, and the plan for execution is examined and modified by the cerebellum so that adequate force can be applied by the muscles to complete the motor act.

Speech is one of the most complex motor acts that we, as humans, engage in, and some of the great minds of our time have taken on the task of explaining how we manage such an enormous task. (See the short discussion of the DIVA model in the box that follows.)

Some components have to be included in any model: a perceptual target, a motor plan, and a feedback system. The target in speech, of course, is the phoneme, and the plan will involve identifying precisely how much to contract each of the muscles involved in respiration, articulation, and phonation to create the target phoneme. Of course, it isn't enough just to contract muscles: The duration of phonemes is a critical component, and, of course, we put a lot of phonemes together to make words!

Feedback is an error-correction system. We listen to what we say and judge how close we were to achieving our goal, and then we correct our production on the next attempt. We pay attention to how it feels when we speak, and alter our production if there is a mismatch between what we expect and what we feel.

Needless to say, the bottom line of all this planning and monitoring is actual production, so the critical element of nerve conduction and muscle contraction composes a great deal of the "execution" component of speech.

Modeling is not just an academic exercise, however. By modeling we can look at how the system can break down and better understand interventions to overcome problems. For instance, I know that auditory feedback is important, but if I lose auditory feedback (lose my hearing) can I compensate for this by using vibrotactile stimulation of my arm to receive feedback of my speech production? These sorts of questions give rise to new and alternative methods of helping people compensate for loss of components of their speech production and perception systems.

To put structures to theory, realize that the motor plan arises in the premotor region of the brain. It is here, specifically in the insular cortex and Broca's area, that the motor plan for phonemes and for the grammatical context is developed. This plan is forwarded to the motor strip (precentral gyrus) for execution. If the plan calls for contraction of the orbicularis oris to purse the lips, for instance, the timing of that contraction will be built into the plan, and the muscles will be contracted according to the timing of that plan.

As the motor plan is being developed, a copy of the plan is sent to the cerebellum, which is responsible for comparing the plan with the current condition of the muscles of the body. So, if the lips are currently retracted, a different amount of force and rate of contraction will be required than if the mouth is wide open. The cerebellum "knows" all about the condition of every muscle, joint, and tendon in the body, and if you plan to make a change in that condition the cerebellum will help you make sure the motor act will achieve the target behavior.

The cerebellum sends its revised motor plan to the cerebral cortex, and execution of muscle contraction can take place. The command for contraction passes from the precentral gyrus by means of upper motor neurons whose axons pass through the internal capsule, and whose output is modified by the subcortical structures of the basal ganglia. These upper motor neurons pass through the brainstem, decussating in the medulla at the pyramidal decussation, and course into the spinal cord, where they terminate at the level of the spinal nerve they are going to activate. That spinal nerve is the "final common pathway" or lower motor neuron, and represents the last neuron in the chain of activation of a muscle. We have ignored the important role that the basal ganglia and the "indirect pathway" can have in maintaining muscle tone and in producing stereotyped repetitive movements, and have neatly sidestepped the fact that sometimes muscles need to be silenced (inhibited) rather than activated in order to successfully complete a task. This is not to say that these are not critically important components, but rather to say that the story of motor activation in speech production is amazingly complex, and worth some very intense study!

Clearly, the execution of speech involves extensive interaction of the areas of the brain in rapid coordination. Humans are amazingly versatile in overcoming obstacles to speech production, which is good news for the speech-language pathology assistant. Try this: Say "Sammy is a friend of mine." Now place your pencil between your molars on one side of your mouth, bite down lightly, and say it again a few times. Were you able to produce intelligible speech? Although the pencil interfered with some dental or labial productions, on the whole you were probably not only intelligible, but accurate. If the program for the individual articulators were "written in stone," you would not have been able to tolerate this aberration (use of a "bite block"), and your speech would have been unintelligible. Through this sort of examination, we realize that we probably develop an internal standard of what we want our speech to sound like, and then we do whatever is necessary to match that standard. Thus, your role as a speech-language pathology assistant could well include helping your client develop that internal standard and take steps to improve his or her communication.

The DIVA Model of Speech Production

Models of speech production must include some forms of feedback about the accuracy of articulation. This feedback may take the form of auditory information (hearing your own production to determine how accurate your attempt at speech was), tactile and kinesthetic feedback (perceiving how accurately your physical target was achieved in articulation), or even feedback from external sources. Guenther, Hampson, and Johnson (1998) and Callan, Kent, Guenther, and Vorperian (2000) proposed the DIVA (Directions Into Velocities of Articulation) model, which utilizes auditory feedback and feedforward as the dominant inputs. The Guenther, Ghosh, and Tourville (2006) model includes both a learning component based upon feedback and a means of allowing the speech system to produce accurate speech without requiring the same level of monitoring that occurs during the learning process. The model is designed to control output commands that represent muscles of speech. The initial input to the system is the auditory model that the articulatory system is supposed to attempt, such as the phoneme /i/. The input /i/ activates "sound map cells" in the modeled premotor cortex, which are themselves modeled after mirror neurons that have been found in the frontal and temporal lobes, and which provide a match-to-model feedback mechanism within the real human brain. Upon activating a sound map cell, an "image" of the sound target is sent to the auditory and somatosensory regions responsible for monitoring accuracy of speech production, representing areas of both the cerebellum and cerebral cortex. The auditory and somatosensory monitoring regions receive input from the cortical planning region as well as real-world input from the auditory mechanism (hearing) and the somatosensory system (tactile and kinesthetic input related to the state of the articulators at a given moment). This input is a reality check for the system itself, and if the command coming from the premotor region results in a distorted acoustic production, the auditory error map will compare the ideal that the premotor region "desired" with the reality that the motor system produced and cause a change in the articulator velocity and position maps. This change will result in the muscles being activated differently on the next trial. If the change in muscle function results in the acoustic signal being closer to the target, another change in the same direction will be made, and the production tried again. Guenther hypothesizes that mirror neurons in the cerebrum may play an important role in the process of learning and maintenance of learned skills. Mirror neurons fire when we perform an action, but they also fire when we see someone else perform the action. They are, in effect, a sort of environmental monitoring system that could be responsible for a number of phenomena, including empathy and motor learning. Guenther's hypothesis is that these neurons may play a role in the match system between the model and the output of the speaker.

Lesions and the Indirect Efferent System

To appreciate the effects of lesions to the indirect motor system, it might help to do a quick exercise: Reach across the desktop to pick up a pencil. As you do this, pay attention to what your muscles are doing. Even as you reach for the pencil, your elbow rotates to accommodate the needs of your arm and hand to make contact with the object. As you get close to the target, your fingers start to close and the rate of movement of your arm slows down. For all of this to happen, your brain must know how fast your muscles are changing length as well as where the target is located in space relative to your hand and body. Contraction of extensors obviously is important, but your brain must also contract flexors to help control extensor contraction lest the movement be ballistic.

Damage to the cerebellum reduces activation of the fusimotor system. Because this system maintains muscle tone through mild, constant muscle contraction, muscles in a person with lesions in the cerebellum lose tone and become flaccid. In contrast, loss of the moderating control by the cerebrum through lesion causes hypertonia in antigravity musculature and extensors because the stretch reflexes are unrestrained.

Lesions and conditions of the basal ganglia have various effects, among them the rigidity of Parkinson's disease. In this condition, intrafusal systems for both extensors and flexors are unrestrained, resulting in simultaneous contraction of antagonists and rigidity. Other basal ganglia lesions result in general hypertonicity.

Impact of Aphasia

The life of an individual with aphasia caused by a stroke is significantly changed by the cerebrovascular event. With the brain lesion comes an instant change in how the individual can interact with his or her environment, with how readily linguistic information can be used to process information and to communicate, and with how easily cognitive processes can be performed.

The individual with left-hemisphere stroke of the frontal lobe faces dysfluency while being very aware of the jumble of verbal output. If the lesion is in the posterior regions, speech will be more fluent but may be "empty" of content, and the person may have difficulty with comprehension, not realizing that his or her speech is not doing what was intended.

It is extremely important that a speech-language pathology assistant enlist the help of a client's family or close friends very early in the process. These significant others will be most able to extend the therapy into every aspect of the person's life, and they will become the individual's most valuable communication partners. Including a partner early in treatment affords the opportunity to move the client back into the world of communication.

SENSATION AND REFLEXES IN MASTICATION AND DEGLUTITION

Natural drives related to hunger bring you to the process of acquiring nutrition, but the food must be palatable for it to be consumed in sufficient quantities to properly nourish you. Further, there must be an adequate neuroanatomical substrate that supports the stages of swallowing. Let us discuss these substrates in turn, and then see how they integrate into the acts of mastication and deglutition.

Sensation Associated with Mastication and Deglutition

Numerous receptors of stimuli are critical for completion of the chewing, sucking, and swallowing (CSS) elements associated with mastication and deglutition. Among these are the gustatory (taste), tactile (touch), temperature (thermal), and pressure senses. Here is a brief discussion of each of these senses as they relate to chewing, sucking and swallowing.

Gustation

Gustation (taste) is a complex and critical component of CSS. Taste drives the desire to continue eating, which fulfills the nutritional requirements of the body. Taste receptors (taste buds, or taste cells) are chemoreceptors in that they respond when specific chemicals come in contact with them. There are five basic tastes: sweet, salty, sour, bitter, and umami. We are familiar with the first four terms, but you may have never run across umami, though you most certainly have tasted it. Umami is the taste of monosodium glutamate, which tastes "meaty," or protein-like. For over a century, we believed that taste receptors were restricted to zones of the tongue, with sweet tastes being sensed at the tip, salty at the sides in front, and sour at the sides in the back. Bitterness was thought to be sensed on the posterior tongue. We know now that all the tastes can be sensed all over the tongue, although there is some truth to the localized preponderance of taste sensors. Taste is mediated by means of three cranial nerves. The facial nerve (CN VII) mediates taste from the anterior two thirds of the tongue, specifically involving sweet, salty, and sour sensations, whereas the glossopharyngeal nerve (CN IX) transmits primarily bitterness information from the posterior one third of the tongue. Taste receptors of the palate are innervated by the facial nerve. Taste receptors of the epiglottis and esophagus are innervated by the vagus nerve (CN X).

Our nutritional needs govern our selection of sweet and umami tastes, as these indicate the presence of carbohydrates (sweet) and protein (umami). Salt is also a necessary mineral, so we "crave" that taste as well. These tastes will elicit salivation, as well as ingestive responses, including tongue protrusion to receive the food, release of insulin, mastication, and deglutition. In contrast, bitter and sour tastes typify poisons, and they will often elicit protective responses that include gagging, coughing, apnea, and salivation (salivation in this case encapsulates the material and protects the oral cavity). Admittedly, we do eat sour and bitter foods, but notice next time you encounter a particularly bitter taste how you find it difficult to swallow, or at least become wary of it! This underscores a critically important point. Tastes can elicit motor responses that may or may not be under volitional (or even conscious) control.

Olfaction

olfaction: *Sense of smell.*

Olfaction (the sense of smell) plays a vital role in appetite and taste. Molecules arising from food pass over olfactory chemoreceptors to increase the strength of the taste perception, a fact to which you can relate if you remember how "flat" your favorite food tasted when you had nasal congestion. In fact, if you tightly occlude your nares and blindly take a bite of apple and then a bite of onion, you will not be able to taste the difference!

Olfactory sensors arise from the olfactory bulb, and cilia protruding from the olfactory sensor transduce the molecular stimulant into the perception of smell that is transmitted to the olfactory bulb located within the cranial space. Information from the receptor is transmitted to the olfactory bulb, which resides within the braincase, and then is transmitted by means of the olfactory tract to the olfactory region of the cortex, which includes the amygdala, the anterior olfactory nucleus, the piriform cortex, the olfactory tubercle, and a portion of the entorhinal cortex. Olfactory sensation arrives at the cerebral cortex through multiple pathways, including the thalamus, and the information serves as a stimulus to emotion and motivation (amygdala), physiological responses (hypothalamus), and memory encoding (hippocampus). The information reaching the orbitofrontal region of the cerebral cortex appears to be involved in olfactory discrimination (i.e., conscious, discriminative processing of smell), and there are even motor responses that are mediated by olfactory stimulation (e.g., salivation, gagging, or even vomiting).

Tactile Sense

The sense of touch is mediated by a number of mechanoreceptors, which are sensors that are sensitive to physical contact. Skin receptors involved in mastication and deglutition are of one of four basic varieties, depending on location and function. Meissner's corpuscles respond to minute mechanical movement in the superficial tissue of the tongue, while Merkel disk receptors transmit the sense of pressure in the superficial region. Pacinian corpuscles are deeply embedded in the tongue and respond to rapid deep pressure to the outer epithelium. Ruffini endings sense stretch within the deep tissues and are critical to our perception of the shape of objects perceived by touch. Vibration sense is a subclass of tactile sense, and may be considered as either deep or superficial pressure, depending on the amplitude of the vibration.

Thermal Receptors

Four classes of thermal stimulation are differentiated by human senses: warm, hot, cool, and cold. Thermal receptors are actually the same as pain sensors, in that they are bare nerve endings. Although it is convenient to group pain and thermal sense, the reality is that thermal sensors are functionally different from pain sensors, with different nerve endings responding to these two broad classes of stimulation.

Pain Sense (Nociception)

Nociceptors (pain sensors) respond directly to a noxious stimulus (e.g., chemical burn), to noxious molecules released by injured tissue (such as positive potassium ions, serotonin, and acetylcholine), to acidity caused by injury, or to direct contact with a traumatic source. Some nociceptors respond to mechanical trauma, whereas others respond to thermal stimulation. Most nociceptors respond to general destruction of tissue rather than to the specific quality of a stimulus, and the perception arising from the stimulation of these receptors (termed polymodal nociceptors) is a burning sensation.

Muscle Stretch and Tension Sense

Muscle stretch is sensed by muscle spindle fibers, which are found predominantly in larger muscles, such as the antigravity muscles of the legs, but are also found within oral musculature. The mandibular elevators (masseter, temporalis, and lateral and medial pterygoid muscles) are richly endowed with stretch receptors, as are the deep tongue fibers of the genioglossus and the palatoglossus muscles. Muscle spindle fibers return a muscle to its original position following passive stretching. As an example, if you were to pull sharply down on your relaxed mandible, the mandible would quickly elevate thereafter, to the point that your teeth might make contact. This sensor system is designed to maintain a muscle at a preset length, so that the monitored muscle group contracts in response to passive stretching. The spindle function is normally inhibited during active contraction, although damage to the upper motor neuron can cause hyperactive stretch reflexes and spasticity. Muscle tension is sensed by Golgi tendon organs (GTOs), found within the tendons and fascia. These organs respond to the active contraction of muscles and serve to inhibit the muscle spindle fibers. Muscle tone is regulated partially through the interaction of muscle spindles and GTOs. Muscle tone refers to the perception of resistance to the passive movement of stretching.

Salivation Response

Salivation is the product of three major glands: the parotid, submandibular, and sublingual. In addition, mucus-secreting accessory salivary glands are present throughout the oral cavity, embedded within the mucosa. These glands are activated by the stimulation of taste receptors (the anterior two thirds of the tongue), mediated by the facial nerve (sublingual and submandibular glands) and glossopharyngeal nerve (parotid gland). The submandibular gland is found behind the free margin of the mylohyoid muscle, between the mylohyoid muscle and the submandibular fossa of the inner mandible. It extends as far posteriorly as the second molar and extends forward as the submandibular duct to open just lateral to the lingual frenulum. The sublingual gland is above the mylohyoid muscle and empties into the mouth through ducts within the sublingual fold. The parotid gland is located posterior to the mandibular ramus and superior to the sternocleidomastoid muscle, and secretions from it empty into the pharynx.

Summary

- Gustation (taste) is mediated by chemoreceptors that transmit information to the brain via the glossopharyngeal, vagus, and facial nerves. Taste sensors are specialized for sweet, sour, salty, bitter, and umami sense.
- Olfaction (the sense of smell) is mediated by chemoreceptors within the nasal mucosa.
- The sense of touch (tactile sense) is mediated by means of mechanoreceptors that respond to deep or shallow touch.
- Four classes of thermal stimulation are differentiated by human senses: warm, hot, cool, and cold.
- Pain sense (nociception) is a response to a noxious stimulus.
- Muscle stretch is sensed by muscle spindle fibers, and muscle tension is sensed by Golgi tendon organs (GTOs), found within tendons and fascia.

- Tactile sense, thermal sense, pain sense, and joint and tendon sense of the face and oral cavity are mediated by the trigeminal, glossopharyngeal, and vagus nerves.
- Salivation occurs because of the stimulation of salivary glands.
- The type of saliva varies between glands. The sublingual gland produces thick mucus secretions, the submandibular gland produces both thin serous and mucus secretions, and the parotid gland secretes only serous saliva.

Reflexes in Mastication and Deglutition

The individual reflex circuits associated with mastication and deglutition are the building blocks for the normal processes associated with the intake of food and drink. These reflexes are mediated at the level of the brainstem and do not require cortical involvement. We have included expulsive reflexes here as well (gag, retch) because of their close association with the systems of mastication and deglutition.

Chewing Reflex

Chewing is a complex reflex that can be triggered by deep pressure on the roof of the mouth, as when you bite a cracker. It involves alternating left-side and right-side contraction of the muscles of mandibular elevation (masseter and medial pterygoid muscles), such that a rotatory motion of the mandible is produced. The alternating contraction of these mandibular elevators is interspersed with the depression of the mandible, which allows the lingual musculature to move the bolus onto and off the molars. The chewing center is located within the midbrain. This center is also involved in the reflexive movements of the tongue for sucking and licking (Baehr & Frotscher, 2012).

Rooting and Sucking Reflexes

The rooting and sucking reflexes—very functional for neonates and infants—rely on tactile stimulation of the perioral region. Lightly stroking the lips or cheek on one side will cause the infant's mouth to open and its head to turn toward the stimulus; this is termed the *rooting reflex*. Light contact within the inner margin of the lips will initiate a sucking response, which involves generating a labial seal (contraction of the upper and lower orbicularis oris), and alternatively protruding and retracting the tongue. Tactile stimulation of the perioral region is mediated by the trigeminal nerve (CN V), and central mediation of sucking is within the midbrain reticular formation.

Uvular (Palatal) Reflex

Uvular elevation occurs in response to excitation of the glossopharyngeal nerve (CN IX) through tactile stimulation in the posterior mouth, particularly on the posterior tongue or fauces.

Gag (Pharyngeal) Reflex

The gag reflex is elicited by tactile stimulation of the faucial pillars, posterior pharyngeal wall, or posterior tongue near the lingual tonsils, which is mediated by the glossopharyngeal nerve. Connection with the vagus nerve via interneurons activates abdominal muscles and muscles of the velum and pharynx, causing the soft palate to elevate and the pharynx to elevate and constrict.

Retch and Vomit Reflex

Retching is an involuntary attempt at vomiting. Vomiting refers to the oral expulsion of gastrointestinal contents. The retching reflex is a complex response mediated by noxious smells (olfactory), tastes (glossopharyngeal), gastrointestinal distress (vagus), vestibular dysfunction (vestibulocochlear), or even a distressing visual or mental stimulation. Stimulation by one or more of these sensory systems, apparently, activates a retching center located near the swallow center in the reticular formation of the medulla oblongata, near the motor nuclei associated with the complex of responses associated with vomiting. The vomit response includes multiple simultaneous or synchronous reflexes, including occlusion of the airway by vocal fold adduction, extreme contraction of abdominal muscles, relaxation of the upper and lower esophageal sphincters, elevation of the larynx and velum, depression of the epiglottis, elevation of the pharynx, and tongue protrusion.

Cough Reflex

The cough reflex is typically initiated by noxious stimulation of the pharynx, larynx, or bronchial passageway. The sensory portion of the vagus nerve transmits information concerning this stimulation to the nucleus solitarius of the medulla. Interneurons activate the expiration center of the medullary reticular formation, which causes the abdominal muscles to contract. The nucleus ambiguus, the motor nucleus of the vagus nerve, causes laryngeal adduction before exhalation, permitting sufficient subglottal pressure to be generated to dislodge the irritating substance from the airway.

Pain Reflex

Although not technically a reflex associated with mastication or deglutition, the pain withdrawal reflex can have an effect on mastication and swallowing. You may remember the unpleasant sensation of having a lesion on your tongue or oral mucosa. When you masticate, you become very aware of the area and tend to avoid it if possible. This response represents a conscious version of the withdrawal response, a natural response to noxious stimuli. The classic withdrawal reflex involves rapid, total removal of a limb from a noxious stimulus, such as removing your hand from a hot stove. Oral and pharyngeal pain responses include the removal of noxious bolus (spicy or excessively hot food), either by expectoration or by swallowing.

Respiration Reflexes

Respiration occurs reflexively but can be voluntarily controlled to a degree. A sensor system near the carotid sinus (the carotid body) responds to the quantity of oxygen and carbon dioxide in the blood, as well as to blood acidity. When oxygen levels decline below a specific criterion level, or when carbon dioxide or acidity increases beyond a specific level, a signal mediated by the glossopharyngeal nerve via the nucleus solitarius is relayed to the respiratory center, which increases the respiration rate. There are individual inspiratory and expiratory centers: excitation of inspiration inhibits expiratory musculature, and vice versa. The two respiratory centers are located in the lower medulla (the inspiratory and expiratory controls are separate).

Summary

- Chewing, sucking, and swallowing (CSS) are the products of numerous individual reflex patterns executed in a synchronous sequence.
- The chewing reflex involves rotatory movement of the mandible, coordinated with movement of the bolus by the tongue.
- The rooting reflex involves orientation to light tactile stimulation of the cheek area, which causes the infant's head to turn toward the stimulus.
- The sucking reflex is elicited by soft contact with the inner margin of the lips, causing protrusion and retraction of the tongue, as well as closing of the lips.
- Uvular elevation occurs in response to the tactile stimulation of faucial pillars, lingual tonsils, or upper pharynx.
- The gag reflex is elicited by the tactile stimulation of faucial pillars, posterior faucial wall, or posterior tongue near the lingual tonsils. It results in the termination of respiration and elevation of the larynx.
- The retching and vomiting reflexes are complex responses that are similar to the gag.

- The cough reflex involves laryngeal adduction, abdominal contraction to develop increased subglottal pressure, and forceful exhalation.
- The pain withdrawal reflex causes withdrawal from a noxious stimulus.
- Respiration occurs because of inadequate oxygenation of or excessive carbon dioxide in the blood or blood acidity.

CHAPTER SUMMARY

The nervous system is a complex, hierarchical structure. Voluntary movement, sensory awareness, and cognitive function are the domain of the cerebral cortex. The communication links of the nervous system are spinal nerves, cranial nerves, and tracts of the brainstem and spinal cord. Several organizational schemes characterize the nervous system. It can be divided functionally into the autonomic and somatic nervous systems. The nervous system can also be divided anatomically into the central and peripheral nervous systems. Neurons communicate through synapses by means of neurotransmitter substances. Effects on the receiving neurons are excitatory or inhibitory. Glial cells provide the fatty sheath for myelinated axons, as well as support structure for neurons.

The cerebral cortex is protected from physical insult by cerebrospinal fluid and the meningeal linings—the dura, pia, and arachnoid maters.

The cerebrum is divided into two hemispheres connected by the corpus callosum. The gyri and sulci of the hemisphere provide important landmarks for lobes and other regions of the cerebrum. The temporal lobe is the site of auditory reception. The frontal lobe is responsible for most voluntary motor activation and is the site of the important speech region known as Broca's area. The parietal lobe is the region of somatic sensory reception. The occipital lobe is the site of visual input to the cerebrum. The insular lobe lies deep in the lateral sulcus and is revealed by deflecting the temporal lobe. The operculum overlies the insula. The functionally defined limbic system includes the cingulate gyrus, uncus, parahippocampal gyrus, and other deep structures.

The basal ganglia are subcortical structures involved in control of movement, and the hippocampal formation of the inferior temporal lobe is deeply implicated in memory function. The thalamus of the diencephalon is the final relay for somatic sensation directed toward the cerebrum and other diencephalic structures. The hypothalamus controls many bodily functions and desires. The regions of the cerebral cortex are interconnected by means of a complex network of projection fibers, connecting the cortex with other structures; association fibers, which connect regions of the same hemisphere; and commissural fibers, which provide communication between corresponding regions of the two hemispheres.

The anterior cerebral arteries serve the medial surfaces of the brain, and the middle cerebral artery serves the lateral cortex, including the temporal lobe, motor strip, Wernicke's area, and much of the parietal lobe. The vertebral arteries branch to form the anterior and posterior spinal arteries, with ascending components serving the ventral brainstem. The basilar artery gives rise to the superior and anterior inferior cerebellar arteries to serve the cerebellum, while the posterior inferior cerebellar artery arises from the vertebral artery. The basilar artery divides to become the posterior cerebral arteries, serving the inferior temporal and occipital lobes, upper midbrain, and diencephalon. The circle of Willis is a series of communicating arteries that provide redundant pathways for blood flow to regions of the cerebral cortex, equalizing pressure and flow rate of blood.

The cerebellum coordinates motor and sensory information, communicating with the brainstem, cerebrum, and spinal cord. It communicates with the rest of the nervous system via the superior, middle, and inferior cerebral peduncles. Position in space, adjustment against gravity, and fine motor adjustments are mediated by the cerebellum. The superior cerebellar peduncle enters the pons and serves the dentate nucleus, red nucleus, and thalamus.

The brainstem is divided into medulla, pons, and midbrain. It is more highly organized than the spinal cord and mediates higher-level body functions such as vestibular responses. The pyramidal decussation of the medulla is the point at which the motor commands originating in one hemisphere of the cerebral cortex cross to serve the opposite side of the body. The reticular formation is a phylogenetically old set of nuclei essential for life function. The pons and midbrain set the stage for communication with the higher levels of the brain, including the cerebellum and cerebrum. This communication link permits not only complex motor acts, but also consciousness, awareness, and volitional acts.

Cranial nerves mediate articulatory, phonatory, and auditory functions. Cranial nerves are sensory, motor, or mixed sensorimotor, and are categorized based on function as general or specialized and as serving visceral or somatic organs or structures. Cranial nerve V, the trigeminal nerve, innervates muscles of mastication and the tensor veli palatini, and it communicates sensation from the face, mouth, teeth, mucosal lining, and tongue. The facial nerve (cranial nerve VII) innervates muscles of facial expression, and the sensory component serves taste of the anterior two thirds of the tongue. The vestibulocochlear nerve (cranial nerve VIII) mediates auditory and vestibular sensation. The glossopharyngeal nerve (IX) serves the posterior tongue taste receptors, as well as somatic sense from the tongue, fauces, pharynx, and eustachian tube. The stylopharyngeus and superior pharyngeal constrictor muscles receive motor innervation via this nerve. The vagus nerve (X) serves autonomic and somatic functions, mediating pain, touch, and temperature from the eardrum and pain from the pharynx, larynx, and esophagus. The recurrent laryngeal nerve and superior laryngeal nerves supply motor innervation for the intrinsic muscles of the larynx. The accessory nerve (XI) innervates the sternocleidomastoid and trapezius muscles, and it collaborates with the vagus nerve in activation of palatal, laryngeal, and pharyngeal muscles. The hypoglossal nerve (XII) innervates the muscles of the tongue with the exception of the palatoglossus.

Communication between neurons of the nervous system occurs at the synapse, and neurotransmitter passing through the synaptic cleft either excites or inhibits the postsynaptic neuron. When a neuron is sufficiently stimulated, an action potential is generated, which causes membrane depolarization and exchange of ions between the extracellular and intracellular spaces. Ion movement results in a change in voltage across the membrane. Resting membrane potential is the relatively stable state of the neuron at rest, whereas the absolute refractory period after excitation is an interval during which the neuron cannot be excited to fire. Neurons are capable of representing differences in input only through rate of response. Myelinated fibers conduct the wave of depolarization more rapidly than demyelinated fibers, primarily due to saltatory conduction.

Higher function of the brain defies a strict localization approach to functional organization. Brain function is classified into regions of primary, higher-order, and association regions. Primary sensory and motor regions include the primary reception area for somatic sense, primary motor area, primary auditory cortex, and primary region of visual reception. Higher-order areas of processing are apparently responsible for extracting features of the stimulus. Association areas are the regions of highest cognitive processing, integrating sensory information with memory. The prefrontal area appears to be involved in higher function related to motor output, and the temporal-occipital-parietal association is involved in spoken and written language function. The limbic association area integrates information relating to affect, motivation, and emotion.

The hemispheres of the brain display clear functional differences. Language and speech, brief duration stimuli, and detailed information are processed in the left hemisphere in most individuals. The right hemisphere appears to process information in a more holistic fashion, preferring spatial and tonal information.

Movement is initiated at the motor strip, but there is a great deal of planning that occurs prior to that point. The premotor regions, including Broca's area, are involved in planning for the motor act, and project that plan to the motor strip. The prefrontal association area also provides input to the motor strip concerning higher cognitive elements of the speech act, and the lowest levels of information (information about muscle stretch and tension) are also fed to the motor strip.

Sensation is mediated by stimulus-specific sensors, including mechanical and chemical, to name two. Taste and smell are mediated by chemosensors, while perception of touch, pressure, and movement on the surface of the body are mediated by mechanoceptors. Stretch receptors monitor muscle length, and Golgi tendon organs control muscle tension. Nociceptors alert us to painful stimuli.

Reflexes are "hard-wired" responses to stimuli in the environment. The chewing reflex is stimulated by pressure on the hard palate, while the gag, retch, and vomit reflexes are stimulated by a number of noxious stimuli, particularly in the posterior mouth and superior pharynx. The pharyngeal reflex is involved in movement of the bolus through the pharyngeal stage of swallowing, and involves many of the protective gestures associated with the gag, retch, and vomit reflexes.

A Story with a Happy Ending

Here is a story of aneurysm and hemorrhage that has a happy ending. While at a public event one Saturday a dear friend (S) developed a debilitating headache. When her headache didn't improve after an hour of nursing it in the cab of her truck, her husband began the long drive home. Her husband wisely decided that a stop by the local hospital was in order, and the emergency physician suggested magnetic resonance imaging (MRI) to help determine the source of the pain. As the MRI was activated, S became unconscious.

As we later learned, S had a history of aneurysms in her family and had been examined frequently to ensure that there were no surprises in her future. Despite these precautions, an aneurysm had developed at the base of her brain and hemorrhaged as the MRI was activated. A Life-Flight helicopter took her to a metropolitan center that specialized in management of hemorrhage, and friends and family watched anxiously as S slowly became aware of her surroundings. To everyone's great joy and relief her recovery was remarkably complete so that she was able to return to her life and work unencumbered. The quick action of the emergency room medical team and the stroke unit at the receiving hospital gave S the chance to be called the "miracle woman" by all who know her.

We should mention here that those of you entering the field of speech-language pathology will have the opportunity to work with people who have had these types of cerebrovascular accidents, and to help them overcome the effects, which can include aphasia (acquired language disorder), dysarthria (motor speech disorder), and cognitive impairments (deficits in cognitive function), to name a few.

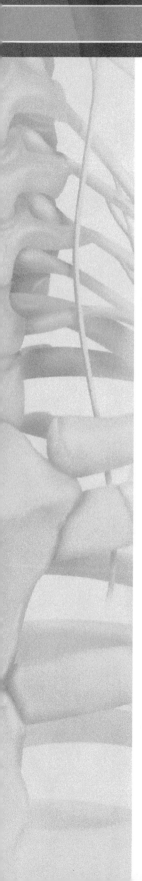

STUDY QUESTIONS

1. The _____ governs voluntary actions.

2. The _____ is responsible for coordinating movement.

3. _____ are groups of cell bodies in the PNS with functional unity.

4. The _____ system includes the cerebrum, cerebellum, subcortical structures, brainstem, and spinal cord.

5. The _____ system consists of the 12 pairs of cranial nerves and 31 pairs of spinal nerves, as well as the sensory receptors.

6. The _____ system governs involuntary activities of involuntary muscles.

7. The _____ system governs voluntary activities.

8. Information directed toward the brain is termed _____ and information directed from the brain is termed _____.

9. On the accompanying figure identify the indicated parts of the neuron.

A. _____

B. _____

C. _____

D. _____

E. _____

F. _____

G. _____

H. _____

I. _____

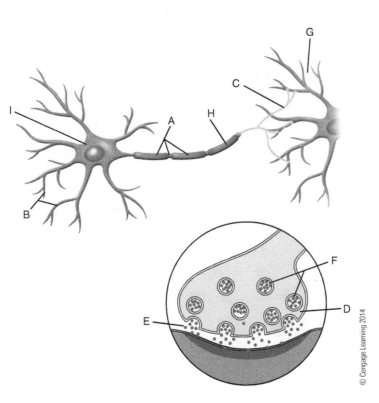

© Cengage Learning 2014

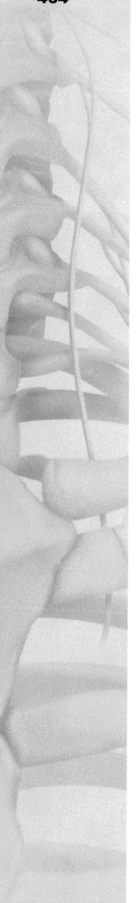

10. On the accompanying figure identify the indicated parts of the cerebrum.

A. _____ lobe

B. _____ lobe

C. _____ lobe

D. _____ lobe

E. _____ gyrus

F. _____ gyrus

G. _____ sulcus

H. _____ sulcus

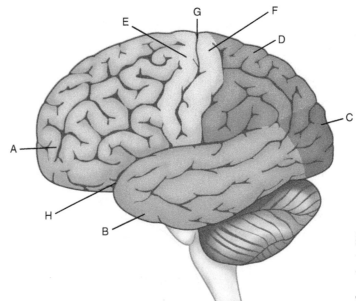

11. On the accompanying figure identify the parts of the surface of the
    cerebrum.

A. _____ gyrus

B. _____

C. _____ gyrus

D. _____ area

E. _____ area

F. _____ gyrus

G. _____ gyrus

H. _____ sulcus

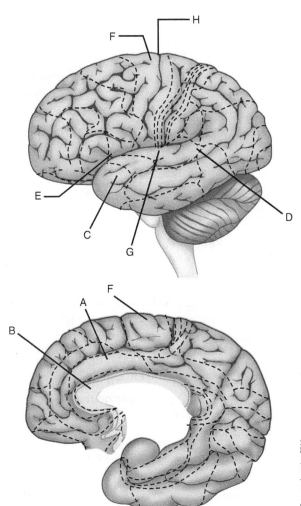

12. On the accompanying figure identify the indicated arteries and structures.

A. _____ artery

B. _____ artery

C. _____ artery

D. _____ artery

E. _____ artery

F. _____ artery

G. _____ artery

H. _____ artery

I. _____

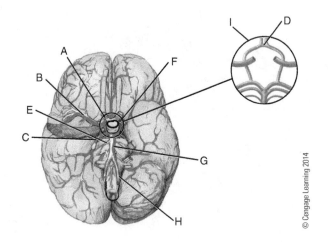

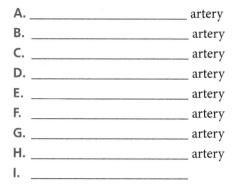

© Cengage Learning 2014

13. _____is a change in electrical potential that occurs when a cell membrane is stimulated adequately to permit ion exchange between intracellular and extracellular spaces.

14. The _____ period is the time during which the cell membrane cannot be stimulated to depolarize.

15. The _____ is a period during which the cell membrane can be stimulated to excitation again, but only with greater than typical stimulation.

16. The _____ of the axon myelin promote saltatory conduction.

17. The substance known as _____ is discharged into the synaptic cleft, stimulating the postsynaptic neuron.

18. Higher cognitive processing occurs generally in _____ areas.

19. The _____ area is involved in language function.

20. The _____ area of the cerebrum appears to be involved in higher function related to motor output (such as inhibition of motor function and the ability to change motor responses), whereas the temporal-occipital-parietal association area is involved in language function.

21. The _____ area integrates information relating to affect, motivation, and emotion.

22. The _____ hemisphere in most individuals is dominant for language and speech, processes brief duration stimuli, and performs detailed analysis.

23. The _____ hemisphere appears to process information in a more holistic fashion, preferring spatial and tonal information.

24. The _____ reflex is involved in mastication of the food bolus.

25. The _____ (type of sensor) is involved in monitoring muscle length.

26. Chemosensors are involved in the senses of _____ and _____.

REFERENCES

Akshoomoff, N. A., & Courchesne, E. (1992). A new role for the cerebellum in cognitive operations. *Behavioral Neuroscience, 106*(5), 731–738.

Albom, M. (1997). *Tuesdays with Morrie.* New York: Broadway Books.

Amaral, D., & Lavenex, P. (2007). Hippocampal anatomy. In P. Andersen, R. Morris, D. Amaral, et al. (Eds.), *The hippocampus book* (pp. 37–114). New York: Oxford University Press.

Andersen, P., Morris, R., Amaral, D., et al. (2007). The hippocampal formation. In P. Anderson, R. Morris, D. Amaral, et al. (Eds.), *The hippocampus book* (pp. 3–6). New York: Oxford University Press.

Bach, P., Peelen, M. V., & Tipper, S. P. (2010). On the role of object information in action observation: An fMRI study. *Cerebral Cortex, 20*(12), 2798–2809.

Baehr, M. & Frotscher, M. (2012). *Duus' topical diagnosis in neurology: Anatomy, physiology, signs and symptoms.* New York: Thieme.

Basha, M. R., Wei, W., Bakheet, S. A., Benitez, N., Siddiqi, H. K., Ge, Y. W., Lahiri, D. K., & Zawia, N. H. (2005). The fetal basis of amyloidogenesis: exposure to lead and latent overexpression of amyloid precursor protein and-amyloid in the aging brain. *Journal of Neuroscience, 25*, 823– 829.

Bateman, H. E., & Mason, R. M. (1984). *Applied anatomy and physiology of the speech and hearing mechanism.* Springfield, IL: Charles C. Thomas.

Bear, M. F., Connors, B. W., & Paradiso, M. A. (1996). *Neuroscience: Exploring the brain.* Baltimore: Williams & Wilkins.

Belmonte, M. K., Allen, G., Beckel-Mitchener, A., Boulanger, L. M., Carper, R. A., & Webb, S. J. (2004). Autism and abnormal development of brain connectivity. *Journal of Neuroscience, 24,* 9228–9231.

Bhatnagar, S. C., & Andy, O. J. (2002). *Neuroscience for the study of communicative disorders* (2nd ed.). Baltimore: Williams & Wilkins.

Bly, L. (1994). *Motor skills acquisition in the first year.* Tucson, AZ: Therapy Skill Builders.

Bowman, J. P. (1971). *The muscle spindle and neural control of the tongue.* Springfield, IL: Charles C. Thomas.

Callan, D. E., Kent, R. D., Gunther, F. H., & Vorperian, H. K. (2000). An auditory-feedback-based neural network model of speech production that is robust to developmental changes in the size and shape of the articulatory system. *Journal of Speech, Language & Hearing Research, 43*(3), 721–736.

Carpenter, M. B. (1991). *Core text of neuroanatomy* (4th ed.). Baltimore: Williams & Wilkins.

Chun, J., & Schatz, D.G. (1999). Rearranging views on neurogenesis: Neuronal death in the absence of DNA end-joining proteins. *Neuron, 22,* 7–10.

Church, J. A., Coalson, R. S., Lugar, H. M., et al. (2008). A developmental fMRI study of reading and repetition reveals changes in phonological and visual mechanisms over age. *Cerebral Cortex, 18,* 2054–2065.

Chusid, J. G. (1985). *Correlative neuroanatomy and functional neurology* (17th ed.). Los Altos, CA: Lange Medical Publications.

Cotman, C. W., & McGaugh, J. L. (1980). *Behavioral neuroscience.* New York: Academic.

Darley, F. L., Aronson, A. E., & Brown, J. R. (1975). *Motor speech disorders.* Philadelphia: Saunders.

Edvinsson, L., & Krause, D. N. (2002). *Cerebral blood flow and metabolism.* Philadelphia: Williams & Wilkins.

Farrer, C., Frey, S. H., Van Horn, J. D., et al. (2007). The angular gyrus computes action awareness representations. *Cerebral Cortex, 18,* 254–261.

Ffytch, D. H. (2005). Perisylvian language networks of the human brain. *Annals of Neurology, 57,* 8–16.

Fields, D. (2004, April). The other half of the brain. *Scientific American,* 53–61.

Filskov, S. B., & Boll, T. J. (1981). *Handbook of clinical neuropsychology.* New York: Wiley.

Fiorentino, M. R. (1973). *Reflex testing methods for evaluating CNS development.* Springfield, IL: Charles C. Thomas.

Flege, J. E. (1988). Anticipatory and carry-over nasal coarticulation in the speech of children and adults. *Journal of Speech and Hearing Research, 31,* 525–536.

Fuller, G. N., & Burger, P. C. (1990). Nervus terminalis (cranial nerve zero) in the adult human. *Clinical Neuropathology, 9*(6), 279–283.

Ganong, W. F. (2003). *Review of medical physiology* (21st ed.). New York: McGraw-Hill/ Appleton & Lange.

Gelfand, S. A. (2001). *Essentials of audiology* (2nd ed.). New York: Thieme Medical.

Guenther, F. H., Ghosh, S. S., & Tourville, J. A. (2006). Neural modeling and imaging of the cortical interactions underlying syllable production. *Brain & Language, 96,* 280–301.

Guenther, F. H., Hampson, M., and Johnson, D. (1998). A theoretical investigation of reference frames for the planning of speech movements. *Psychological Review, 105,* 611–633.

Kandel, E. R. (1991). Brain and behavior. In E. R. Kandel, J. R. Schwartz, & T. M. Jessell (Eds.), *Principles of neural science* (3rd ed.), pp. 9–48. Norwalk, CT: Appleton & Lange.

Kandel, E. R., Schwartz, J. H., & Jessell, T. M. (2000). *Principles of neural science* (4th ed.). New York: McGraw Hill.

Kaufman, D. M. (2000). *Clinical neurology for psychiatrists* (5th ed.). Philadelphia: W. B. Saunders.

Kuehn, D. P., Lemme, M. L., & Baumgartner, J. M. (1991). *Neural bases of speech, hearing, and language.* Boston: Little, Brown.

MacKay, L. E., Chapman, P. E., & Morgan, A. S. (1997). *Maximizing brain injury recovery.* Gaithersburg, MD: Aspen.

McMinn, R. M. H., Hutchings, R. T., & Logan, B. M. (1994). *Color atlas of head and neck anatomy.* London: Mosby-Wolfe.

Moore, K. L. (1988). *The developing human.* Philadelphia: W. B. Saunders.

Netsell, R. (1986). A neurobiologic view of speech production and the dysarthrias. San Diego: College-Hill.

Netter, F. H. (1983a). *The CIBA collection of medical illustrations* (Vol. 1). *Nervous system.* Part I. *Anatomy and physiology.* West Caldwell, NJ: CIBA Pharmaceutical Company.

Netter, F. H. (1983b). *The CIBA collection of medical illustrations* (Vol. 1). *Nervous system.* Part II. *Neurologic and neuromuscular disorders.* West Caldwell, NJ: CIBA Pharmaceutical Company.

Netter, F. H. (1997). *Atlas of human anatomy.* Los Angeles: Icon Learning Systems.

Noback, C. R., Demarest, R. J., & Strominger, N. L. (1991). *The nervous system: Introduction and review.* Philadelphia: Williams & Wilkins.

Nolte, J. (2002). *The human brain* (5th ed.). St. Louis: Mosby.

Parker, J., Mitchell. A., Kalpakidou, A., et al. (2008). Cerebellar growth and behavioural and neuropsychological outcome in preterm adolescents. *Brain, 131*(5), 1344–1351.

Poritsky, R. (1992). *Neuroanatomy: A functional atlas of parts and pathways.* St. Louis: Mosby-Year Book.

Rohen, J. W., & Yokochi, C. (1993). *Color atlas of anatomy.* New York: Igaku-Shoin.

Spirduso, W. W. (1995). *Physical dimensions of aging.* Champaign, IL: Human Kinetics.

Saper CB, Iverson S, Frackowiak R. Integration of sensory and motor system. In: Kandel ER, Schwartz JH, Jessel TM, editors. *Principles of neural science.* New York: McGraw Hill; 2000. p. 350.

Sugiura, L., Ojima, S., Matsuba-Kurita, H., et al. (2011). Sound to language: Different cortical processing of the first and second language in elementary school children as revealed by a large scale study using fNIRS. *Cerebral Cortex, 21*(10), 2374–2393.

Tsao, D. Y., Freiwald, W. A., Tootell, R. B. H., & Livingstone, M. S. (2006). A cortical region consisting entirely of face-selective cells. *Science, 311,* 670–674.

Twietmeyer, A., & McCracken, T. D. (1992). *Coloring guide to regional human anatomy* (2nd ed.). Philadelphia: Lea & Febiger.

Whitlock, K. E. (2004). Development of the nervus terminalis: Origin and migration. *Microscopic Research Techniques, 65*(1–2), 2–12.

Winans, S. S., Gilman, S., Manter, J. T., & Gatz, A. J. (2002). *Manter and Gatz's essentials of clinical neuroanatomy and neurophysiology* (10th ed.). Philadelphia: Davis.

Wood, P. J., & Criss, W. R. (1975). *Normal and abnormal development of the human nervous system.* Hagerstown, MD: Harper & Row.

Yost, W. A. (2000). *Fundamentals of hearing: An introduction* (4th ed). New York: Academic.

Zemlin, W. R. (1998). *Speech and hearing science. Anatomy and physiology* (4th ed.). Needham Heights, MA: Allyn & Bacon.

Appendix

STUDY QUESTION ANSWERS

CHAPTER 1

1. ANATOMY is the study of the structure of an organism.
2. PHYSIOLOGY is the study of the function of a living organism and its parts.
3. CLINICAL, or APPLIED, anatomy is anatomical study for diagnosis and treatment of disease.
4. SYSTEMIC ANATOMY is involved in the description of individual parts of the body without reference to disease, viewing the body as a composite of systems that function together.
5. Skin and mucous membrane are made up of EPITHELIAL tissue.
6. CARTILAGE is a particularly important connective tissue because it is both strong and elastic.
7. MUSCLE is contractile tissue.
8. LIGAMENTS bind organs together or hold bones to bone or cartilage.
9. FASCIA is a sheetlike membrane surrounding organs.
10. TENDONS attach muscle to bone or to cartilage.
11. The relatively immobile point of attachment of a muscle is the ORIGIN.
12. The relatively mobile point of attachment of a muscle is the INSERTION.
13. Identify the systems from their definitions:
    a. MUSCULAR SYSTEM This system includes smooth, striated, and cardiac muscles of the body.
    b. SKELETAL SYSTEM This system includes the bones and cartilages that form the structure of the body.
    c. RESPIRATORY SYSTEM This system includes the passageways and tissues involved in gas exchange with the environment, including the oral, nasal, and pharyngeal cavities, the trachea and bronchial passageway, and the lungs.

d. DIGESTIVE SYSTEM This system includes the esophagus, liver, intestines, and associated glands.
    e. NERVOUS SYSTEM This system includes the nerve tissue and structures of the central and peripheral nervous systems.

14. Identify the systems of speech from their definitions:
    a. RESPIRATORY SYSTEM This system includes the passageways and tissues involved in gas exchange with the environment, including the oral, nasal, and pharyngeal cavities, the trachea and bronchial passageway, and the lungs.
    b. PHONATORY SYSTEM This system is involved in production of voiced sound and uses components of the respiratory system (the laryngeal structures).
    c. ARTICULATORY SYSTEM This system is the combination of structures used to alter the sounds of speech, including parts of the anatomically defined digestive and respiratory systems (the tongue, lips, teeth, soft palate, etc.).
    d. RESONATORY SYSTEM This system includes the nasal cavity and soft palate and portions of the anatomically defined respiratory and digestive systems.

15. On the figure, identify the descriptive terms indicated.
    a. TRANSVERSE plane
    b. SAGITTAL plane
    c. CORONAL, or FRONTAL, plane
    d. ANTERIOR, or VENTRAL, aspect
    e. POSTERIOR, or DORSAL, aspect
    f. ABDUCT (movement away from midline)
    g. ADDUCT (movement toward midline)
    h. DISTAL (located away from midline)
    i. MEDIAL (located near midline)
    j. LATERAL (related to the side)
    k. SUPERIOR (above)
    l. INFERIOR (below)

16. Pathology is the study of diseased tissue. By extension, a speech-language pathologist is one who studies the "pathology" of our field, communication disorders.

CHAPTER 2

1. PRESSURE is defined as force distributed over area.

2. NEGATIVE pressure causes air to enter the container until the pressure is equalized.

3. How many of each of the following vertebrae are there?

   7 cervical vertebrae

   12 thoracic vertebrae

   5 lumbar vertebrae

   5 sacral vertebrae (fused)

4. On the figure, identify the indicated landmarks.
   a. SPINOUS process
   b. TRANSVERSE process
   c. CORPUS
   d. SUPERIOR ARTICULAR facet
   e. INFERIOR COSTAL facet
   f. SUPERIOR COSTAL facet
   g. VERTEBRAL foramen

5. The SPINAL CORD passes through the vertebral foramen.

6. On the figure, identify the indicated landmarks.
   a. ILIUM
   b. ISCHIUM
   c. PUBIC BONE
   d. SACRUM
   e. ILIAC CREST
   f. PUBIC SYMPHYSIS
   g. COCCYX
   h. CLAVICLE
   i. SCAPULA
   j. MANUBRIUM STERNI
   k. XIPHOID or ENSIFORM PROCESS
   l. CORPUS STERNI
   m. STERNAL NOTCH

7. On the figure, identify the indicated landmarks.
   a. TRACHEA
   b. MAINSTEM BRONCHUS
   c. SECONDARY BRONCHUS
   d. TERTIARY BRONCHUS

8. On the figure, identify the indicated muscles and structures.
   a. EXTERNAL OBLIQUE ABDOMINIS
   b. INTERNAL OBLIQUE ABDOMINIS
   c. RECTUS ABDOMINIS
   d. TRANSVERSUS ABDOMINIS
   e. LINEA ALBA
   f. INGUINAL LIGAMENT
   g. LINEA SEMILUNARIS

9. On the figure, identify the indicated muscles.
   a. SERRATUS POSTERIOR SUPERIOR
   b. LEVATOR COSTARUM BREVIS
   c. LEVATOR COSTARUM LONGUS

10. Identify the muscles indicated in the figure.
    a. SCALENUS ANTERIOR
    b. SCALENUS MEDIUS
    c. SCALENUS POSTERIOR

11. Identify the muscles and portions of muscles indicated in the figure.
    a. STERNOCLEIDOMASTOID
    b. CLAVICULAR head
    c. STERNAL head
    d. PECTORALIS MAJOR
    e. PECTORALIS MINOR

12. Contraction of the diaphragm increases the VERTICAL dimension of the thorax.

13. Contraction of the accessory muscles of inspiration increase the TRANSVERSE dimension of the thorax.

14. Contraction of the muscles of expiration DECREASES the volume of the thorax.

15. Passive expiration involves the forces of ELASTICITY and GRAVITY.

16. Identify the described volumes and capacities.
    a. TIDAL VOLUME
    b. INSPIRATORY RESERVE volume
    c. EXPIRATORY RESERVE volume
    d. RESIDUAL volume
    e. VITAL capacity
    f. FUNCTIONAL RESIDUAL capacity
    g. TOTAL LUNG capacity

17. DEAD AIR SPACE is the volume of air that cannot undergo gas exchange.

18. INTRAORAL pressure is the air pressure in the oral cavity.

19. SUBGLOTTAL pressure is the air pressure below the vocal folds.

20. ALVEOLAR, or PULMONIC, pressure is the pressure in the alveolus.
21. INTRAPLEURAL, or PLEURAL, pressure is the pressure between the visceral and parietal pleural membranes.
22. When the diaphragm contracts, pressure in the alveolus DECREASES.
23. When air pressure in the lungs is lower than that of the atmosphere, air will ENTER the lungs.
24. When the body is reclining, the resting lung volume DECREASES.
25. Use of the muscles of inspiration to impede the outward flow of air during speech is termed CHECKING ACTION.
26. In advanced emphysema the diaphragm is pulled down and stretched relatively flat by the flaring of the rib cage. In normal inspiration contraction of the diaphragm causes the central tendon to pull down, causing air to enter the lungs (Boyle's law dictates that a drop in alveolar pressure causes airflow into the lungs). When the diaphragm of an individual with advanced emphysema contracts, it pulls the ribs closer together because they were distended by the "barrel chest." As a result, the alveoli are compressed, causing an increase in alveolar pressure and causing air to leave the lungs. Thus, the inspiratory gesture of the diaphragm causes expiration. The single inspiratory avenue left to the individual is to elevate the sternum and clavicle using clavicular breathing.

CHAPTER 3

1. Identify the structures indicated on the figure.
   a. EPIGLOTTIS cartilage
   b. THYROID cartilage
   c. CRICOID cartilage
   d. ARYTENOID cartilage
   e. CORNICULATE cartilage
   f. HYOID bone
2. Identify the landmarks indicated on the figure.
   a. SUPERIOR CORNU
   b. INFERIOR CORNU
   c. OBLIQUE LINE
   d. THYROID NOTCH
   e. ANGLE OF THYROID
   f. LAMINA
3. Identify the landmarks indicated on the figure.
   a. MUSCULAR process
   b. VOCAL process

4. Identify the muscles indicated in the figure.
   a. TRANSVERSE ARYTENOID
   b. OBLIQUE ARYTENOID
   c. POSTERIOR CRICOARYTENOID
5. Identify the muscles indicated in the figure.
   a. MYLOHYOID
   b. DIGASTRICUS ANTERIOR
   c. DIGASTRICUS POSTERIOR
   d. STYLOHYOID
6. Identify the muscles indicated in the figure.
   a. GENIOHYOID
   b. DIGASTRICUS ANTERIOR
   c. DIGASTRICUS POSTERIOR
   d. MYLOHYOID
7. This is a view of the laryngeal opening from above. Identify the indicated structures.
   a. ARYEPIGLOTTIC FOLD
   b. TRUE VOCAL FOLDS
   c. VALLECULAE
   d. EPIGLOTTIS
8. Identify the two muscles in the figure.
   a. THYROVOCALIS
   b. THYROMUSCULARIS
9. The CRICOTHYROID muscle is the primary muscle responsible for change of vocal fundamental frequency.
10. The space between the vocal folds is the GLOTTIS.
11. The BERNOULLI effect states that given a constant volume flow of air or fluid, at a point of constriction there will be a decrease in air pressure perpendicular to the flow and an increase in velocity of the flow.
12. Removal of the larynx would leave the airway unprotected from intrusion of foreign matter during swallowing. To avoid this danger, the airway is sealed off surgically, and a stoma is surgically opened up through the trachea to permit unhampered respiration.
13. ABDOMINAL FIXATION is the process of capturing air in the thorax to provide the muscles with a structure upon which to push or pull.
14. In GLOTTAL attack, the vocal folds are adducted before initiation of expiratory flow.
15. In BREATHY attack, the vocal folds are adducted after the initiation of expiratory flow.
16. In SIMULTANEOUS attack, the vocal folds are adducted simultaneous with initiation of expiratory flow.

17. During modal phonation, the vocal folds open from INFERIOR to SUPERIOR. The folds close from INFERIOR to SUPERIOR.

18. The minimum subglottal driving pressure for speech is 3 to 5 cm H_2O.

19. In the mode of vibration known as GLOTTAL FRY, the vocal folds vibrate at a much lower rate than in modal phonation, and the folds exhibit a syncopated vibratory pattern.

20. In the mode of vibration known as FALSETTO, the vocal folds lengthen and become extremely thin and reedlike.

21. Presence of vocal nodules or other space-occupying laryngeal pathology may result in BREATHY phonation.

22. To increase vocal intensity, one must INCREASE subglottal pressure and INCREASE medial compression.

23. To increase vocal fundamental frequency, one must INCREASE vocal fold tension by LENGTHENING the vocal folds.

24. OPTIMAL PITCH is the pitch of phonation that is optimal or most appropriate for an individual.

25. HABITUAL PITCH is the vocal pitch habitually used during speech.

26. As vocal intensity increases, the closed phase of the vibratory cycle INCREASES.

27. The vocal folds vibrate as a function of the transglottal pressure drop: The subglottal pressure is higher than the supraglottal (oral) pressure, so air flows through the glottis and the vocal folds vibrate. When the fistula was unoccluded, the transglottal pressure drop increased markedly, making control of the vocal folds difficult and causing the aperiodicity we saw. We have seen the same phenomenon in individuals with neurological diseases such as multiple sclerosis. In that case, we saw increased aperiodicity as a function of open vowel position, but the principle still holds.

CHAPTER 4

1. The SOURCE-FILTER theory of vowel production states that the voicing source is routed through the vocal tract where it is shaped into the sounds of speech by the articulators.

2. On the figure, identify the indicated bones and landmarks.
   a. MAXILLA (bone)
   b. MANDIBLE (bone)
   c. ZYGOMATIC bone
   d. NASAL bone
   e. FRONTAL bone
   f. FRONTAL process
   g. ALVEOLAR process
   h. SYMPHYSIS MENTI

3. On the figure, identify the indicated bones and landmarks.
   a. SPHENOID bone
   b. OCCIPITAL bone
   c. TEMPORAL bone
   d. CRISTA GALLI
   e. CRIBRIFORM PLATE
   f. FORAMEN MAGNUM

4. On the figure, identify the indicated bones and landmarks.
   a. ZYGOMATIC bone
   b. TEMPORAL bone
   c. MAXILLAE (bone)
   d. MANDIBLE (bone)
   e. NASAL bone
   f. FRONTAL bone
   g. PARIETAL bone
   h. OCCIPITAL bone
   i. RAMUS
   j. ANGLE
   k. ZYGOMATIC process
   l. CONDYLAR process
   m. CORONOID process
   n. CORPUS
   o. MASTOID process
   p. STYLOID process
   q. EXTERNAL AUDITORY MEATUS

5. On the figure, identify the indicated structures.
   a. PALATINE process
   b. MAXILLAE (bone)
   c. PALATINE bone
   d. PREMAXILLA
   e. INCISIVE foramen
   f. INTERMAXILLARY suture
   g. STYLOID process
   h. MEDIAL PTERYGOID plate
   i. LATERAL PTERYGOID plate
   j. MASTOID process
   k. FORAMEN MAGNUM
   l. PTERYGOID HAMULUS

6. On the figure, identify the indicated muscles.
   a. TENSOR VELI PALATINI
   b. LEVATOR VELI PALATINI
   c. PALATOGLOSSUS
   d. PALATOPHARYNGEUS

7. On the figure, identify the indicated muscles.
   a. BUCCINATOR
   b. ORBICULARIS ORIS SUPERIORIS
   c. ORBICULARIS ORIS INFERIORIS
   d. DEPRESSOR ANGULI ORIS
   e. DEPRESSOR LABII INFERIORIS
   f. ZYGOMATIC MAJOR
   g. ZYGOMATIC MINOR
   h. LEVATOR LABII SUPERIORIS ALAEQUE NASI
   i. LEVATOR ANGULI ORIS
   j. LEVATOR LABII SUPERIORIS
   k. RISORIUS
   l. PLATYSMA

8. On the figure, identify the indicated muscles.
   a. MASSETER
   b. TEMPORALIS
   c. LATERAL PTERYGOID
   d. MEDIAL PTERYGOID

9. On the figure, identify the indicated muscles.
   a. GENIOGLOSSUS
   b. HYOGLOSSUS
   c. DIGASTRICUS POSTERIOR
   d. STYLOGLOSSUS
   e. STYLOHYOID
   f. PALATOGLOSSUS
   g. INFERIOR LONGITUDINAL
   h. SUPERIOR LONGITUDINAL

10. On the figure, identify structures the indicated muscles.
    a. VOMER (bone)
    b. PALATINE process
    c. HORIZONTAL plate
    d. PERPENDICULAR plate
    e. CARTILAGINOUS SEPTUM
    f. NASAL bone

11. MASTICATION refers to the processes involved in food preparation, such as chewing food, moving the food onto the molars, and so forth.

12. DEGLUTITION refers to swallowing.

13. In the ORAL PREPARATORY stage of swallowing, food is prepared for swallowing.

14. In the ORAL stage of swallowing, mastication ceases, the tongue drops down and pulls posteriorly, and the anterior tongue elevates to the hard palate and squeezes the bolus back toward the faucial pillars.

15. In the PHARYNGEAL stage of swallowing, the bolus contacts the anterior faucial pillars, the soft palate elevates, respiration stops, the vocal folds tightly adduct, the larynx elevates and moves forward, and the cricopharyngeus relaxes as food enters the pharynx.

16. During the ESOPHAGEAL stage of swallowing, the bolus is transported through the esophagus.

17. Identify the muscle that best fits the statement. (In some cases more than one muscle fills the bill.)
    a. SUPERIOR LONGITUDINAL INTRINSIC elevates tongue tip.
    b. INFERIOR LONGITUDINAL INTRINSIC depresses tongue tip.
    c. GENIOGLOSSUS, POSTERIOR PORTION protrudes tongue.
    d. GENIOGLOSSUS, ANTERIOR PORTION; STYLOGLOSSUS retracts tongue.
    e. PALATOGLOSSUS elevates posterior tongue.
    f. TRANSVERSE INTRINSIC narrows tongue.
    g. VERTICAL INTRINSIC; GENIOGLOSSUS flattens tongue.
    h. PALATOGLOSSUS; PALATOPHARYNGEUS depresses soft palate.
    i. TENSOR VELI PALATINI tenses soft palate.
    j. CRICOPHARYNGEUS constricts esophageal opening.
    k. SUPERIOR PHARYNGEAL CONSTRICTOR constricts upper pharynx.
    l. LEVATOR VELI PALATINI elevates velum.

18. Motor control in the body develops from HEAD to TAIL and from PROXIMAL to DISTAL.

19. Elevation of the posterior tongue requires active contraction of the palatoglossus, perhaps the styloglossus, and the vertical intrinsic muscle. In addition, the tongue is pulling against the soft palate to achieve elevation because the palatoglossus is a velar depressor as well. When the palatoglossus contracts to elevate the tongue, the tensor and levator veli palatine must contract to keep the soft palate elevated.

CHAPTER 5

1. The PINNA of the outer ear is important for localization of sound in space.

2. Resistance to flow of energy is called IMPEDANCE.

3. The area ratio between the tympanic membrane and the oval window provides a 25-DB gain, and the level advantage gives a 2-DB gain.

4. The cochlea performs both SPECTRAL analysis and TEMPORAL analysis.

5. Compression in the fluid of the scala vestibuli is translated directly to the basilar membrane, and the disturbance at the basilar membrane causes the initiation of TRAVELING wave.

6. High-frequency sounds are resolved at the base of the cochlea, with progressively lower sounds processed at progressively higher positions on the cochlea. This array is called TONOTOPIC.

7. The frequency analysis ability of the basilar membrane is determined by graded WIDTH, STIFFNESSS, and THICKNESS.

8. At the apex, the basilar membrane is THICKER than at the base.

9. At the apex, the basilar membrane is WIDER than at the base.

10. F—The cilia of the outer hair cells are embedded in the tectorial membrane.

11. T—The cilia of the inner hair cells are embedded in the tectorial membrane.

12. HIGH-THRESHOLD neurons require a higher intensity and encompass the higher end of our auditory range of signal intensity, whereas LOW-THRESHOLD neurons respond at very low signal levels and display random firing even when there is no stimulus.

13. FREQUENCY SPECIFICITY refers to the ability of the cochlea to differentiate spectral components of a signal.

14. The CHARACTERISTIC frequency of a neuron is the frequency to which it responds best.

15. Tuning curves are composites of the responses of a single fiber at each frequency of presentation. The sharper the tuning curve is, the greater is the FREQUENCY SPECIFICITY of the basilar membrane.

16. Rate of firing of neurons increases as the INTENSITY increases.

17. Stimulation of the CROSSED-OLIVOCOCHLEAR bundle and the UNCROSSED-OLIVOCOCHLEAR bundle reduces the firing rate of neurons innervated by them.

18. The EXTERNAL AUDITORY meatus is a conduit for sound reaching the tympanic membrane.

19. The INTERNAL AUDITORY meatus is a conduit for the CRANIAL NERVE VIII nerve fibers coursing to the brainstem.

20. The tympanic membrane (or eardrum) is made up of THREE layers of tissue.

21. The outer layer of the tympanic membrane is continuous with the EPITHELIUM OF EXTERNAL AUDITORY MEATUS.

22. The INTERMEDIATE layer of the tympanic membrane is made up primarily of radiating fibers.

23. The UMBO is a landmark produced by the most distal part of the manubrium malli.

24. The MALLEUS is the bone of the middle ear directly attached to the tympanic membrane.

25. The STAPES is the bone of the middle ear directly communicating with the oval window.

26. The MANUBRIUM of the malleus attaches to the tympanic membrane.

27. The FOOTPLATE of the stapes articulates with the oval window.

28. The STAPEDIUS muscle pulls the stapes posteriorly.

29. The TENSOR TYMPANI muscle pulls the malleus anteromedially.

30. The entryway to the cochlea and vestibular system is via the space known as the VESTIBULE.

31. The OSSEOUS LABYRINTH is the system of cavities within bone that houses the membranous labyrinth.

32. The scala VESTIBULI and scala TYMPANI are incomplete spaces in the osseous labyrinth.

33. The ROUND window provides communication between the scala tympani and the middle ear.

34. The OVAL window permits communication between the scala vestibuli and the middle ear space.

35. The MEMBRANOUS LABYRINTH is a fluid-filled sac attached to the walls of the osseous labyrinth and is filled with endolymph.

36. REISSNER'S membrane separates the scala vestibuli and the scala media; the BASILAR membrane separates the scala media from the scala tympani.

37. The TUNNEL OF CORTI separates the outer and inner hair cells.

38. The hair cells are innervated by the VIII VESTIBULOCOCHLEAR nerve.

39. As with any other body structure, the ossicles are subject to trauma. A frequent cause of disarticulation of the ossicles is head trauma that involves the temporal bone (this may also cause a perilymph fistula, which is a tear in the basilar or Reissner's membrane that allows perilymph and endolymph to mingle). Another cause of disarticulation is noise or high-pressure trauma: The high-pressure forces associated with explosions can easily cause disarticulation.

40. The fruit bat cochlea is, naturally enough, smaller than that of the human. In addition, the cochlea of the bat is extremely sensitive to ultra-high frequencies (above human range of hearing), because high-frequency sounds are more efficient for echolocation. Elephants, on the other hand, have larger cochleas than humans. They process sounds that are lower than those we can hear!

CHAPTER 6

1. The CEREBRUM governs voluntary actions.
2. The CEREBELLUM is responsible for coordinating movement.
3. GANGLIA are groups of cell bodies in the PERIPHERAL NERVOUS SYSTEM with functional unity.
4. The CENTRAL NERVOUS SYSTEM includes the cerebrum, cerebellum, subcortical structures, brainstem, and spinal cord.
5. The PERIPHERAL NERVOUS SYSTEM consists of the 12 pairs of cranial nerves and 31 pairs of spinal nerves, as well as the sensory receptors.
6. The AUTONOMIC NERVOUS SYSTEM governs involuntary activities of involuntary muscles.
7. The SOMATIC NERVOUS SYSTEM governs voluntary activities.
8. Information directed toward the brain is termed AFFERENT and information directed from the brain is termed EFFERENT.
9. On the figure, identify the indicated parts of the neuron.
   a. AXON
   b. DENDRITE
   c. TELODENDRIA
   d. TERMINAL END BOUTON
   e. SYNAPTIC CLEFT
   f. SYNAPTIC VESICLES
   g. POSTSYNAPTIC NEURON
   h. MYELIN SHEATH
   i. SOMA
10. On the figure, identify the indicated parts of the cerebrum.
    a. FRONTAL lobe
    b. TEMPORAL lobe
    c. OCCIPITAL lobe
    d. PARIETAL lobe
    e. PRECENTRAL gyrus
    f. POSTCENTRAL gyrus
    g. CENTRAL sulcus
    h. LATERAL sulcus
11. On the figure, identify the parts of the surface of the cerebrum.
    a. CINGULATE GYRUS
    b. CORPUS CALLOSUM
    c. SUPERIOR TEMPORAL GYRUS
    d. WERNICKE'S AREA
    e. BROCA'S AREA
    f. PRECENTRAL GYRUS
    g. HESCHL'S GYRUS
    h. CENTRAL SULCUS
12. On the figure, identify the indicated arteries and structures.
    a. ANTERIOR CEREBRAL ARTERY
    b. MIDDLE CEREBRAL ARTERY
    c. POSTERIOR CEREBRAL ARTERY
    d. ANTERIOR COMMUNICATING ARTERY
    e. SUPERIOR CEREBELLAR ARTERY
    f. INTERNAL CAROTID ARTERY
    g. BASILAR ARTERY
    h. VERTEBRAL ARTERY
    i. CIRCLE OF WILLIS
13. ACTION POTENTIAL is a change in electrical potential that occurs when a cell membrane is stimulated adequately to permit ion exchange between intracellular and extracellular spaces.
14. The ABSOLUTELY REFRACTORY period is the time during which the cell membrane cannot be stimulated to depolarize.
15. The RELATIVELY REFRACTORY PERIOD is a period during which the membrane can be stimulated to excitation again, but only with greater than typical stimulation.
16. The NODES OF RANVIER of the axon myelin promote saltatory conduction.
17. The substance known as NEUROTRANSMITTER is discharged into the synaptic cleft, stimulating the postsynaptic neuron.

18. Higher cognitive processing occurs generally in ASSOCIATION areas.

19. The TEMPORO-OCCIPITAL-PARIETAL ASSOCIATION area is involved in language function.

20. The FRONTAL ASSOCIATION area of the cerebrum appears to be involved in higher function related to motor output (such as inhibition of motor function and the ability to change motor responses), whereas the temporal-occipital-parietal association area is involved in language function.

21. The LIMBIC ASSOCIATION area integrates information relating to affect, motivation, and emotion.

22. The LEFT hemisphere in most individuals is dominant for language and speech, processes brief duration stimuli, and performs detailed analysis.

23. The RIGHT hemisphere appears to process information in a more holistic fashion, preferring spatial and tonal information.

24. The CHEWING reflex is involved in mastication of the food bolus.

25. The MUSCLE SPINDLE (type of sensor) is involved in monitoring muscle length.

26. Chemosnsors are involved in the senses of OLFACTION and GUSTATION.

Glossary

Abdomen: The region represented externally as the front (anterior) abdominal wall.

Abduction: The process of moving two structures farther apart.

Absolute refractory period: The time during depolarization when the cell membrane cannot be stimulated to depolarize again.

Adduction: The process of moving two structures closer together.

Adipose tissue: Areolar tissue that is richly impregnated with fat cells.

Aditus: The entrance of the larynx.

Agonists (prime movers): Muscles that move a structure.

Alveolar pressure (P_{al}): Pressure in the alveolus. Also referred to as pulmonic pressure.

Alveoli: Air sacs in the lungs.

Anastomoses: Points of communication among arteries.

Anatomical position: The body is erect and the palms and arms face forward.

Anatomy: The study of structure of an organism.

Antagonists: Muscles that oppose a prime mover or agonist.

Anterior: In front of.

Anterior commissure of glottis: The anterior-most region of the glottis.

Aphonia: Loss of voicing.

Aplasia: Lack of development.

Aponeurosis: Sheetlike tendon.

Appendicular skeleton: The portion of the skeleton that includes only the lower and upper limbs.

Applied anatomy: The subdiscipline of anatomy concerned with diagnosis, treatment, and surgical intervention. Also referred to as *clinical anatomy*.

Approximation: When referring to vocal folds, making contact.

Areolar tissue: Supportive connective tissue. Also referred to as *loose connective tissue*.

Arm: The region from the shoulder to the elbow.

Articulate: Join.

Articulation: The process of bringing the mobile and immobile articulators into contact for the purpose of shaping the sounds of speech.

Atmospheric pressure (P_{atm}): Pressure generated as a result of the weight of atmospheric gases.

Atresia: Absence.

Auditory physiology: The study of auditory function.

Autonomic nervous system: The division of the central nervous system that is responsible for involuntary functions.

Average fundamental frequency: The average frequency of vibration taken over a given time period of phonation.

Axial skeleton: The portion of the skeleton that is the head and trunk, with the spinal column being the axis.

Axis: The real or imaginary line running through the center of a body or structure.

Axon: The terminal point of a neuron, through which information passes.

Baseplate membrane: Thin, membranous subsurface of epithelial tissue that serves structural, functional, and developmental purposes depending on its location. Also referred to *basement membrane*.

Beating ciliated epithelia: Cells with hairlike protrusions that actively beat to remove contaminants from the epithelial surface.

Bernoulli effect (principle): Given a constant volume flow of air or liquid, at a point of constriction there will be a decrease in air pressure perpendicular to the flow and an increase in velocity of flow.

Bifurcates: Divides into two parts.

Blood: Connective tissue that contains plasma and blood cells.

Bolus: A mass of masticated food ready to be swallowed.

Bone: Dense, inelastic connective tissue.

Boyle's law: Given a gas of constant temperature, increasing the volume of the chamber in which the gas is contained will cause a corresponding decrease in pressure, and vice versa.

Breaths per minute (bpm): The number of complete inhalations and exhalations performed in 1 minute.

Breathy phonation: The mode of phonation produced with extra airflow through the partially adducted vocal folds. Also referred to as *pressed phonation*.

Breathy vocal attack: Phonation by expiration before adduction of the vocal folds.

Broca's area: The region of the third frontal convolution of the dominant hemisphere responsible for speech motor planning.

Buccoversion: Tilted toward the cheek.

Capacity: Functional unit that is a combination of respiratory volumes, used to express physiological limits.

Cardiac muscle: Muscle of the heart, composed of cells that interconnect like a net.

Cartilage: Connective tissue that is elastic.

Caudal: Toward the tail.

Central nervous system (CNS): The division of the nervous system that contains the brain and spinal cord.

Cephalo-caudal: Development occurs from head to tail.

Cerebrovascular system: The vascular supply of the central and peripheral nervous systems.

Checking action: Using the muscles of inspiration to impede the outflow of air during expiration.

Class I occlusal relationship: The normal occlusal relationship characterized by the maxillary and mandibular molar relationship in which the maxillary first molar is retracted one-half tooth relative to the mandibular first molar. Also referred to as *neutroclusion*.

Class II malocclusion: The occlusal relationship characterized by the maxillary and mandibular molar relationship in which the maxillary first molar is retracted at least one tooth relative to the mandibular first molar.

Class III malocclusion: The occlusal relationship characterized by the maxillary and mandibular molar relationship in which the maxillary first molar is advanced at least one tooth relative to the mandibular first molar.

Clinical eruption: Eruption of dentition through the gum.

Compact bone: Sheetlike bone.

Comparative anatomy: The study of anatomical structures across species.

Compressive strength: The ability of a material to resist crushing.

Connective tissue: Tissue that supports and connects other tissue.

Convergence: The neural process in which outputs of many neurons contribute to the depolarization of a single neuron.

Cornu: Horn.

Corpus: Body.

Cough: Forceful expiration of air following tight adduction of the vocal folds, for the purpose of expelling foreign matter from the airway.

Cranium: The part of the skull that houses the brain.

Cubic centimeter (cc): A milliliter, or one thousandth of a liter.

Dead air space: The space, representing the conductive passageway of the respiratory system, that contains a volume of air that never undergoes gas exchange (approximately 150 cc in adults).

Deciduous (shedding) teeth: The primary set of teeth.

Deep: Closer to the central axis of the body.

Deglutition: The process of swallowing.

Dendrite: The component of a neuron that generally receives input from another neuron or sensor.

Descriptive anatomy: The description of individual parts of the body without reference to disease. Also referred to as *systemic* or *systematic anatomy*.

Developmental anatomy: The study of development of the organism's anatomy from conception to adulthood.

Diarthrodial joints: Highly mobile joints lubricated with synovial fluid. Also referred to as *synovial joints*.

Direct motor system: The motor system under voluntary control. Also referred to as *pyramidal motor system*.

Distal: Away from midline.

Distoversion: Tilted away from the midline of the dental arch.

Divergence: The neural process in which one neuron passes information to many other neurons.

Dorsal: Referring to the back surface of a body.

Dorsal trunk: The region commonly referred to as "the back."

Dorsiflexion: Hyperextension.

Dysphagia: Disorder of swallowing.

Elasticity: Having the ability and tendency to return to original position.

Electromyography: The study of forces exerted by muscles.

Electrophysiology: Measurement and study of the electrical activity of cells.

Epithelial tissue: Tissue that provides a protective lining for the surface of the body and internal surfaces of cavities.

Eversion: Turning the foot outward.

Expiration: The process of eliminating air from the lungs for respiration.

Expiratory reserve volume (ERV): The volume of air that can be expired following passive, tidal expiration (approximately 1000 cc for adults).

Extension: The act of pulling two ends farther apart; the opposite of flexion.

External: Outside a cavity or body.

Extrinsic laryngeal muscles: Muscles with one attachment in the larynx and one attachment outside the larynx.

Falsetto: Phonation high in frequency, which is produced by significant increase in laryngeal tension that results in thinned vocal fold margins.

Fascia: Sheetlike membrane of connective tissue that surrounds organs.

Fibrocartilage: Smooth cartilage made up of a mixture of white fibrous and collagen tissue.

Fibrous tissue: Tissue that binds structures together.

Fissure: Significant infolding or complete separation of two structures of the cerebral or cerebellar cortex.

Flexion: Bending at a joint, usually toward the ventral surface.

Force physiology: The study of forces exerted by muscles.

Fossa: Indentation or cavity.

Frontal section: Section that divides the body into front and back portions.

Functional residual capacity (FRC): The volume of air in the thorax after a passive exhalation (approximately 2100 cc for adults).

Functional unity: Groups of tissues working for a single functional purpose.

Fundamental frequency: The lowest component of a harmonic series. In phonation, the lowest frequency of the voiced source.

Glandular epithelium: Epithelium that secretes fluids.

Glia (glial cells): Nervous system tissue that provides support and nutrients in the nervous system.

Glottal attack: Phonatory onset that occurs with the adduction of the vocal folds before expiration.

Glottal fry: A low-frequency mode of vibration characterized by syncopated rhythm and generated by low subglottal air pressure.

Glottis: The space between the vocal folds.

Gross anatomy: The study of structures visible without the aid of microscopy.

Gustation: Sense of taste.

Gyri: Outfolding of tissue on the cerebral or cerebellar cortex.

Habitual pitch: The frequency of vibration of the vocal folds habitually used by an individual during speech.

Hyaline cartilage: Smooth, glassy, blue cartilage for surfaces of bones that come together in joints.

Hyperextension: Extension that continues to the point where the dorsal surfaces approach each other.

Hypertonus: Abnormal increase in muscle tone.

Indirect (extrapyramidal) motor system: The motor system that provides background support for the direct motor system.

Inferior: Below, closer to the ground.

Infraversion: Inadequate eruption relative to the other teeth in the arch.

Innervation: Process of communication of muscles from and to the brain.

Insertion: The point of attachment of a muscle that is mobile when a muscle contracts.

Inspiration: The process of bringing air into the lungs for respiration.

Inspiratory capacity: The maximum inspiratory volume possible after tidal expiration (approximately 3000 cc in adults).

Inspiratory reserve volume (IRV): The volume of air that can be inhaled after a tidal inspiration (approximately 2475 cc for adults).

Internal: Within a cavity or body.

Intonation: The changes in pitch in continuous speech.

Intraoral pressure (P_m): Pressure in the oral cavity.

Intraosseous eruption: Eruption of dentition through bone.

Intrapleural pressure (P_{pl}): Pressure between the visceral and parietal pleurae.

Intrinsic laryngeal muscles: Muscles with both origin and insertion in the larynx.

Inversion: Turning the sole of the foot inward.

Labioversion: Tilted toward the lip.

Laryngeal stridor: Harsh sound produced upon inhalation or exhalation.

Lateral: To the side.

Leg: Portion of the lower extremity from the knee to the ankle.

Lesion: Damage to tissue.

Ligament: Band of connective tissue responsible for binding structures together.

Linguaversion: Tilted toward the tongue.

Loudness: The perceptual correlate of intensity.

Lower extremity: The region that includes the thigh, calf, ankle, and foot.

Lymphoid tissue: Specialized connective tissue in tonsils and adenoids.

Manometer: Device that measures pressure.

Mastication: The process of chewing.

Matrix: Intercellular material of connective tissue.

Medial: Toward midline. Also referred to as *mesial*.

Mediastinal: Referring to the mediastinum, or "middle space" of the thorax, which contains the heart.

Mesioversion: Tilted toward the midline of the dental arch.

Micrognathia: Small mandible relative to the maxillae.

Microscopic anatomy: The study of structures not visible to the unaided eye.

Microtia: Small ear.

Midsagittal section: Section that cuts the body into left and right halves.

Milliliter (mL): One thousandth of a liter.

Modal register: The mode of vibration used for daily speaking.

Monoloud: Of unvarying vocal loudness.

Monopitch: Speech with little or no perceived variation in pitch.

Morphology: Form.

Motor (efferent/excitatory) innervation: Innervation that causes muscles to contract or glands to secrete.

Motor nerve: Nerve that activates muscle or gland.

Motor unit: Tissue consisting of one motor nerve fiber and the muscle fibers to which it attaches.

Muscular tissue: Tissue that is capable of contraction.

Nares: Nostrils.

Nasal regurgitation: Loss of masticated food through the nasal cavity.

Necrotic tissue: Dead tissue.

Neural tissue: Tissue that is specialized to transmit information.

Neuraxis: The axis of the nervous system, including spinal cord, brainstem, and cerebrum.

Neuromuscular junction: The point of synapse between muscle fiber and motor fiber.

Neurons (nerve cells): Tissue specialized for communication.

Neutroclusion: The normal occlusal relationship characterized by the maxillary and mandibular molar relationship in which the maxillary first molar is retracted one-half tooth relative to the mandibular first molar.

Occlusion: Closing.

Olfaction: Sense of smell.

Optimal pitch: The most efficient frequency of vibration of the vocal folds.

Origin: The point of attachment of a muscle that is immobile when a muscle contracts.

Oscillation: Repeated vibration of a body at the same frequency.

Overjet: Condition of normal dentition in which the upper incisors overlap and hide the lower incisors.

Palmar: Referring to the palm of hand.

Palmar grasp reflex: Reaction of stimulation of the palm that causes the fingers to grasp.

Palpation: Feeling a structure using one's hands.

Paralysis: Loss of voluntary motor function due to lesion in the nervous system.

Parasternal: Near the sternum.

Parasympathetic nervous system: The component of the autonomic nervous system responsible for reducing sympathetic (fight or flight) responses of the body, as well as other functions when the body is at rest.

Paresis: Weakness arising from lesion in the nervous system.

Pathological anatomy: The area of study concerned with diseased tissue.

Pelvis: The area of the hip bones.

Pericardium: The membranous sac enclosing the heart.

Perimysium: Special fascia surrounding muscle.

Periosteum: Fibrous membrane covering of a bone.

Peripheral: Away from the center of the body.

Peripheral nervous system (PNS): The division of the nervous system that contains cranial and spinal nerves.

Persistent closed bite: The posterior dentition fails to occlude properly as a result of supraversion of the anterior teeth.

Persistent open bite: Anterior dentition fails to occlude properly as a result of supraversion of the posterior teeth.

Pharyngeal recesses: Valleculae and piriform sinuses.

Physiology: The study of an organism's function.

Pitch: The perceptual correlate of frequency of vibration.

Pitch range: The range of phonation possible, calculated as the highest frequency of vibration minus the lowest frequency of vibration.

Plane: A flat or relatively smooth surface.

Plantar: Referring to the sole of the foot, the flexor surface.

Plantar flexion: Extension of the toes.

Plantar grasp reflex: Reaction to stimulation of the sole of the foot that causes the toe of the feet to "grasp."

Plasma: Fluid component of blood.

Posterior: Toward the back; behind.

Posterior commissure of glottis: The posterior-most region of the glottis.

Process: An anatomical structure protruding from a surface.

Pronation: Rotation of the hand so the palmar surface is directed inferiorly.

Prone: Lying on the belly.

Propagation: The spreading effect of wave action; in neural responses, the communication of information through the nervous system.

Prosody: Combination of changes in fundamental frequency and vocal intensity that provides linguistically relevant information (e.g., vocal pitch, intonation, loudness, duration, and rhythm).

Proximal: Near a body or structure.

Proximo-distal: Development occurs from medial to distal structures.

Quiet tidal volume: Tidal volume at rest.

Residual volume (RV): The volume of air in the lungs after a maximum exhalation; the volume of air that cannot be expelled (approximately 1100 cc in adults).

Respiration: Exchange of gas between an organism and its environment.

Respiratory physiology: The study of all processes involved in breathing.

Resting membrane potential (RMP): The condition of a neuron at rest, in which it is polarized and ready to discharge.

Rostral: Toward the head.

Sagittal plane: Plane created by a sagittal section.

Sagittal section: Section that divides the body into left and right parts.

Saltatory conduction: The process in a neural response in which information in the axon passes from node to node, thereby greatly increasing conduction speed.

Sensory (afferent) innervation: Innervation that provides the central nervous system with information about the state of the body or tissues.

Sign: Measurable or objective component of illness or condition.

Simultaneous vocal attack: Phonation initiated through simultaneous adduction of the vocal folds and respiratory expiration.

Skeletal ligaments: Connective tissue that binds bone to bone.

Smooth muscle: Muscular tissue not under voluntary control, especially of the digestive tract and blood vessels.

Soma: The cell body of a neuron.

Somatic nervous system: The subdivision of the nervous system responsible for voluntary motor function and nonvisceral sensation.

Spatial summation: The quality of some neurons wherein they require multiple synaptic inputs from a broad array of neurons in order to be stimulated to depolarize.

Spectral analysis: Analysis of a signal that identifies frequency components of that signal.

Spirometer: Device that measures volume of air expelled or inspired.

Spongy bone: Porous bone.

Stenosis: Narrowing.

Stress: The emphasis on a word produced in continuous speech, relative to the emphasis of the entire utterance.

Striated muscle: Skeletal muscle, voluntary muscle.

Subglottal pressure (P_s): Pressure beneath the level of the vocal folds.

Successional teeth: Teeth in the mature dental arch that replace corresponding teeth of the deciduous arch.

Sulci: Minor infolding of tissue on the cerebral or cerebellar cortex.

Superficial: Confined to the surface.

Superior: Above; farther from the ground.

Supination: Rotation of the hand so the palmar surface is directed superiorly.

Supine: Lying on the back.

Supraglottal: The region above the vocal folds.

Suprasegmental: Information in the speech signal that spans two or more phonemes; generally called prosodic elements.

Supraversion: Excessive eruption relative to the majority of teeth in the arch.

Surface anatomy: The study of the form and structure of the surface of the body, especially with reference to the organs beneath the surface.

Sympathetic nervous system: The component of the autonomic nervous system responsible for body system responses that prepare the body to cope with stressful situations.

Synergists: Muscles used to stabilize structures.

Temporal summation: The quality of some neurons wherein the neuron requires virtually simultaneous inputs from other neurons before it can be stimulated to depolarize.

Tendons: Connective tissue bands that are part of the muscle and attach muscle to bone or cartilage.

Tensile strength: The ability of a material to resist being pulled apart.

Thorax: The chest region.

Tidal volume: The volume of air exchanged during one cycle of respiration.

Torquing: Twisting of a shaft while one end does not move.

Torsiversion: Twisted on the long axis.

Total lung capacity (TLC): The total volume of the respiratory system that can undergo gas exchange, equaling the sum of tidal volume, inspiratory reserve volume, expiratory reserve volume, and residual volume (approximately 5100 cc in adults).

Transverse section: Section that divides the body into upper and lower halves.

Upper extremity: The region consisting of the arm, forearm, wrist, and hand.

Valleculae: Pair of small indentations between the tongue and epiglottis.

Ventral: Referring to the front surface of a body.

Ventricular: Referring to cavities or passageways to structures.

Visceral ligaments: Connective tissue that binds organs together or holds structures in place.

Vital capacity (VC): The combination of inspiratory reserve volume, expiratory reserve volume, and tidal volume, representing the capacity of air available for speech (approximately 4000 cc in adults).

Vocal folds (vocal cords): The vibrating component of the larynx used to produce sound.

Vocal tract: The oral cavity, the pharynx, and the nasal cavity.

Volume: In respiration, the displacement of air that represents specifically partitioned components of the respiratory system, measured in cubic centimeters or cubic inches.

Whispered speech: Speech produced without vocal fold vibration by causing air to pass along the edges of the tensed vocal folds, thus producing a friction sound source.

White fibrous tissue: Connective tissue that is strong, dense, and highly organized.

Yellow (elastic) cartilage: Cartilage that has greater elasticity than other forms of cartilage.

Yellow elastic tissue: Connective tissue in cartilage.

Index